OXFORD MEDICAL PUBLICATIONS

Essentials of microbiology
for dental students

Essentials of microbiology for dental students

Jeremy Bagg

Senior Lecturer in Oral Microbiology
University of Glasgow Dental School
Glasgow, UK

T. Wallace MacFarlane

Professor of Oral Microbiology
University of Glasgow Dental School
Glasgow, UK

Ian R. Poxton

Professor of Microbial Infection and Immunity
University of Edinburgh Medical School
Edinburgh, UK

Chris H. Miller

Associate Dean for Research and Graduate Education
Indiana University School of Dentistry
Indianapolis, USA

with a contribution from
Andrew J. Smith

Lecturer in Oral Microbiology
University of Glasgow Dental School
Glasgow, UK

Illustrated by Simon Bagg

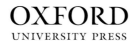

OXFORD
UNIVERSITY PRESS

OXFORD
UNIVERSITY PRESS

Great Clarendon Street, Oxford OX2 6DP

Oxford University Press is a department of the University of Oxford.
It furthers the University's objective of excellence in research, scholarship,
and education by publishing worldwide in

Oxford New York

Auckland Bangkok Buenos Aires Cape Town Chennai
Dar es Salaam Delhi Hong Kong Istanbul Karachi Kolkata
Kuala Lumpur Madrid Melbourne Mexico City Mumbai
Nairobi São Paulo Shanghai Taipei Tokyo Toronto

Oxford is a registered trade mark of Oxford University Press
in the UK and in certain other countries

Published in the United States
by Oxford University Press Inc., New York

First published 1999
Reprinted 2002, 2003

A catalogue record for this book is available from the British Library

Library of Congress Cataloging in Publication Data
Essentials of microbiology for dental students / Jeremy Bagg . . .
[et al.]; with a contribution from Andrew J. Smith; illustrated
by Simon Bagg.
1. Mouth—Microbiology. 2. Medical microbiology. I. Bagg, Jeremy.
QR47.E87 1999 616′.01–dc21 99–10433
ISBN 0 19 263076 8 (Pbk)

Typeset by EXPO Holdings, Malaysia
Printed in Hong Kong, China

Preface

The oral cavity is inhabited by a very complex microbial flora. This flora interacts with the host and contributes to the health of the individual, although in certain circumstances it can also cause disease. Many of the conditions that dental surgeons diagnose and treat, for example dental caries and periodontal disease, are caused by micro-organisms that are predominantly members of the normal oral flora. In addition, members of the oral microflora are involved in some systemic infections, for example infective endocarditis. There are also a number of systemic infections that have important implications in dental practice, for example those with blood-borne viruses. A thorough knowledge of microbiology and its clinical implications is, therefore, essential for all practising dentists.

The experience of the authors, who are all involved in teaching microbiology to dental students, is that there is a need for a highly illustrated textbook which links the science of microbiology and immunology with those clinical aspects directly relevant to dentistry. In particular, students need to be presented with those key facts that are of particular importance to dentists, rather than extensive coverage of all aspects of the ever-enlarging field of microbiology. This book aims to fulfil that role and to be appropriate for use at all stages of the dental curriculum. It is hoped that it will also be of value to qualified dentists undertaking postgraduate study.

The first section describes the fundamental principles of microbiology and immunology, defining the nature of micro-organisms and host–parasite interactions. Applied clinical aspects, such as immunization, antimicrobial drugs, and instrument sterilization are also covered in this part of the book. The second section describes a range of systemic infections relevant to dental professionals. Following the two general introductory chapters in this section, a 'systems' approach has been employed, whereby infections have been classified on the basis of the organ system involved. This has allowed the material to be presented in a clinically relevant context. The final section contains nine chapters on specialized oral microbiology, including a final chapter on the control of cross-infection in dentistry.

In addition to the extensive use of colour illustrations and tables to clarify the subject matter, the team of British and American authors has taken care to ensure that the material is suitable for use internationally. We hope that the nature and quality of the presentation will make this an invaluable resource for the teaching of microbiology to dental students and will foster an understanding of the ever-increasing importance of infectious agents in modern clinical practice.

Glasgow, Edinburgh, Indianapolis JB, TWMacF, IRP, CM
1999

Contents

Acknowledgements

The authors would like to thank their families and friends whose patience and forbearance have made the writing of this book possible. The comments and advice of many colleagues and students has been of great value as the manuscript has developed. Special thanks are due to Dr Peter Stewart and Mr Simon Bagg for their expert proof-reading skills and constructive comments. We also wish to record our thanks to all those who kindly provided illustrative material, in particular Laetitia Brocklebank, Stephen Creanor, Curtiss Gemmell, Mette Kjeldsen, Michael Lewis, Duncan MacKenzie, Gordon MacDonald, Ian Miller, Sheila Patrick, Lionel Rawle, and Malcolm Richardson. A huge debt of gratitude is due to Oxford University Press for their efficiency, professionalism, support, and cheerfulness, which have helped us to meet the inevitable deadlines.

List of abbreviations

5-HT	5-hydoxytryptamine (also known as serotonin)
A	adenine
Ab	antibody
ADA	American Dental Association
ADP	adenosine diphosphate
AFB	acid-fast bacilli
AFLP	amplified fragment length polymorphism
Ag	antigen
AHA	American Heart Association
AIDS	acquired immune deficiency syndrome
APC	antigen-presenting cell
ARDRA	amplified rDNA restriction analysis
ARDS	adult respiratory distress syndrome
ASOT	antistreptolysin O titre
ATP	adenosine triphosphate
AUG	acute ulcerative gingivitis
AZT	azidothymidine
BANA	benzoyl-DL-arginine-naphthylamide
BCG	bacille Calmette–Guérin
BI	biological indicators (of sterility)
bp	base pair
C	cytosine
CD	cluster of differentiation
CDC	Centers for Disease Control and Prevention (USA)
CFA	colonization factor antigen
CGD	chronic granulomatous disease
CJD	Creutzfeldt–Jakob disease
CMC	chronic mucocutaneous candidosis
CMV	cytomegalovirus
CNS	central nervous system
CSF	cerebrospinal fluid
DNA	deoxyribonucleic acid
DTH	delayed-type hypersensitivity
DTP	mixed vaccine containing diphtheria toxoid, tetanus toxoid, and pertussis vaccine (also known as DPT)
EA	early antigen
EB	elementary body
EBV	Epstein–Barr virus
EF-G	elongation factor-G
Eh	redox potential
EIEC	enteroinvasive *Escherichia coli*
ELISA	enzyme-linked immunosorbent assay
EPEC	enteropathogenic *Escherichia coli*
ETEC	enterotoxigenic *Escherichia coli*
Fab	antigen-binding fragment
Fc	crystallizable fragment
FTA	fluorescent treponema antibody
FTA(Abs)	fluorescent treponema antibody absorbed
G	guanine
GCF	gingival crevicular fluid
GM-CSF	granulocyte–monocyte colony-stimulating factor
gp	glycoprotein (gene product)
HAT	hypoxanthine aminopterin and thymidine
HAV	hepatitis A virus
HBcAg	hepatitis B core antigen
HBeAg	hepatitis Be antigen (proteolytic cleavage product of HBcAg)
HBsAg	hepatitis B surface antigen
HBV	hepatitis B virus
HCV	hepatitis C virus
HDV	hepatitis D virus
HEV	hepatitis E virus
Hfr	high-frequency recombination
HGV	hepatitis G virus
HHV	human herpesvirus
HHV-6	human herpesvirus 6
Hib	*Haemophilus influenzae* serotype b (vaccine)
HIV	human immunodeficiency virus
HPV	human papillomavirus
HSV	herpes simplex virus
HTLV	human T-lymphotropic virus (also known as human T-cell leukaemia virus)
HUS	haemolytic uraemia syndrome
ICAM	intercellular adhesion molecule
IFN	interferon
Ig	immunoglobulin
IL	interleukin
INH	isoniazid
IPS	intracellular polysaccharides
IV	intravenous
K	killer cells (*not* the same as NK cells)

kDa	kilodalton
KDO	keto-deoxy-octonic acid
kPa	kilopascal
LFA	lymphocyte functional antigen
LGL	large granular lymphocyte
LOS	lipo-oligosaccharide
LPS	lipopolysaccharide (endotoxin)
LT	(heat-) labile toxin
mAb	monoclonal antibody
MAC	membrane-attack complex
MALT	mucosa-associated lymphoid tissue
MBC	minimal bactericidal concentration
MDRTB	multiple drug-resistant (strains of) *Mycobacterium tuberculosis*
MHC	major histocompatibility complex
MIC	minimal inhibitory concentration
MMR	measles, mumps, rubella (vaccine)
mRNA	messenger RNA
MRSA	methicillin-resistant *Staphylococcus aureus*
MSB	Mitis Salivarius Bacitracin (growth medium)
MSH	Melanophore Stimulating Hormone
mV	millivolts
NAD$^+$	nicotinamide–adenine dinucleotide (i.e. the oxidized form)
NK	natural killer cells (*not* the same as K cells)
NSU	non-specific urethritis
NTM	non-tuberculous mycobacteria
OM	outer membrane
OMPs	outer membrane proteins
PABA	para-amino benzoic acid
PAGE	polyacrylamide gel electrophoresis
PCP	*Pneumocystis carinii* pneumonia
PCR	polymerase chain reaction
PFGE	pulsed-field gel electrophoresis
PMC	pseudomembranous candidosis

PPD	purified protein derivative
R-LPS	rough-form LPS (see also S-LPS)
RAPD	randomly amplified polymorphic DNA
RB	reticulate body
rDNA	DNA coding for rRNA
RFLP	restriction fragment length polymorphism
RNA	ribonucleic acid
rRNA	ribosomal RNA
RT	reverse transcription
S-LPS	smooth-form LPS (i.e. normal configuration of LPS)
SCID	severe combined immunodeficiency
SIRS	systemic inflammatory response syndrome
S_j	similarity coefficient
ST	(heat-) stable toxin
STD	sexually transmitted disease
T	thymine
TB	tuberculosis
TCR	T-cell receptor
T_{DTH}	delayed-type hypersensitivity T-cell (now known as TH1 cells)
T_H	T-helper cell
TNF	tumour necrosis factor
TPHA	*Treponema pallidum* haemagglutination
tRNA	transfer RNA
TSST	toxic shock syndrome toxin
U	uridine
UTI	urinary tract infection
VCA	viral capsid antigen
VDRL	Venereal Disease Reference Laboratory
VRE	vancomycin-resistant enterococci
VTEC	verotoxin-producing *Escherichia coli*
VZV	varicella zoster virus
WHO	World Health Organization

Section 1

1

The concept of micro-organisms

- Introduction
- The diversity of micro-organisms and their habitats

The concept of micro-organisms

Introduction

The history of microbiology and immunology

Before the development of the light microscope all living organisms could be divided empirically, without too much debate, into two Kingdoms: the Plants and the Animals. In the 1660s, Robert Hooke, using a crude compound microscope, was probably the first person to see cells; a few years later Antonie van Leeuwenhoek, using the first high-resolution, single lens microscope, saw micro-organisms for the first time. These microscopic living creatures, some of which were seen to move, were described as small animals or 'animalcules'. From Leeuwenhoek's drawings we know them to be bacteria and protozoa. It is of interest to note that his specimens included material scraped from his own teeth.

There was a gap of almost two centuries before the development of the first high-quality compound microscope, together with the pioneering work of Pasteur, Koch, and Lister, established the importance of micro-organisms as agents of disease, and the science of bacteriology (or the more modern microbiology) was born (Fig. 1.1). Following the discovery of penicillin by Fleming, the development of antimicrobial chemotherapy slowly began, and is now the driving force behind a large and important branch of microbiology. Much of modern immunology had its roots in the study of micro-organisms by such key players as Metchnikoff and Erhlich (Fig. 1.1).

Robert Koch was the first person to prove that micro-organisms caused disease. Absolute proof can be established by fulfilling the following postulates, though this raises ethical problems in studies of human disease.

Koch's postulates

1. The specific micro-organism should be isolated from all cases of a specific disease, and should not be found in healthy individuals.

2. The specific micro-organism should be isolated from the diseased individual and grown in pure culture on artificial medium.

3. The isolated micro-organism should reproduce the specific disease when inoculated into a healthy individual.

4. The specific micro-organism should be re-isolated in pure culture from the experimental infection.

Early studies on unicellular, microscopic organisms established that there were several different morphological types. Those resembling animals were referred to as protozoa and those resembling plants were termed algae. The yeasts, moulds, and other microscopic forms which resembled plants but did not possess photosynthetic pigments were the fungi, while the bacteria tended to be smaller agents, simpler than the other

EARLY MICROBIOLOGISTS AND IMMUNOLOGISTS		
Louis Pasteur	1822–1895	'Father of microbiology' Widespread interests. Disproved the theory of spontaneous generation
Robert Koch	1843–1910	Established the Germ Theory of Disease — see his postulates in the text
Joseph Lister	1827–1912	First to use antiseptics in surgery
Alexander Fleming	1881–1955	Discovered penicillin in 1928
Elie Metchnikoff	1845–1916	Described phagocytosis
Paul Ehrlich	1854–1915	Described the concept of humoral immunity

Fig. 1.1 Some key players in early microbiology and immunology.

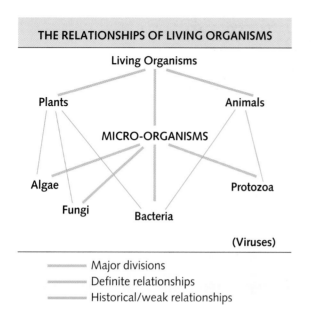

THE RELATIONSHIPS OF LIVING ORGANISMS

Living Organisms

Plants

Animals

MICRO-ORGANISMS

Algae

Protozoa

Fungi

Bacteria

(Viruses)

Major divisions
Definite relationships
Historical/weak relationships

Fig. 1.2 The relationships between living organisms.

types, and recognized as causing a range of infectious diseases (Fig. 1.2). The viruses are a special group of acellular structures which were discovered much later and which cannot be readily termed living organisms. Viruses are described in detail in Chapter 5.

Prokaryotic and eukaryotic cells

With the development of the electron microscope in the 1950s it was possible for the first time to explore the internal architecture of cells. It soon became apparent that in the whole spectrum of living creatures – from the simplest bacterium to the most complex higher organism – there are only two basic types of cell, the prokaryotic cell and the eukaryotic cell. The prokaryotic cell (Fig. 1.3) is small and simple in structure without any internal membrane-bound structures or organelles; while the eukaryotic cell (Fig. 1.4) is larger and more complex, with an obvious membrane-bound nucleus and other internal organelles such as mitochondria. Bacteria, together with other similar micro-organisms classified as rickettsiae, chlamydiae, mycoplasmas, Archaebacteria (primitive bacteria, often found in extremes of environment), and cyanobacteria (formerly blue-green algae), are prokaryotic. All other unicellular and all multicellular organisms are eukaryotic. The fundamental differences in cell structure (Fig. 1.5) have important consequences when considering antimicrobial action, as many antimicrobial agents target prokaryotic-specific structures or metabolic pathways.

On examining the structure of mitochondria (and chloroplasts in plant cells) it soon becomes apparent that they have many similarities to prokaryotes: size; 70S ribosomes; undergo binary fission; and have circular DNA. It is therefore assumed that the eukaryotic cell originally evolved from a symbiotic relationship between a primitive precursor cell and intracellular prokaryotic micro-organisms.

The diversity of micro-organisms and their habitats

Micro-organisms were the earliest forms of life on the planet, and many such primitive types still inhabit the harsh environments which must resemble those which existed when life first

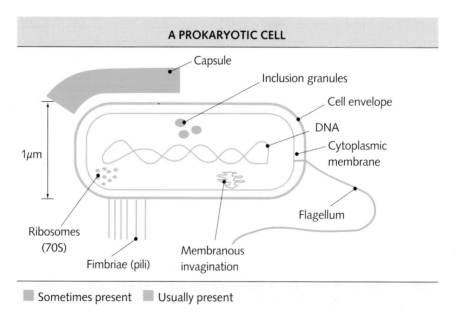

A PROKARYOTIC CELL

Capsule

Inclusion granules

Cell envelope

DNA

Cytoplasmic membrane

1μm

Flagellum

Ribosomes (70S)

Fimbriae (pili)

Membranous invagination

Sometimes present   Usually present

Fig. 1.3 Diagram of an idealized prokaryotic cell.

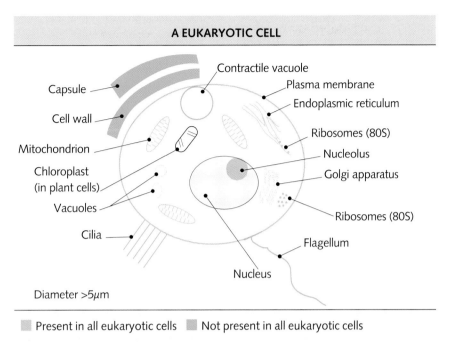

Fig. 1.4 Diagram of an idealized eukaryotic cell.

COMPARISON OF PROKARYOTIC AND EUKARYOTIC CELLS

Character	Prokaryotic	Eukaryotic
Appearance in electron microscope	Simple	Complex
Size	<5µm	>5µm
Arrangement of DNA	Circular double-stranded chromosome No nuclear membrane	Linear chromosomes complexed with basic proteins Contained within nuclear membrane
Internal membranes	None, although invaginations of cytoplasmic membrane may be extensive	Endoplasmic reticulum and Golgi apparatus
Membrane-bound organelles	None	Mitochondria, chloroplasts
Envelope structure	Peptidoglycan normally present	Peptidoglycan never found
Ribosomes	Small (70S)	Large (80S)
Reproduction	Asexual by binary fission	Sexual and asexual Meiosis and mitosis
Antibiotic action	Targets prokaryote-specific structures or pathways	Largely inactive

Fig. 1.5 Table comparing key features of prokaryotic and eukaryotic cells.

began. Virtually every ecological niche is colonized by micro-organisms, and each species is adapted to the specific habitat. The vast majority of micro-organisms do not cause disease and are saprophytic, obtaining their nutrition from the breakdown of organic matter. Their primary role is in the various natural cycles such as the carbon, nitrogen, oxygen, and sulphur cycles which are concerned with the decomposition of living matter and recycling of elements vital for the well-being of life on earth.

Atmospheric requirements

Many micro-organisms obtain their energy by fermentation (substrate-level phosphorylation), a process which does not require oxygen. The smallest amount of oxygen is toxic to some of these micro-organisms, or at least inhibits their growth, and these are termed strict anaerobes. Other micro-organisms perform respiration (oxidative phosphorylation), and are aerobes. A few species of bacteria can respire anaerobically, utilizing CO_2 or NO_3^- instead of O_2 as the final electron acceptor. Thus, *Pseudomonas aeruginosa*, usually considered to be an aerobe, can grow anaerobically if nitrate is present in the growth medium. Many micro-organisms can both ferment and respire and are known as facultative anaerobes. The microaerophilic bacteria, typified by the genus *Campylobacter* (see Chapter 15), are unusual in that they require subnormal levels of oxygen for their growth; while others, the capnophilic bacteria, which are commonly found in the oral ecosystem, have a requirement for carbon dioxide.

As well as the atmospheric requirements of micro-organisms, other chemical and physical parameters such as temperature, pH, and osmolarity are important (Chapter 2) and some species, notably the Archaebacteria, can exist under extreme conditions (Fig. 1.6).

The normal flora and pathogens

Many sites in the body, for example the skin and the gut, are colonized by large numbers of micro-organisms in health. This normal human microbiota, or the normal flora of the human body, is often referred to erroneously as the commensal flora. The host certainly derives some benefit from these populations, not least by the colonization resistance conferred (Chapter 7).

ANTIMICROBIAL FACTORS IN HEALTH	
Mechanical	Flushing action of liquids: saliva, urine
	Peristalsis of gut
	Skin — an impermeable barrier
	Cough/sneeze reflex
	Mucus
	Cilia
	Shedding of epithelial cells
(Bio)chemical	Anaerobicity
	Acidity
	Sebaceous secretions
	Sweat (high salt)
	Lysozyme — antibacterial enzyme
	Digestive enzymes
	Bile — detergent action
	Colonization resistance
Immunological	Complement
	Phagocytosis
	Inflammation
	Acute phase response
	Antibodies
	Cell-mediated responses

Fig. 1.7 Factors which normal microbiota must contend with in a healthy host. Defects in these factors may result in opportunist infections.

BACTERIAL SURVIVAL IN EXTREMES	
Chemical/physical condition	**Type of micro-organism**
High temperature	**Thermophilic** – optimum growth temperature >45°C, with life up to 100+°C in conditions of high pressure
Low temperature	**Psychrophilic** – optimum growth below 20°C, with some well below 0°C
High osmotic pressure	**Halophilic** – important in high salt environments in nature and in food spoilage of salted foods
Acidic	**Acidophilic** – important in acidic environments in nature, including pickled foods and the stomach
Alkaline	**Basophilic** – most notably in environments with high levels of ammonia

Fig. 1.6 Extremes of physicochemical environments in which bacteria can grow.

Throughout the outside surface and most of the mucosal surfaces of the human body there are niches of considerable diversity, ranging from the dry, salty conditions of the skin to the acidic stomach. In health, micro-organisms exist in a stable equilibrium with the host, and the innate and acquired immune defences (Chapter 7) have evolved in parallel with the micro-organisms to maintain this equilibrium (Fig. 1.7).

Those micro-organisms which cause disease are termed pathogens. These may be primary pathogens which, as part of their normal life cycle, cause harm to the host, and are examples of true biological parasites. Many pathogens, however, are part of the normal microbiota where they exist in a symbiotic or commensal relationship, or are environmental saprophytes. These may, if the opportunity presents, become opportunist pathogens. Typically, it is when the normal host defences break down and the individual becomes immunologically compromised (for example in AIDS) that the host becomes susceptible to diseases caused by these opportunist pathogens. Pathogenesis will be covered in detail in Chapter 4.

Further reading

Mims, C, Playfair, J, Roitt, I, Wakelin, D, and Williams, R (1998). Microbes and parasites; and The host–parasite response. In *Medical microbiology* (2nd edn), Chapters 1 and 2. Mosby, London.

Key facts

- The main groups of micro-organisms are bacteria, fungi, protozoa, and algae.

- Most are microscopic (<10 μm) and unicellular.

- All living cells are either prokaryotic or eukaryotic.

- Prokaryotes are simple cells with no internal membranes or organelles, for example bacteria.

- Eukaryotes are complex cells with a nucleus, internal organelles, and extensive internal membranes, for example protozoa, fungi, and human cells.

- Micro-organisms are found in extremely diverse habitats.

- Most bacteria are saprophytic, involved in recycling elements, but some cause disease (pathogens).

- The human microbiota (normal flora) is found throughout the skin and mucosal surfaces of the body and is in equilibrium with the host defence mechanisms.

- Micro-organisms that cause disease are either primary pathogens or opportunist pathogens.

2

Bacterial structure and physiology

- Bacterial cell structure
- Structure and function of the bacterial cell envelope
- The cytoplasm
- Sporulation
- Bacterial physiology

Bacterial structure and physiology

Bacterial cell structure

Size and shape

Most bacteria are either spherical (coccus) or rod-shaped (bacillus), and are usually arranged in a manner characteristic of the genus, growing either singly, in clusters, or in chains. The dimensions of a bacterium are typically in the order of 1 μm (Fig. 2.1).

The Gram stain

As described in the previous chapter, bacteria are typical prokaryotes. Most bacteria can be divided into one of two types, Gram-positive and Gram-negative, by means of the Gram stain, which is summarized in Fig. 2.2. Although developed empirically by Christian Gram, a Danish microbiologist, in the 1880s, as a convenient method for classifying bacteria, it also gives a great deal of information on the structure of the bacterial cell envelope.

Gram-positive bacteria have a relatively thick amorphous wall (Figs 2.3(a), (b)) which retains the fixed violet dye within the cell. Gram-negative bacteria have a layered appearance due to the presence of two membranes: the inner or cytoplasmic membrane and the outer membrane (Figs 2.4(a), (b)). The organic solvent used in Step 4 of the Gram-staining process disrupts this membranous envelope and the stain is washed out of Gram-negative bacteria.

Some groups of bacteria cannot be considered typical Gram-positive or Gram-negative organisms, as they either do not take up the Gram stain, or they have a different type of envelope entirely. The mycobacteria, such as *Mycobacterium tuberculosis* and *M. leprae* (the causative agent of tuberculosis and leprosy, respectively), are perhaps the best-known examples. These mycobacteria have a waxy envelope containing complex glycolipids, which renders them impervious to the Gram stains. Traditionally, mycobacteria are stained by the Ziehl–Neelsen stain, which involves driving a carbol (phenolic) fuchsin stain into the bacteria with heating, and then decolorizing the background with dilute acid in alcohol (3% HCl in 95% ethanol) – giving rise to the term acid-fast bacilli or AFB; AFB stain bright red.

SHAPES AND ARRANGEMENTS OF BACTERIA	
Cocci	**Rods (bacilli)**
Single coccus	Single rod
Pair of cocci (diplococci)	Chain of rods
Cluster of cocci (staphylococci)	Curved rod (vibrio)
Chains of cocci (streptococci)	Spiral

Fig. 2.1 The various shapes and arrangements of bacteria (not drawn to scale).

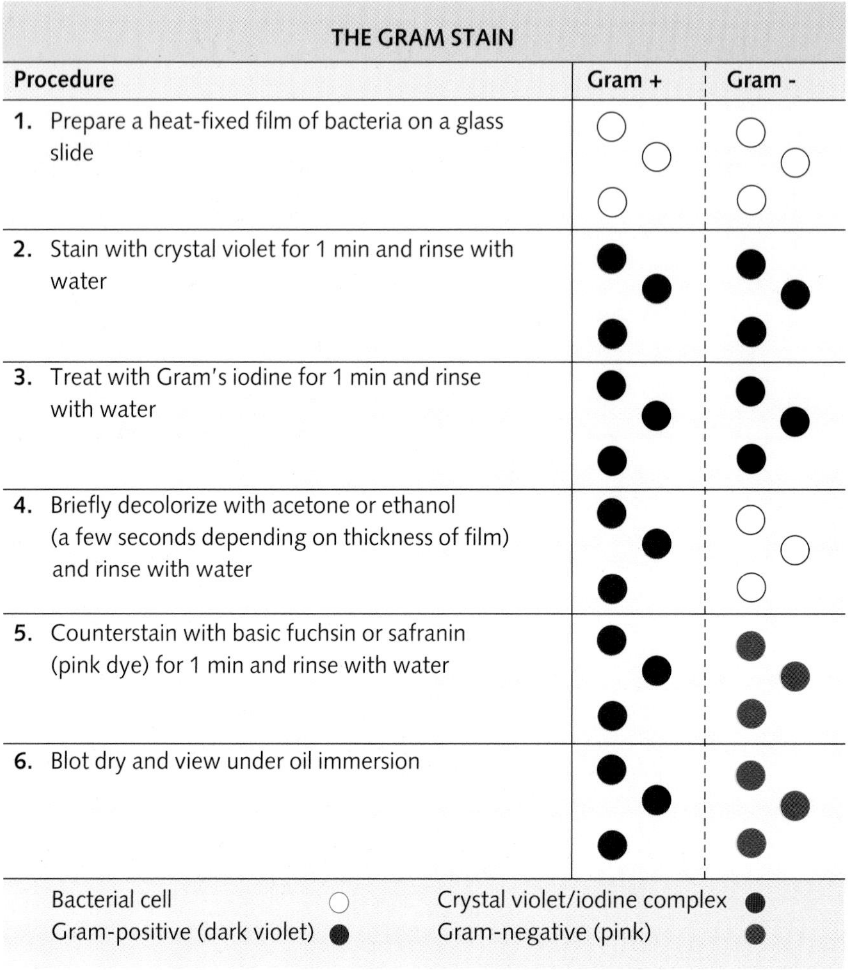

THE GRAM STAIN		
Procedure	**Gram +**	**Gram -**
1. Prepare a heat-fixed film of bacteria on a glass slide	○ ○ ○	○ ○ ○
2. Stain with crystal violet for 1 min and rinse with water	● ● ●	● ● ●
3. Treat with Gram's iodine for 1 min and rinse with water	● ● ●	● ● ●
4. Briefly decolorize with acetone or ethanol (a few seconds depending on thickness of film) and rinse with water	● ● ●	○ ○ ○
5. Counterstain with basic fuchsin or safranin (pink dye) for 1 min and rinse with water	● ● ●	● ● ●
6. Blot dry and view under oil immersion	● ● ●	● ● ●

Bacterial cell	○	Crystal violet/iodine complex	●
Gram-positive (dark violet)	●	Gram-negative (pink)	●

Fig. 2.2 The method for Gram staining a bacterial film.

Structure and function of the bacterial cell envelope

The bacterial cell envelope provides a structural and physiological barrier between the cytoplasm (inside) of the cell and the external environment. The cytoplasmic membrane is a typical membrane consisting of a phospholipid bilayer into which are embedded proteins, some of them crossing the whole width of the membrane: the fluid mosaic model (Fig. 2.5). It is a semi-permeable membrane and osmosis takes place across it. The result is that the inside of the cell is at a high osmotic pressure compared to the outside environment. One of the major functions of the layers outside the cytoplasmic membrane is therefore to withhold this extreme osmotic pressure, thus giving the cell its strength and shape. The functions of the bacterial envelope are listed in Fig. 2.6. Many of these will be covered in detail in later sections of the book.

The Gram-positive bacterium possesses a structure outside of the cytoplasmic membrane that could be termed a wall. This consists of two major polymers: peptidoglycan and a secondary wall polymer which is often a teichoic acid. Many Gram-positive bacteria often also have a protein layer on the surface of the wall. These proteins are sometimes arranged as fibrils perpendicular to the wall and are involved in adhesion, or they may also be present in crystalline surface layers (S-layers) or regular arrays with more of a structural function.

The Gram-negative surface layers are best described as an envelope rather than a wall, as the outer membrane (OM) structure does not readily equate with the wall of Gram-positive bacteria or plant or fungal cells. In the electron microscope the OM appears as a classical membrane, but in chemical terms it is very different from the typical structure: it is asymmetric. The inner leaflet consists of the usual phospholipids, but the sole lipid component of the outer leaflet is the lipopolysaccharide (LPS) molecule, resulting in a relatively non-fluid membrane and a major permeability barrier. There are a small number of major outer membrane proteins (OMPs), but these are fewer in number than in the cytoplasmic membrane. Some of the OMPs form transmembrane diffusion channels and are termed porins.

GRAM-POSITIVE CELL WALL

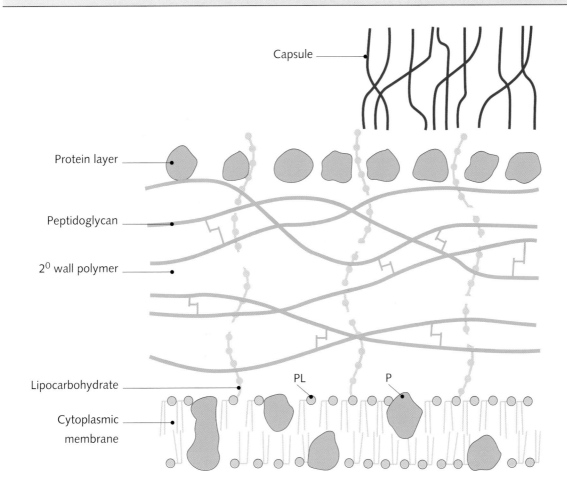

Capsule

Protein layer

Peptidoglycan

2^0 wall polymer

Lipocarbohydrate

Cytoplasmic membrane

PL

P

(a)

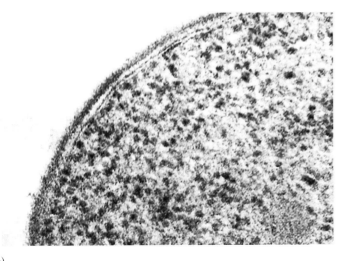

(b)

Fig. 2.3 (a) Diagram of the envelope of Gram-positive bacteria. PL, phospholipid; P, protein. (b) Electron micrograph of the envelope of Gram-positive bacteria.

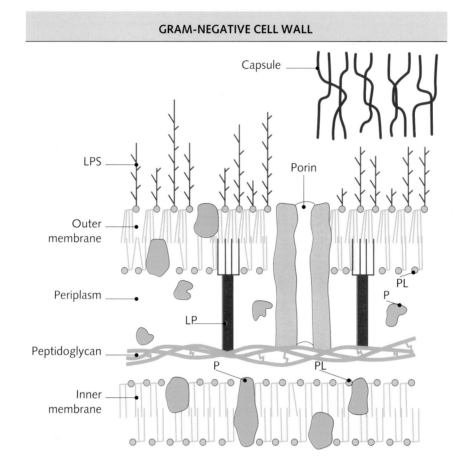

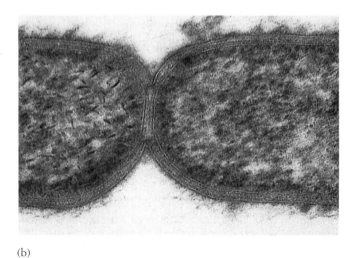

Fig. 2.4 (a) Diagram of the envelope of Gram-negative bacteria. LPS, lipopolysaccharide; LP, lipoprotein; PL, phospholipid; P, protein. (b) Electron micrograph of the envelope of Gram-negative bacteria.

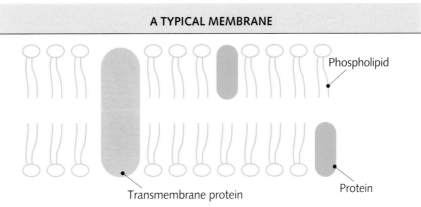

Fig. 2.5 Diagram of a typical membrane (fluid mosaic model).

FUNCTIONS OF THE BACTERIAL CELL ENVELOPE

- Protects against osmotic lysis
- Gives bacterium rigidity and shape
- Acts as permeability barrier which can be selective
- Maintains ionic balance between inside of cell and the growth environment
- Carries the transport machinery which operates across the membrane
- Senses the environment
- Supports the flagellar motors
- Supports fimbriae and other adhesins
- Is involved in invasion/penetration of cells
- Acts as matrix of biosynthetic processes
- Is involved in cell division
- Protects against host defence mechanisms
- Protects against antibacterial substances

Fig. 2.6 Summary of functions of the bacterial cell envelope.

Outside the envelopes of many Gram-positive and Gram-negative bacteria there is often a capsule or slime layer, which is described later.

Macromolecules of the envelope

Peptidoglycan

Peptidoglycan is the major structural molecule of the envelope and is responsible for the shape and strength of the cell. It can be considered as a single molecule which covers the whole three-dimensional surface of the bacterium. Peptidoglycan consists of long, parallel chains of *N*-acetylated amino sugars (alternating *N*-Ac glucosamine and *N*-Ac muramic acid) which are cross-linked

by short peptide chains (Fig. 2.7). There is a greater amount of peptidoglycan in the Gram-positive wall than in the Gram-negative envelope.

Some species, notably *Chlamydia* spp., appear Gram-negative in the electron microscope but they have no peptidoglycan layer between the cytoplasmic (inner) and outer membrane. Instead they have their major outer membrane proteins cross-linked through disulphide bridges, giving the OM a degree of strength.

Teichoic acids and other secondary cell-wall molecules

In the strictest sense, teichoic acids are polymers of poly(ribitol phosphate) or poly(glycerol phosphate) which are found in the cell walls of Gram-positive bacteria (Fig. 2.8). These polymers may have sugar or amino acid substituents, either as side chains or within the chain of the polymer. The phosphate group confers an overall negative charge to the polymers, and one of the main functions of the macromolecule is thought to be in the scavenging of divalent cations, particularly calcium and magnesium, from the growth environment of the bacterium. These polymers are also the substrate for autolytic enzymes, and they are also exploited as antigens for the serological classification of certain genera.

Some Gram-positive bacteria have analogous, negatively charged, wall polymers which are not true teichoic acids – i.e. they do not contain glycerol or ribitol phosphate. They do, however, contain charged groups such as uronic acids or phosphates and functionally they are the same as teichoic acids.

The membrane-bound analogues, the lipoteichoic acids and other membrane-bound lipocarbohydrates, are anchored in the cytoplasmic membrane through a glycolipid. They also have a role in sequestering divalent cations and channelling them down to the membrane, together with a possible role in bacterial adhesion.

Lipopolysaccharides

Lipopolysaccharides (LPS) are complex, amphipathic molecules located as the sole lipid in the outer membrane of Gram-negative bacteria. Structurally, LPS molecules are divided into three

THE STRUCTURE OF PEPTIDOGLYCAN

Unit structure

M — G — M — G — M — G — M — G —
|
L-ala
|
D-glu
|
L-lys ← peptide cross-link → D-ala
| |
D-ala   L-lys
                                  |
                                 D-glu
                                  |
                                 L-ala

G — M — G — M — G — M — G — M — G —

Three-dimensional structure

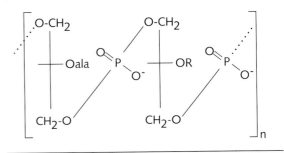

——— Peptide side chain   ——— Cross-bridge

M	=	*N*-acetyl muramic acid
G	=	*N*-acetyl glucosamine
ala	=	alanine
lys	=	lysine
glu	=	glutamic acid
L	=	usual L isomer
D	=	unusual D isomer

Fig. 2.7 The chemical structure of peptidoglycan.

TEICHOIC ACIDS

Ribitol type

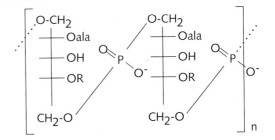

Glycerol type

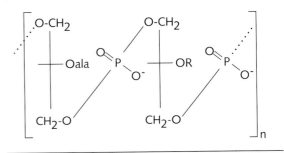

R = a sugar substituent
ala = an O-substituted D-alanine
n = 30-40

Fig. 2.8 Chemical structure of typical teichoic acids.

ance. Mutant bacteria lacking the O-polysaccharide appear 'rough' and have a rough-form or R-LPS. Some species of bacteria naturally produce an R-LPS and these molecules are sometimes termed lipo-oligosaccharides (LOS) (Fig. 2.9).

The lipid A molecule consists of a disaccharide backbone (usually bis-glucosamine) which is substituted with five or six fatty acids and two phosphates. Between different species of Gram-negative bacteria, there is little variation in the structure of the lipid A part of the molecule, whereas related species have identical structures. In the core region, there are several unusual sugars which are found only in bacteria, for example 3-deoxy-D-*manno*-2-octulosonic acid, which is still more commonly known by the initial letters of its previous name, KDO (keto-deoxy-octonic acid). The inner part of the core is, like lipid A, highly conserved within related species, but some variation can occur in the outer part. However, it is in the O-polysaccharide that the real variation occurs. The many different possible combinations of sugars and the configuration of the linkages between them give rise to an infinite number of different oligosaccharide-repeating units. In the species *Escherichia coli* alone there are approximately 160 different structures recognized, giving rise to the distinct O-serogroups.

main sections: the lipid A; the core oligosaccharide; and the O-polysaccharide or O-antigen (Fig. 2.9). The O-polysaccharide is made up of a chain of repeating oligosaccharide units of heterogeneous length. This normal configuration of LPS is usually referred to as smooth-form LPS (S-LPS), since wild-type bacteria possessing this molecule produce colonies with a 'smooth' appear-

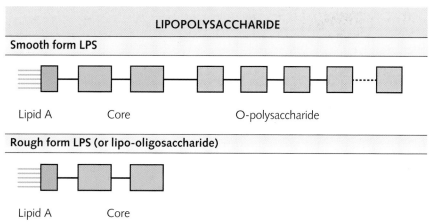

Fig. 2.9 Diagrammatic representation of lipopolysaccharide.

LPS is an essential component of the Gram-negative bacterium. Its functions include a structural role, where the fatty acid chains pack tightly in the OM resulting in a relatively non-fluid structure which forms an impervious barrier. As described earlier for teichoic acids, LPS molecules are negatively charged, and the long sugar chains confer a degree of hydrophilicity on the bacterial surface. In pathogenic bacteria, LPS is considered to be one of the most important virulence determinants. It has a role in protecting the organism from the effects of serum complement. The lipid A region is extremely biologically active, giving rise to the synonym for LPS of endotoxin. These properties of LPS/endotoxin will be covered in more detail in Chapter 4.

Capsule/slime

Many bacteria, both Gram-positive and Gram-negative, possess a gel-like layer outside the envelope. This may be in the form of a discrete capsule which can extend from the envelope for a distance several times the diameter of the cell. Alternatively, this gel material may not be firmly attached but forms a slime which is released into the surrounding environment. Most of these materials are polysaccharide in nature, and are often referred to collectively as exopolysaccharides. However, some species, for example *Bacillus* spp., produce a capsule consisting of poly-amino acids. The capsule of *Bacillus anthracis*, the causative organism of anthrax, has a capsule of poly(D-glutamic acid). Exopolysaccharides are sometimes neutral homopolysaccharides, for example the glucans and fructans of many oral streptococci, or negatively charged heteropolysaccharides, where uronic acids are common constituents. The poly(D-glutamic acid) capsule with its negative charge is probably physiologically analogous to the negatively charged polysaccharide capsule.

The capsule is a highly hydrated gel and under the microscope, with both living or stained bacteria, it is invisible. The simplest way to demonstrate the capsule is by mixing a suspension of bacteria with an equal volume of Indian Ink on a slide, covering with a coverslip, pressing down firmly to create an extremely thin film, and then viewing it under the microscope. The capsule is

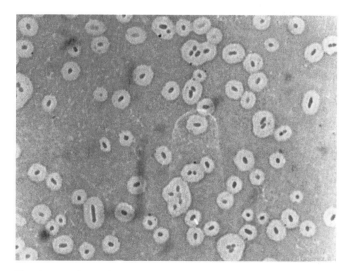

Fig. 2.10 Indian Ink stain to demonstrate the bacterial capsule. (Courtesy of Sheila Patrick.)

'negatively' stained, appearing as a clear zone around the cell where the microscopic Indian Ink (carbon) particles have not penetrated (Fig. 2.10).

The capsule has various functions, and perhaps the most universal of these is its involvement in adhesion to surfaces. Many bacteria colonize both inert and living surfaces, and grow in microcolonies or as a consortium in a biofilm. Dental plaque is an excellent example of this. Other functions can be considered as protective and in the pathogen include protection from, and evasion of, the immune system. These will be covered in detail in Chapter 4.

Surface appendages

The surface appendages can be divided into two main types: those involved in motility (flagella), and those involved in adhesion (fimbriae/pili).

Flagella (singular: flagellum)

Many species of bacteria can move actively through an aqueous environment. This motility can be governed by several different mechanisms, including the poorly understood gliding motility of *Cytophaga* spp. However, the mechanisms involving flagella are the most common and the best understood. The arrangement of flagella varies between different species, but is the same for a given species. Flagella can be found singly (monotrichous) or in bundles (lophotrichous) at one or both poles of the cell, or they can be arranged over the whole cell surface (peritrichous) (Fig. 2.11). The flagellum consists of a long thin filament projecting for up to several micrometres from the cell surface. The main part of the filament is made up of protein subunits (flagellin) arranged in several helices around a central hollow core. At the base of the flagellum, a 'motor' is located in the cell envelope. It consists of a series of rings through which the base of the filament can rotate in either a clockwise or an anticlockwise direction. Above the base of the filament there is a short bent region which produces a propeller-like propulsion from the revolving flagellum (Fig. 2.11). A motile bacterium is able to perform chemotaxis or phototaxis, that is move towards or away from stimuli such as chemicals or light, respectively. Receptors which are sensitive to such stimuli are located on the bacterial surface and respond by making the flagellum rotate in one or other direction. The resultant motility, which varies between a tumbling and a directional mode, depending on the direction of rotation, allows the bacterium to swim by means of a 'random walk' towards or away from the source of the stimulus.

Spirochaetes move in a corkscrew manner by means of an axial filament. This consists of a bundle of flagellum-like structures, which lies between the cell surface and an outer sheath and connects one end of the cell to the other (see Fig. 14.2).

Fimbriae/pili (singular: fimbria/pilus)

The terms fimbriae and pili (see Fig. 1.3) are synonymous for most purposes. These appendages tend to be found only on Gram-negative bacteria, and are shorter and straighter than flagella (see Fig. 2.11), although the basic structure is the same: helices of the protein (always called pilin) arranged around a hollow core, but without a motor. The term fimbria originated in the UK where it was first recognized and studied in enterobacteria, while pilus was coined in the USA for the appendage on the gonococcus organism. Because of the abundance of American textbooks, pilus is perhaps more commonly used, though many microbiologists would like to have some consensus as to when each term should be used. There is a view that fimbriae should be used for those structures having a role in adhesion, the commonest property of these appendages, while pilus be restricted to the sex pilus, the appendage which connects mating cells and through which the DNA passes during the process of conjugation (Chapter 6).

Fimbriae usually bind to a surface through a specific recognition mechanism. The end of the fimbria carries a molecule (peptide) which recognizes a specific receptor on the surface to

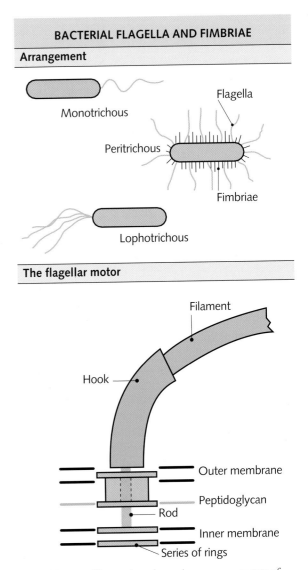

BACTERIAL FLAGELLA AND FIMBRIAE

Arrangement

The flagellar motor

Fig. 2.11 Diagram illustrating the various arrangements of bacterial flagellae, fimbriae, and the structure of the flagellar motor.

which it binds. The host cell receptor is usually a sugar residue, and the recognition molecule on the bacterium is termed a lectin.

Gram-positive bacteria do not have classical fimbriae, but many possess a fine fibrillar arrangement of proteins on their surface, sometimes termed fibrillae, which bind to host molecules. This is best exemplified by the M-protein of *Streptococcus pyogenes*.

The cytoplasm

The cytoplasm of bacteria contains all the biosynthetic machinery required by the bacterium for growth and cell division, together with the genetic material. The latter consists of a double helix of DNA arranged in a supercoiled circular structure. It is not enclosed in a nuclear membrane, but is often referred to as the 'bacterial chromosome' because of the analogy with the eukaryotic structures. In growing bacteria the DNA can account for up to 20% of the volume of the bacterium. Smaller circles of 'extra-chromosomal' DNA are often present in bacteria and these are termed plasmids (Chapter 6). They carry genes which may confer the bacterium with properties such as antibiotic resistance or the capacity to produce toxins or enzymes.

The ribosomes used for protein synthesis are smaller than their eukaryotic counterpart, with a sedimentation coefficient of 70S (compared with 80S in eukaryotes). They consist of two subunits of 30S and 50S, giving a net 70S. They are the site of action of several antibiotics such as the aminoglycosides, macrolides, and tetracyclines (Chapter 9).

Many bacteria possess inclusion granules within their cytoplasm, and in some species they are utilized as characteristics which can serve as markers for identification purposes. Their main function is thought to be one of storage, being produced when their main constituent element is present in excess in the culture medium. Metachromatic granules, or volutin, are deposits of inorganic polyphosphate, which can be dyed with methylene blue and are characteristic of *Corynebacterium diphtheriae*. Starch and glycogen granules are commonly revealed in many bacteria when stained with iodine. Lipid inclusions are found in mycobacteria and are visualized with Sudan Black dye. Some bacterial toxins characteristically form as crystalline cytoplasmic inclusions.

Sporulation

Bacterial cells, unlike all higher and many lower eukaryotic cells, are unable to differentiate or undergo morphogenesis. However, some bacterial species, i.e.. the aerobic *Bacillus* spp. and the anaerobic *Clostridium* spp., can perform a primitive process of differentiation termed sporulation. The bacterium on encountering stressful conditions, such as dehydration or nutrient limitation, can convert to a resting or dormant endospore. This endospore is then highly resistant to many harsh physical and chemical conditions such as heat (some can withstand boiling), dryness, toxic chemicals, and radiation. From a practical point of view, spore-forming bacteria can be very difficult to eradicate during sterilization procedures.

During the process of sporulation, before the spore is free of the 'parent' cell, it often has a characteristic appearance within the bacterial cell. This can be defined on the basis of the spore's location in the cell (terminal/subterminal/central), its diameter (smaller/same/greater than vegetative cell), and its shape (spherical/oval) and can be used to assist in diagnosis.

On returning to favourable conditions, spores can germinate and form new vegetative cells.

Bacterial physiology

Nutrition

The nutritional requirements of bacteria vary enormously. At the simplest extreme, *Escherichia coli* and related enterobacteria can grow in a simple synthetic medium containing the inorganic salts which are necessary to supply the major essential elements of carbon, hydrogen, oxygen, nitrogen, phosphorus, and sulphur, together with a source of energy – the simplest being glucose. Trace elements are not usually added specifically since they typically occur at adequate levels as contaminants in commercial chemicals. Some bacteria release extracellular hydrolytic enzymes into the environment for nutritional purposes, and such enzymes, for example proteases, may play a role in disease production.

Conventionally, bacteria are cultured in liquid media (broths) or on the surfaces of solid media which have agar added as a gelling agent. Agar, a polysaccharide extracted from seaweed, is relatively inert (is not metabolized by most bacteria), gels below 50°C (heat-labile ingredients can be added after sterilization by filtration) and melts at 100°C (does not melt when incubated). Agar media are usually contained in flat, circular plates (Petri dishes).

Many bacteria require certain amino acids, vitamins, and other growth factors which can be supplied by adding yeast extracts and meat digests to the media. These are available commercially as various forms of nutrient broths and nutrient agars. Other bacteria require more extensive additions, and for many clinically important bacteria these requirements can be fulfilled by the addition of blood or serum (from horses).

Some bacteria require living cells for their growth, and these can be supplied by tissue culture methods. However, a few species, notably *Mycobacterium leprae* and *Treponema pallidum*, the causative agents of leprosy and syphilis, respectively, can only be cultured when inoculated into a living animal.

Energy production

Production of energy can be considered as the processes by which bacteria produce adenosine triphosphate (ATP) by the phosphorylation of adenosine diphosphate:

$$\text{Adenosine–P–P} + \text{energy} + \text{P} \rightarrow \text{Adenosine–P–P–P}$$

As described briefly in Chapter 1, this is achieved mainly by fermentative or respiratory processes. The large group of photosynthetic bacteria produce ATP by harnessing energy from light, but these will not be discussed further.

The anaerobic bacteria, which produce energy only by fermentation, use substrate-level phosphorylation, and can utilize carbohydrates or amino acids as fermentable substrates. Aerobic and facultative organisms utilize both substrate-level and oxidative phosphorylation, producing much more ATP per mole of substrate if the oxidative process is used (Fig. 2.12). Glycolysis is the central pathway for carbohydrate metabolism, but many bacteria have alternative pathways such as the pentose phosphate and Entner–Doudoroff pathways, which are outside the scope of this book. The end products of fermentation are typically ethanol, carbon dioxide, lactic acid, and volatile, short-chained fatty acids, the latter giving some anaerobic bacteria their characteristic foul smell.

BACTERIAL ENERGY PRODUCTION AND ASSOCIATED METABOLIC PATHWAYS

PROTEIN	CARBOHYDRATE	LIPID

Amino acids · Sugars · Glycerol · Fatty acids

GLYCOLYSIS

Glyceraldehyde-3-P

ATP

Pyruvic acid

Acetyl Co-A

Lactic acid · **Ethanol +CO$_2$**

KREBS' CYCLE

ATP

CO$_2$

ELECTRON TRANSPORT

O$_2$ · H$_2$O

(or NO$_3^-$ or SO$_4^{2-}$ or CO$_3^{2-}$) (or NO$_2^-$/N$_2$O/N$_2$ or H$_2$S or CH$_4$)

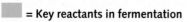 = Key reactants in fermentation

Atmospheric growth conditions	Energy production by	Final electron acceptor	Type of phosphorylation	Moles ATP produced per glucose equivalent
Aerobic	Aerobic respiration	Molecular oxygen	Substrate level and oxidative	38
Anaerobic	Anaerobic respiration	Inorganic molecule e.g. NO$_3^-$ or SO$_4^{2-}$ or CO$_3^{2-}$	Substrate level and oxidative	>2 <38
Aerobic or anaerobic	Fermentation	Organic molecule	Oxidative	2

Fig. 2.12 Summary of energy production and associated metabolic pathways in bacteria.

Biosynthesis of macromolecules

The various macromolecules (nucleic acids, proteins, carbohydrates, and lipids) required for the structure and biosynthetic machinery of the bacterial cell must be assembled from the nutrients supplied from the growth medium. As described previously, the nutritional requirements of different bacteria range from being extremely simple to complex. Consequently, there is a range of biosynthetic capabilities in different bacteria. Some, such as *E. coli*, can synthesize their macromolecules from simple inorganic molecules, while other bacteria have requirements for amino acids, peptides, vitamins, and growth factors. Although bacteria have some pathways peculiar to themselves, the basic pathways which they possess for their biosynthetic processes are similar to those of their eukaryotic counterparts. The reader is referred to a standard biochemistry textbook if more information is required.

Growth of bacteria

Growth can be defined as the orderly increase of all the chemical components of the cell. Bacteria fulfil this definition, and when they have grown to a certain size (length) they undergo cell division to produce two daughter cells identical to the parent cell. The process is termed binary fission (Fig. 2.13). Bacterial growth can be equated to cell number: one bacterium divides into two, these two produce four, and then eight, and so on. The growth rate of a bacterium is therefore measured by measuring the change in bacterial number per unit time. The time between cell divisions can be as short as 10–20 minutes for many common bacteria growing in laboratory media.

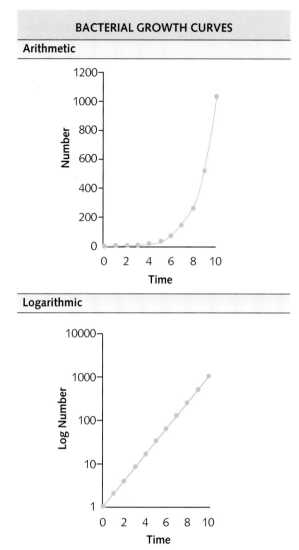

BACTERIAL GROWTH CURVES

Fig. 2.14 Arithmetic and logarithmic graphs illustrating changes in bacterial number per unit time.

The number of bacteria at a given time can be estimated by taking a small sample and counting the number of organisms directly using a counting chamber (haemocytometer-type) and a microscope, or by diluting a sample and spreading small volumes over the surface of an agar plate and counting the number of colonies after a suitable incubation time (one bacterium produces one colony).

If bacterial number is plotted against time the shape of the curve will show an exponential increase (Fig. 2.14). However, if the number of bacteria is plotted as a log value, a straight line graph is obtained (Fig. 2.14).

The bacterial growth curve

If a broth culture of bacteria is set up from a small inoculum, the population size increases following a classical pattern (Fig. 2.15). There are three distinct phases:

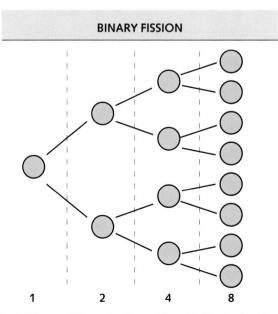

BINARY FISSION

Fig. 2.13 Diagram illustrating bacterial multiplication by binary fission. Each circle represents a bacterial cell.

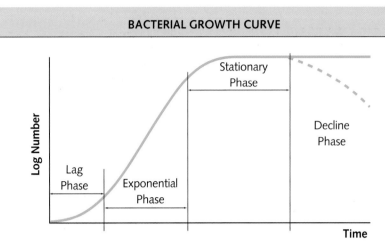

Fig. 2.15 The classic bacterial growth curve for a batch culture.

1. *The lag phase*: the inoculated bacteria are becoming acclimatized to the environment, switching on enzymes, adjusting to the temperature and atmospheric conditions.

2. *The logarithmic, or exponential phase*: there are no restraints on the bacteria, and they are dividing exponentially: 1 to 2 to 4 to 8 to 16....

3. *The stationary phase*: an essential nutrient becomes limited, or there is a build-up of a toxic metabolite (for example an acid or alcohol) which stops the growth. At this stage some bacterial species die and there is a decline phase, while other bacteria may remain viable for an extended time. Spore-formers often sporulate at this time.

This is the type of culture that is typically set up in the laboratory to investigate the identity of a bacterium, or its susceptibility to an antibiotic. It is termed a batch culture and has some parallels in Nature, for example the contamination of a sterile fluid or the formation of an abscess or lung infection. Obviously many other parameters must be considered, not least the response of the host when the 'culture' is an active infection.

Another way of culturing bacteria, which is commonly used industrially, is by means of continuous culture, a process whereby medium is constantly added, with the excess medium plus culture draining away. The growth rate can be controlled by altering the dilution rate of the culture. This type of culture also has parallels in Nature, for example the normal flora of the mouth and gastrointestinal tract, diarrhoeal disease, and urinary tract infections.

Key facts

- Shapes and arrangements of bacteria: cocci, rods/bacilli, vibrios, and spirals; these may grow singly, in clusters, or in chains.

- Gram-positive bacteria are dark violet and Gram-negative bacteria are pink after staining. The Gram reaction is related to the structure of the cell envelope. Gram-positive bacteria have a cytoplasmic membrane and wall; Gram-negative bacteria have inner and outer membranes (latter with LPS and porins). Other examples are the waxy envelopes of mycobacteria (acid-fast bacilli).

- The structure and function of typical membranes: lipid bilayer and fluid mosaic model. The process of osmosis.

- The structure and function of peptidoglycan: long parallel chains of alternating *N*-acetyl glucosamine and *N*-acetyl muramic acid are cross-linked through peptide side-chains and cross-bridges. These are responsible for the shape and strength of the bacterium.

- Teichoic acids are present in Gram-positives: they have a negative charge and scavenge divalent cations.

- Lipopolysaccharides are present in the outer membrane of Gram-negative bacteria: S- and R-forms, non-fluid membrane, endotoxin.

- Capsules, slime, exopolysaccharides: these have a role in adhesion/biofilm and in protection.

- Surface appendages: flagella are used for movement, fimbriae/pili for attachment.

- Bacterial cytoplasm contains: DNA supercoiled, circular; 70S ribosomes for protein synthesis; inclusion/storage granules.

Key facts *(cont.)*

- Sporulation is seen in *Bacillus* spp. and *Clostridium* spp., and resistance of bacterial (endo)spores.

- Nutrition: can be simple to complex.

- Energy production: follows fermentation and respiration pathways.

- Binary fission and bacterial growth: exponential. Batch and continuous culture.

Further reading

Murray, PR, Rosenthal, KS, Kobayashi, GS, and Pfaller, MA (1998). Bacterial morphology and cell wall structure and synthesis; and Bacterial metabolism and growth. In *Medical microbiology* (3rd edn), Chapters 3 and 4. Mosby Year Book, St Louis.

3

Bacterial taxonomy

- Bacterial classification and nomenclature
- Different approaches to taxonomic methods
- Bacterial identification

Bacterial taxonomy

Taxonomy is the term given to the systematic classification, naming, and identification of living organisms. Bacterial taxonomy is often thought of as a complex but 'necessary evil', that is uninteresting to learn and overwhelms many students. It is, however, at the very root of biological communication and is essential for describing an organism, whether newly discovered or well known. A working knowledge of taxonomy is also useful for diagnostic microbiology and for studies in epidemiology and pathogenicity. The intricacies of the rapidly moving field of modern taxonomic research and its methodologies are largely beyond the scope of this book. However, sufficient detail will be given to enable the reader to acquire adequate skills in the communication of bacterial names, and to illustrate the reasons why taxonomy is so important.

Traditionally, all living organisms were classified into different hierarchical groups or taxa (singular, taxon), based on a system originally devised by Linnaeus (a Swedish botanist) in 1735. The term kingdom is at the top of the hierarchy, and there are five kingdoms: Prokaryotae (bacteria), Protista (algae and protozoa), Myceteae (the fungi), Plantae, and Animalia. This is followed by phylum (animals and protozoa) or division (plants, algae, fungi, and bacteria), class, order, family, genus, and finally species. This system is still the most widely used for the classification of plants, animals, and most other living organisms, and remains the main method for micro-organisms, with the exception of viruses (chapter 5).

The following scheme is illustrated for the human being:

Kingdom: Animalia
Phylum: Chordata
Class: Mammalia
Order: Primates
Family: Hominoidea
Genus: *Homo*
Species: *sapiens*

The genus and species names are used together to give the scientific name (or Latin binomial) of the organism (although Greek and sometimes modern European words are commonly used and are latinized). This binomial is printed in italics with the genus name beginning with an upper case (capital) letter, and the species name with a lower case (small) letter, for example *Homo sapiens*. In a piece of writing this can be abbreviated to the form *H. sapiens* after it has been written out initially in full.

Bacterial classification and nomenclature

The system described above is commonly abbreviated for bacterial classification. The kingdom Prokaryotae is normally divided into three divisions: Eubacteria, Archaebacteria, and Cyanobacteria. Class and order are usually ignored, being replaced instead by morphological divisions based on cell shape, Gram reaction, and nutritional properties. The next important division is family, followed by genus and species. The use of these terms will now be illustrated for two important medical pathogens, *Escherichia coli* and *Staphylococcus aureus*.

The organism *Escherichia coli* is a Gram-negative, rod-shaped, facultatively anaerobic organism which is tolerant to bile. This places it in the family Enterobacteriaceae. A series of metabolic tests, including the fermentation of various sugars and the production of indole from tryptophan, separates it from other genera of Enterobacteriaceae such as *Salmonella* and *Proteus* and places it in the genus *Escherichia* and the species *coli*. It is commonly abbreviated to *E. coli*.

Staphylococcus aureus is a facultatively anaerobic Gram-positive coccal organism growing in clusters, belonging to the family Micrococcaceae. It is tolerant to 10% sodium chloride, resistant to lysozyme, but sensitive to lysostaphin, and thus belongs to the genus *Staphylococcus*. As it possesses Protein A on its cell surface and produces the enzyme coagulase this places it in the species *aureus*. This can be abbreviated to *S. aureus*.

In writing, where two different species are being discussed which both have the same initial letter for the genus, for example *Staphylococcus aureus* and *Streptococcus mutans*, it is common to use the terms *Staph.* and *Strep.* as the abbreviations, to avoid ambiguity. When bacterial names are used as adjectives, for example staphylococcal toxin or clostridial spore, or are used collectively, for example salmonellae or streptococci, the names are not italicized and do not begin with a capital letter.

Different approaches to taxonomic methods

Traditionally, morphological and biochemical characters have been used in taxonomy. These characters are referred to as phenotypic, and tend to group organisms into structurally and physiologically related organisms. In bacterial taxonomy the shape of the organism, the Gram stain, and its metabolic processes are phenotypic characters of prime importance. Figure 3.1 summarizes the most important phenotypic methods used in bacterial taxonomy. This form of taxonomy can therefore be thought of as a natural system which shows the degree of relatedness of organisms. In order for the organisms to be arranged in a classical taxonomic tree it is necessary to devise a hierarchy of characters, with some characters being more important than others. The relative importance of a character is often very subjective with little or no scientific objectivity. For example, is the shape of an organism more important than its reaction to the Gram stain or its ability to ferment glucose?

Numerical, or Adansonian, taxonomy is significantly different from the classical approach described above and was originally devised about 200 years ago to avoid inherent bias in the classical methods. Every observable character of an organism carries an equal weight and they are considered equally in calculating similarities or differences between organisms. A similarity coefficient can be calculated between two or more organisms. The results of

PHENOTYPIC METHODS IN BACTERIAL TAXONOMY	
Character examined	**Types identified/comment**
Gram reaction	Gram-positive Gram-negative Acid fastness/alcohol fastness
Cell shape	Coccus Rod/bacillus Curved or spiral
Motility/presence of flagellum(a)	Motile, non-motile Flagellar arrangement: single, multiple, polar, peritrichous
Spores	Presence or absence Shape and position in cell
Mode of energy production	Fermentation Aerobic or anaerobic respiration Photosynthesis
Enzyme activities	Biochemical tests Preformed enzyme activities Multilocus enzyme electrophoresis
Cell-wall structures	Peptidoglycan types Teichoic acid types LPS chemotype
Lipid analysis	Whole cell fatty acids Phospholipids and sphingolipids Mycolic acid analysis
Serological analysis	Capsular antigens LPS antigens Other surface antigens: flagella, proteins Use of monoclonal and polyclonal antibodies
Protein analysis by polyacrylamide gel electrophoresis (PAGE)	Whole cell protein Outer membrane proteins Crystalline surface proteins
Phage and bacteriocin typing	Suitable for particular species
Pyrolysis/mass spectrometry	Sophisticated methods which analyse the total chemical composition of bacterial cells

Fig. 3.1 Phenotypic methods used in bacterial taxonomy.

NUMERICAL TAXONOMY AND DENDROGRAMS

In a series of strains, phenotypic characters are recognized and counted

Similarity coefficients (S_J) are calculated for pairs of the series of strains using the following formula:

$$(S_J) = \frac{a}{a + b + c} \; \%$$

Where
- a = number of characters positive in both strains
- b = number of characters positive in strain 1 and negative in strain 2
- c = Number of characters positive in strain 2 and negative in strain 1

Matrices of similarity coefficients can be made up, or dendrograms constructed, as exemplified below for 10 hypothetical strains:

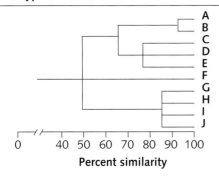

Fig. 3.2 Numerical taxonomy and construction of dendrograms.

such methods do not give rise to the classical genus and species, but to mathematical relationships which are often represented as a dendrogram demonstrating similarities and differences. Modern computer programs can be used to analyse numerical data and construct dendrograms (Fig. 3.2).

Evolution is an important concept to consider in taxonomy, as genetically similar organisms are certainly related and are also likely to be morphologically related. Evolutionary relatedness and similarities in structure and physiology have given rise to the term phylogenetic or natural taxonomy. In the past 10 years the sequencing of ribosomal RNA (rRNA) and the genes coding for rRNA have revolutionized our views on bacterial phylogeny.

The classical and numerical systems could conceivably result in the grouping of organisms which are structurally and physiologically related, but which are genetically distinct, within the same taxon. Again in the last 10 years or so, this problem has led to the wide-scale use of genetic or molecular approaches. Genotypic taxonomy uses the organism's genetic characteristics, which are considered by many to be more important than phenotypic characteristics. Figure 3.3 lists the main genotypic methods in current use. It appears that this modern approach to taxonomy is being led by the rapid advances in nucleic acid-based technology and has placed taxonomy into the 'hi-tech' end of biology, regaining a status which has been absent for the best part of a century. Further details of genotypic methods are given in Chapter 6.

The definition of a species can be described in genotypic taxonomy as 'a group of strains sharing 70% or greater DNA:DNA relatedness, with 5°C or less difference in melting points by stepwise denaturation between homologous and heterologous hybrids formed under standard conditions' (see Chapter 6 for further explanation). Phenotypic taxonomic methods should agree with this definition.

GENOTYPIC METHODS IN BACTERIAL TAXONOMY	
General method	**Specific method**
Mol % G + C	
Restriction enzyme patterns	Restriction fragment length polymorphism (RFLP) Pulsed-field gel electrophoresis (PFGE)
DNA:DNA hybridization	
DNA sequencing	
PCR-based DNA fingerprinting	Ribotyping Amplified rDNA restriction analysis (ARDRA) Randomly amplified polymorphic DNA (RAPD) Amplified fragment length polymorphism (AFLP)
DNA probes	
rRNA sequencing	

Fig. 3.3 Genotypic methods used in bacterial taxonomy. Full details of the methods are beyond the scope of this book, but see Chapter 6 for more information.

As stated earlier, one of the prime uses of taxonomy is in communication. For example, the diagnostic laboratory must be able to communicate with the clinician in terms of bacterial nomenclature. If the system is so confused and rapidly changing then this will be unworkable. This means that there should perhaps be two levels of bacterial classification and nomenclature, one at the research level which is detailed and progressive, the other at the pragmatic level which is changed less frequently. There is an inevitable dichotomy, but there must also be compatibility between the two systems, with the latter being adaptable to change as development proceeds at the research level.

A final term to be introduced here is polyphasic taxonomy. It was coined in 1970, but has recently been reintroduced as a 'Consensus approach to bacterial systematics'. In principle, this method uses all the phenotypic, genotypic, and phylogenetic information available. Databases can be constructed of genotypic, phenotypic, and numerical results, and, assuming that the technology produces reproducible data, access should allow universal use of this data. It is likely that for the foreseeable future, however, nucleic acid sequence data will be the most useful of these facilities.

Bacterial identification

The steps taken in the laboratory to identify a bacterium follow a series of routine procedures which are summarized in Fig. 3.4. This is a practical topic and there are many textbooks and laboratory manuals dedicated to the subject of bacterial identification. As demonstrated in Fig. 3.4, the major techniques employed are traditional, based on culture and identification by classical methods such as microscopy, colonial appearance, growth characteristics, and biochemical/metabolic tests. For some bacteria, simple Gram staining and colonial appearance on a selective medium are sufficient for presumptive species identification by an experienced microbiologist. For other species, a more extensive battery of tests would be required. A myriad of commercial test kits are now available for the rapid identification of many clinically important bacteria. However, they should be used with caution, and a skilled technician is still required to ensure that pure cultures are being used and that correct interpretations of the tests are made.

Semi-systematic lists of clinically important bacteria are given in Figs 3.5, 3.6, and 3.7.

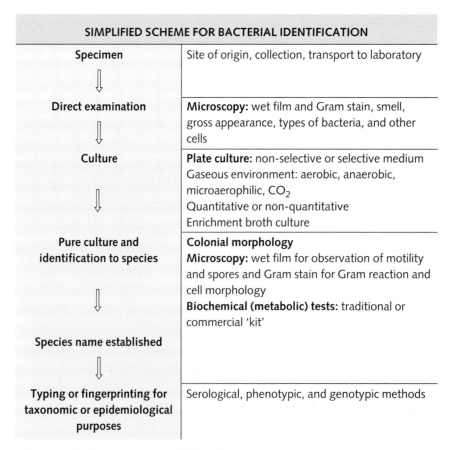

SIMPLIFIED SCHEME FOR BACTERIAL IDENTIFICATION

Specimen	Site of origin, collection, transport to laboratory
⇩	
Direct examination	**Microscopy:** wet film and Gram stain, smell, gross appearance, types of bacteria, and other cells
⇩	
Culture	**Plate culture:** non-selective or selective medium Gaseous environment: aerobic, anaerobic, microaerophilic, CO_2 Quantitative or non-quantitative Enrichment broth culture
⇩	
Pure culture and identification to species	**Colonial morphology** **Microscopy:** wet film for observation of motility and spores and Gram stain for Gram reaction and cell morphology **Biochemical (metabolic) tests:** traditional or commercial 'kit'
⇩	
Species name established	
⇩	
Typing or fingerprinting for taxonomic or epidemiological purposes	Serological, phenotypic, and genotypic methods

Fig. 3.4 A simplified scheme for bacterial identification – major steps and a summary of techniques.

CLINICALLY IMPORTANT GRAM-POSITIVE BACTERIA

Organism	Diseases/other comments
Gram-positive cocci	
Aerobes *Staphylococcus aureus* **(coagulase positive)**	Wound infections, boils, abscesses, septicaemia, food poisoning, toxic-shock syndrome, common skin commensal. Note emergence of antibiotic resistant MRSA (methicillin resistant *S. aureus*)
Coagulase-negative staphylococci	Usually non-pathogenic skin commensals but now associated with colonization of prosthetic devices and bacteraemias
Streptococcus pyogenes **(Group A streptococcus)**	β-haemolytic. Tonsilitis, scarlet fever, wound infections, erysipelas, septicaemia, (also rheumatic fever and glomerulonephritis)
Streptococcus agalactiae **(Group B streptococcus)**	β-haemolytic. Neonatal meningitis and septicaemia. Vaginal carriage
'Viridans' streptococci '*Strep. milleri*' group	α-haemolytic oral commensals
Streptococcus mutans	Non-haemolytic. Dental caries formation
Streptococcus pneumoniae	α-haemolytic. Normal commensal of upper respiratory tract, pneumonia, meningitis, otitis, bronchitis
Enterococcus spp. *E. faecalis* **and** *E. faecium*	Faecal commensals. Endocarditis. Note emergence of VRE (vancomycin resistant enterococci)
Anaerobes *Peptococcus,* *Peptostreptococcus*	Commensals in mouth and faeces. Component of mixed wound infections
Gram-positive rods	
Spore-formers: Anaerobic *Clostridium* spp.	Tetanus, botulism, gas gangrene, other wound infections, colitis, food poisoning
Spore-formers: Aerobic *Bacillus anthracis*	Anthrax
Bacillus cereus	Food poisoning (associated with rice)
Non-spore-formers *Lactobacillus, Bifidobacterium* *Eubacterium* **and** *Propionibacterium* spp.	Common commensals in predominantly anaerobic sites
Actinomyces spp.	Soft tissue infections especially of oral origin Sometimes in mycelial form resembling fungal hyphae
Corynebacterium diphtheriae	Diphtheria. Phage-encoded toxin production
Listeria monocytogenes	Foodborne: abortion, meningitis

Fig. 3.5 Clinically important Gram-positive bacteria.

CLINICALLY IMPORTANT GRAM-NEGATIVE BACTERIA	
Organism	**Diseases/other comments**
Gram-negative cocci	
Aerobic *Neisseria gonorrhoeae*	Gonorrhoea
Neisseria meningitidis	Meningitis, meningococcal sepsis. Relatively common commensal of upper respiratory tract
Anaerobic *Veillonella* spp.	Commensals of the oral cavity. Pathogenic role uncertain, although isolated from various sites of infection, including abscesses with a mixed flora
Gram-negative rods	
Aerobic *Escherichia coli*	Common faecal commensal. Urinary tract infection, gastroenteritis (ETEC, EPEC, EIEC) O157 and haemolytic uraemia syndrome (HUS: renal failure), wound infection, septicaemia
Salmonella spp.	Enteric (typhoid) fever, food poisoning
Shigella spp.	Bacillary dysentery
Proteus, Klebsiella, Enterobacter spp.	Urinary tract infection, wound infection, commensals
Pseudomonas aeruginosa	Wound infections, especially burns, opportunist pathogen, for example in cystic fibrosis
Burkholderia cepacia	A plant pathogen giving serious infections in some cystic fibrosis patients
Haemophilus influenzae	Meningitis (type b), pneumonia, bronchitis
Bordetella pertussis	Whooping cough
Legionella pneumophila	Legionnaires' disease
Yersinia pestis	Plague (flea-borne pathogen)
Brucella abortus	Brucellosis (undulant fever), abortion in cattle
Anaerobic *Bacteroides fragilis* *Bacteroides* spp.	Common faecal commensals, wound infections, abscesses
Porphyromonas gingivalis *Prevotella intermedia* *Prevotella oralis* *Fusobacterium* spp.	Periodontal disease, wound infection

Fig. 3.6 Clinically important Gram-negative bacteria.

Identification beyond species level

For most known bacteria it is possible, using a few key tests, to establish the genus and the species to which a particular bacterium belongs. However, it is often advantageous to go beyond the species level to give important extra information. The terms subspecies, race, and variety, which are used in other classification schemes, are not commonly used in bacterial taxonomy. It is more common to use the suffix '-type'. This can be serotype (based on the presence of certain antigens), biotype (based on certain biochemical reactions which can be used to subdivide a species), phage- or bacteriocin-type, or toxin type. These are phenotypic characters and can give important information in some epidemiological investigations.

MISCELLANEOUS CLINICALLY IMPORTANT BACTERIA	
Organism	**Diseases/other comments**
Miscellaneous bacteria	
Acid-fast bacilli	
Mycobacterium tuberculosis	Tuberculosis
Mycobacterium leprae	Leprosy
Other (atypical) *Mycobacterium* spp.	Tubercular infections of immunocompromised patients, especially HIV-infected patients
Curved Gram-negative bacteria *Campylobacter jejuni*	Microaerophilic. Diarrhoea
Helicobacter pylori	Causal association with gastric and duodenal ulcers
Vibrio cholerae	Cholera
Spiral bacteria *Treponema pallidum*	Syphilis
Oral spirochaetes	Possible role in periodontal disease
Leptospira spp.	Animal pathogen. Weil's disease from rat bites
Borrelia spp.	Lyme Disease: a tick-borne infection caused by *B. burgdorferi*
Obligate intracellular bacteria and mycoplasmas *Chlamydia* spp.	Obligate intracellular parasites. Have structure similar to Gram-negative bacteria but without peptidoglycan
C. trachomatis	Infections of the eye (trachoma) and the genital tract
C. psittaci	Predominantly in birds and animals but is a generalized zoonosis in Man
C. pneumoniae	Pneumonia
Mycoplasma spp.	Extremely small pleomorphic organisms with no rigid cell wall. Not obligate parasites, but require sterols for growth. Cause respiratory tract and genital tract infections
Rickettsia spp.	Small bacteria mainly obligate intracellular parasites. Cause typhus and spotted fevers. Mainly transmitted by arthropod vectors — ticks and lice. Q-fever

Fig. 3.7 Miscellaneous clinically important bacteria.

An example would be the investigation of an outbreak of food poisoning caused by *E. coli*. If *E. coli* serotype O157 were identified it would predict the risk of the haemolytic uraemic syndrome, a major cause of acute renal failure in children suffering from diarrhoea due to this organism. It would then be important to find its source and prevent infection of others.

Another way of showing identity between strains of the same species in epidemiological investigations is to 'fingerprint' them. This usually means genetic fingerprinting, using one of the methods listed in Fig. 3.3. Restriction enzyme digests of whole cell DNA or polymerase chain reaction (PCR)-amplified genes are the usual methods (see Chapter 6). Phenotypic fingerprinting is also possible using polyacrylamide gel electrophoresis (PAGE) of whole cell or envelope proteins, or lipopolysaccharide patterns.

Key facts

- Taxonomy is the systematic classification, naming, and identification of a living organism.

- Bacteria belong to the kingdom Prokaryota.

- The scientific name of an organism is given as a Latin binomial and is printed in italics. The genus name is given first with the initial letter a capital, and the species name in small letters, for example *Escherichia coli*.

- Taxonomic methodologies include phenotypic, numerical, phylogenetic, genotypic, and polyphasic schemes.

- Bacterial identification to species level is performed by following a series of defined steps which may include culture, microscopy, and morphological, biochemical, immunological, and genetic tests.

- At the level below species, typing or fingerprinting may be performed to give extra information for epidemiological or taxonomic studies.

Further reading

Collier, LH (ed.). (1998). *Topley and Wilson's microbiology and microbial infections* (9th edn). Edward Arnold, London.

Murray, PR, Rosenthal, KS, Kobayashi, GS, and Pfaller, MA (1998). Bacterial classification. In *Medical microbiology* (3rd edn), Chapter 2. Mosby Year Book, St Louis.

4

Bacterial pathogenicity

- The relationships between bacteria and host
- Pathogenesis of bacterial disease
- Virulence
- Conclusions

Bacterial pathogenicity

The relationships between bacteria and the host

A bacterial pathogen is simply a bacterium that causes harm to a host, resulting in disease, whilst pathogenicity is the process by which this is brought about. Before describing bacterial pathogenicity, it is useful to consider some of the biological relationships that occur between bacteria and the human body.

The resident microflora

The body is naturally colonized by a vast and complex microflora or microbiota which consists mainly of bacteria. These bacteria are generally considered harmless and are found over the whole outer surface of the body and in much of the gastrointestinal tract, the urogenital tract, and the oropharynx. Thus, most epithelial surfaces, with the exception of the lungs and the upper small intestine, have a resident microflora. This association of bacteria with the host is a relatively stable symbiotic relationship. The bacteria gain obvious benefit from the relationship by being in a fairly constant environment, to which they are adapted.

Commensal and symbiotic relationships

If it is considered that the host does not benefit from the relationship, but is unharmed, the association would be termed a commensal association. However, if the human host also gains from such an association (and this is perhaps more usually the situation), then it is more accurate to describe the relationship as mutualistic or truly symbiotic. This normal microflora, however, is often termed the commensal flora, which is an erroneous description in most cases. It is likely that some of the symbiotic bacteria produce nutrients and vitamins for the host and break down harmful chemicals, but one of the most important benefits that the host derives is protection from harmful micro-organisms. The harmless bacteria that naturally colonize areas prevent access by pathogens, a feature often referred to as colonization resistance. For example, if the normal bacterial flora of the mouth is disturbed as a result of treatment with a broad-spectrum antibiotic, a possible consequence might be the development of a candidal infection such as thrush (see Fig. 26.10). This is because the yeast *Candida albicans* – a eukaryotic fungal pathogen which is naturally resistant to antibacterial agents – is allowed access to sites normally colonized by harmless bacteria.

Parasitism

The final type of biological association that must be considered is parasitism, where the host is harmed by the relationship but the parasite gains. In biological terms an obligate parasite requires a host for all or part of its life cycle. This is summarized in Fig. 4.1. For the parasite to be successful in biological terms it must be able to complete this life cycle, even if the host is ultimately killed. Bacterial parasites of humans are, by definition, pathogens, since they harm the host and cause disease. Furthermore, they are termed obligate or primary pathogens, since causing harm is a necessary part of their life cycle. They are also infectious and can be transmitted from a single individual to one or many others. The organisms *Vibrio cholerae* and *Neisseria gonorrhoeae*, which cause cholera and gonorrhoea, respectively, are both good examples of obligate parasites, that is to say infectious agents requiring a human host. Other bacteria, including some which produce food-poisoning, for example *Salmonella enteritidis*, have their main reservoir in animals where they live parasitically, but they can cause disease in humans following transmission via food or drink.

Not all bacterial pathogens are true parasites, because some do not depend on a host for their life cycle:

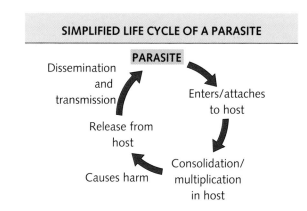

Fig. 4.1 A simplified life cycle of a parasite. There may be more than one host species, and the parasite may have a free-living stage.

- Some bacterial pathogens normally live in the environment, existing saprophytically (gaining their nutrition from dead organic matter) and only causing disease when they inadvertently enter the host. *Clostridium tetani* (which can cause tetanus when it enters a wound from the soil) and *Legionella pneumophila* (which causes Legionnaires' Disease but lives naturally in water) are good examples of pathogens that are not parasites.

- The components of the normally harmless microflora may also become pathogenic. Thus, a bacterium which lives normally and harmlessly on the skin may become a pathogen if it enters a wound, for example *Staphylococcus aureus*. Similarly, oral streptococci, which are harmless in the mouth, can cause infective endocarditis following a bacteraemia in patients with rheumatic heart disease.

Opportunistic infections

A bacterium which normally lives harmlessly with the host, and is non-pathogenic because of a host's normally functioning immune system, may become pathogenic if the immune system is compromised in some way. Such organisms are termed opportunist pathogens. This type of infection has assumed mounting importance in recent years, following the use of powerful immunosuppressive drugs in modern medicine and the emergence of AIDS. A good example of a versatile opportunistic pathogen is *Pseudomonas aeruginosa*, which can cause serious infections of burns or contribute to severe lung disease in cystic fibrosis sufferers, both conditions where innate immune mechanisms have been compromised. Many of the bacteria of the normal oral flora can cause opportunistic infections when they enter sites in which abscesses can develop, both within the mouth (Chapter 24) and elsewhere in the body, for example the brain.

Pathogenesis of bacterial disease

All pathogens, whether parasites or not, go through a series of stages during the pathogenic process. These steps are referred to as pathogenesis and are summarized in Fig. 4.2. Most pathogens possess several different pathogenic mechanisms which operate in concert, and the whole process is often referred to as being multifactorial. It is most unusual for only a single pathogenic factor to be involved in a bacterial disease, though an example is botulism, where the ingestion of a potent toxin produced in food by *Clostridium botulinum* results in a potentially lethal poisoning.

Virulence

An important term, which is used in connection with pathogenesis, is virulence. Virulence is a measure of how harmful a pathogen might be to a host. The determinants that confer, on the bacterium, the potential to cause harm are termed virulence factors. These may either be associated with the cell, usually the cell surface, or be produced extracellularly as exotoxins. Virulence factors may be involved in one or more of the stages of pathogenesis such as adherence, invasion, nutrient acquisition, or evasion of immune mechanisms, as well as contributing to the disease process. Many virulence factors have a role in the primary physiology or structure of the bacterium and their role in virulence may be purely coincidental.

Virulence factors

Surface-associated virulence factors

These factors are summarized in Fig. 4.3. Full details of their structure and physiological function are given in Chapter 2. Many of these surface structures act by allowing the bacterium to evade the immune response by three main mechanisms (see Chapter 7 for details of the host defence mechanisms mentioned below):

- The long O-polysaccharide chains of LPS, or capsular polysaccharides, help to protect against complement-induced lysis by activating complement at a distance from the bacterial cell membrane, thus preventing insertion of the complement–membrane attack complex.

- Bacteria with capsules are often resistant to phagocytosis. The capsule is usually a large hydrated gel with hydrophilic properties surrounding the bacterium. During growth, capsulate bacteria frequently stick together, producing a microcolony, which is often attached to a substratum as a biofilm. This is resistant to phagocytic cells simply because of its large size. Capsulate pneumococci (*Streptococcus pneumoniae*) are the classic example of this type of evasion mechanism.

- Certain bacteria 'hide' from the immune system by having their outer surface covered by a material which mimics host (self) material. This is termed antigenic mimicry or camouflage. There are several well-known examples of this phenomenon, but the most striking is that of the group B capsular type of *Neisseria meningitidis*, the type of meningococcus responsible for most cases of bacterial meningitis in temperate regions of the world. The group B capsular polysaccharide is made up of sialic acid (poly-*N*-acetyl neuraminic acid), a substance commonly found on the cell surface of mammalian cells. Its structure is identical to that of an embryonic neuronal cell coat. Apart from it hiding the bacterium from the immune system, presenting as a self-antigen, it is also non-immunogenic, and thus of no use in vaccine formulation.

Lipopolysaccharide (LPS, endotoxin), and to a lesser extent peptidoglycan, teichoic acids, and some other cell-surface carbohydrates, act in pathogenesis as potent stimulators of the immune system. The resulting responses, which include inflammation (following the release of cytokines such as interleukin (IL)-1, IL-6, and tumour necrosis factor (TNF)), recruitment of leucocytes, and triggering the complement and clotting cascades are beneficial when produced at an optimal level. However, if they are overproduced, because of excessive stimula-

STAGES IN BACTERIAL PATHOGENESIS		
Stage	**Mechanism**	**Comment**
Entry	Via food, water, aerosol or direct contact; through natural orifices; through wound or bite (arthropod or higher animal)	The innate host defence system prevents entry through intact surfaces
Attachment	Adherence via fimbriae/pili, colonization factors, surface/outer membrane proteins, capsular slime or polysaccharide	Avoids flushing action of host body fluids, cilia and peristalsis
Multiplication and consolidation	Expression of mechanisms for acquisition of nutrients, for example iron. Microcolony formation and production of biofilm	Bacteria may exist as either a single species, or a consortium of several species
Evasion of host defences	Anticomplementary, antiphagocytosis, camouflage, IgA protease production, intracellular habit, overcomes colonization resistance	Both the innate and acquired immune defences may be evaded
Cause damage	Exotoxins, endotoxins, invasion of cells/tissues, endproducts of metabolism, immunopathology	Rarely a single mechanism, usually multifactorial, including inflammation and immune – complex damage
Release and spread	Usually a reverse of entry mechanisms, including aerosols, coughs, and sneezes, diarrhoea, faecal – oral, exchange of body fluids, direct contact, animal vectors (zoonosis)	Necessary to complete life cycle of true parasites. Does not occur for all pathogens

Fig. 4.2 The stages in bacterial pathogenesis. Parasites, by definition, complete all these stages, but this is not necessary for all pathogens.

tion, this can result in severe immunopathology (Chapter 17). Endotoxic shock, septic shock, severe sepsis, and the systemic inflammatory response syndrome (SIRS) (see Fig. 17.9) are terms used to describe this condition. It is a major cause of death in severely ill patients.

Bacterial exotoxins

In contrast to endotoxins (LPS) – which are cell-associated during normal growth of the Gram-negative bacterium and heat-stable – exotoxins are extracellular products. They are produced by both Gram-positive and Gram-negative bacteria. Exotoxins are proteins, often enzymes, usually of high molecular mass and are heat-labile. They cause damage to cells, tissues, or can affect the whole animal.

Several different methods are available for the classification of exotoxins. A simple method is to classify them by their site of action within the body. Thus, neurotoxins act on nerves, enterotoxins act on the gastrointestinal tract, and cytotoxins act on cells. Another approach is to describe them by their biochemical mode of action, for example proteases, phospholipases, collagenases, ADP-ribosylating (an ADP-ribose is transferred from NAD^+), and bipartite (two parts: A = active and B = binding). The latter two properties are common to several types of exotoxin. A further method of classification is to group them into their action at the cellular level (Fig. 4.4).

The major benefits endowed on a pathogen by exotoxins include aiding its spread through the body (tissue destruction),

SURFACE-ASSOCIATED VIRULENCE FACTORS	
Virulence factor	**Contribution to virulence**
Fimbriae/pili, fibrillae, colonization factors	Adhesion, antiphagocytic
Capsule/slime, exopolysaccharide, glycocalyx	Adhesion, protection against phagocytosis and complement, camouflage from immune system
Peptidoglycan, muramyl peptides	Immunomodulation, induction of inflammatory mediators
Lipopolysaccharide/LPS/LOS/ endotoxin (active component: Lipid A)	Protection against complement, induction of inflammatory cytokines: endotoxic shock/ systemic inflammatory response syndrome
Teichoic acid, lipoteichoic acid, secondary cell-wall (lipo)carbohydrates	Adhesion, sequestration of divalent cations, induction of inflammatory mediators
Flagella, axial filaments	Chemotaxis, penetration of mucus
Outer membrane proteins	Adhesion. Sequestration of iron. Invasion. Intracellular survival
Surface proteins	Adhesion, binding Fc region of immunoglobulins

Fig. 4.3 Surface-associated bacterial virulence factors. LPS, lipopolysaccharide; LOS, lipo-oligosaccharide.

CLASSIFICATION OF BACTERIAL EXOTOXINS	
Cellular level at which they act	**Examples and modes of action**
Extracellular action on connective tissue	Collagenases, hyaluronidases, proteases
On or within membranes — probably do not enter cells but transmit signals to the inside	Stable toxin (ST) of enterotoxigenic *Escherichia coli*
Traverse host cell membrane and kill cells	Cytotoxin. Diphtheria toxin (an ADP ribosylating bipartite toxin)
Traverse host cell membrane and deregulate cell functions	Cholera toxin (an ADP ribosylating bipartite toxin)
Pore-forming, thiol-activated cytolytic	Staphylococcal alpha, gamma, and theta toxins. Pneumolysin. Interact with cholesterol in membranes to produce pores. Damages cells of the immune system
Damage membranes	Phospholipases (alpha toxin of *Clostridium perfringens*). Surfactant (staphylococcal delta toxin)
Superantigens	Staphylococcal toxic-shock syndrome toxin and staphylococcal enterotoxin. Bind to MHC class II molecules. T-cell proliferation and massive cytokine release (see Chapter 7 for further details)

Fig. 4.4 Classification of bacterial exotoxins by their action at the cellular level.

killing phagocytic cells (diphtheria toxin, and some staphylococcal toxins), and contributing to transmission (diarrhoea, coughing). Others, such as the neurotoxins, for example tetanus and botulinum toxins, seem to have no beneficial role for the pathogen.

Some bacterial metabolites can act as virulence factors and play a role in disease production. These include acids, which are key factors in dental caries.

Genetic regulation of virulence factors

Bacterial pathogenicity is often multifactorial, with several virulence factors working together to cause disease. Some bacteria always (constitutively) produce their full battery of virulence factors in all growth conditions. However, for many bacteria, especially those that can exist in an environment where they are not being pathogenic, it is unnecessary (energetically wasteful) for them to produce virulence factors which would only be required during their pathogenic phase. Many of these bacteria have evolved genetic systems for regulating the phenotypic expression of virulence factors. The expression is often regulated by environmental stimuli and is controlled in a co-ordinated manner, a single stimulus resulting in the co-ordinated expression of two or more virulence factors. An example is the *toxR* gene of *Vibrio cholerae*. A single protein, with both sensing and kinase activity, co-ordinately regulates the expression of both cholera toxin and the 'toxin co-regulated pilus' (which is used for adherence), following stimulation brought about by a change in temperature, pH, amino acid availability, or in osmolarity.

Many genes which code for virulence are carried on plasmids or lysogenic bacteriophage (prophage) within the bacterium. The bacteria become non-pathogenic if they lose their plasmid or prophage. Examples of bacteria carrying virulence plasmids are the enterotoxigenic *E. coli* (diarrhoea-causing *E. coli*) which have plasmid genes encoding both their colonization factors (fimbriae) and enterotoxin. Diphtheria toxin is encoded by lysogenic bacteriophage carried by *Corynebacterium diphtheriae*.

Conclusions

Bacterial pathogenicity is a rapidly growing area of microbiology. It is very amenable to investigation by modern molecular techniques, the cloning of virulence factors, and determination of the DNA sequence of their genes, therefore allowing greater insight into their roles in virulence and to their control.

It should be emphasized that bacterial pathogenicity has to be viewed from two aspects, from that of the pathogen (its virulence) and of the host (the immune system). The host–pathogen relationship is in a state of equilibrium, and pathogenicity is sometimes referred to in terms of the host–pathogen equation. The outcome of the association, whether in favour of the host or the pathogen, can be strongly influenced by clinical intervention. Thus, understanding of pathogenicity forms the basis of many of the strategies employed for the prevention and treatment of bacterial diseases. Bacterial genetics, the immune system, and intervention strategies are described more fully in later chapters.

Key facts

- Bacterial pathogenicity is the process whereby the bacterium (the pathogen) causes harm or disease to the host. It is usually a multifactorial process.

- Three natural associations can exist between bacteria and the host: symbiosis (or mutualism) – both gain; commensalism – bacterium gains, host is unharmed; and parasitism – bacterium gains, host is harmed.

- Pathogens can be primary/obligate pathogens or they can be opportunists.

- There are several stages in pathogenesis, including entry or attachment, evasion of the immune system, cause of harm, and release and spread.

- Virulence is a measure of the potential the bacterium has to cause harm. Virulence factors can be bacterial cell-surface associated, or extracellular exotoxins.

- Harm is brought about by a process which is often multifactorial, involving both bacterial factors and the host response.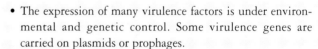

- The expression of many virulence factors is under environmental and genetic control. Some virulence genes are carried on plasmids or prophages.

- The host–pathogen relationship is in a state of equilibrium which can be altered by clinical intervention.

Further reading

Mims, C, Dimmock, N, Nash, A, and Stephen, J. (1995). *Mims' pathogenesis of infectious disease* (4th edn). Academic Press, London.

Mims, C, Playfair, J, Roitt, I, Wakelin, D, and Williams, R (1998). Pathologic consequences of infection. In *Medical microbiology* (2nd edn), Chapter 12. Mosby, London.

Salyers, AA and Whitt, DD (1994). *Bacterial pathogenesis: a molecular approach* (International Student Edition). American Society for Microbiology, Washington DC.

Taussig, MJ (1984). Infection: bacteria. In *Processes in pathology and microbiology* (2nd edn), Section 4. Blackwell, Oxford.

5

Viruses: structure, classification, replication, and pathogenicity

- Characteristics of viruses
- Symmetry of viruses
- Classification of viruses
- Detection of viruses
- Viral replication
- Effects of viruses on host cells
- Routes of viral infection
- Patterns of viral infection
- Host response to viral infection

Viruses: structure, classification, replication, and pathogenicity

Viruses are an important cause of disease in man. They are relevant to dentists because they may cause disease either directly (for example herpes simplex virus) or indirectly (for example oral manifestations of HIV infection) in the oral and perioral regions. In addition, the prevention of cross-infection with viruses during dental treatment (Chapter 28) is an important element of safe dental practice.

Characteristics of viruses

Viruses differ from other groups of micro-organisms such as bacteria in a number of key respects. The important characteristics of viruses are summarized in Fig. 5.1. They are very small agents with a simple chemical composition – comprising the viral genome and an outer protein coat known as the capsid. Each particle has a strict geometric structure, and the capsid is composed of multiple building blocks known as capsomeres. The genome may be either DNA or RNA, but never both, and may be single- or double-stranded, linear, or circular. The particles have no rigid cell wall.

CHARACTERISTICS OF VIRUSES
• Small size (20 – 300nm)
• Simple chemical composition
• Sub-unit construction
• Strict geometric structure
• Genetic information as DNA or RNA
• Replication strictly intracellular
• No intracellular organelles
• No rigid cell wall
• Sensitive to interferon

Fig. 5.1 Summary of the important biological characteristics of viruses.

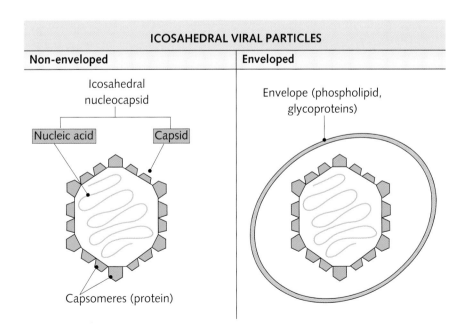

ICOSAHEDRAL VIRAL PARTICLES

Non-enveloped

Icosahedral nucleocapsid

Nucleic acid   Capsid

Capsomeres (protein)

Enveloped

Envelope (phospholipid, glycoproteins)

Fig. 5.2 Diagram illustrating the generalized structure of icosahedral viral particles. (Redrawn from M.J. Taussig 1984; with permission from Blackwell Scientific Publications.)

Viruses are unable to synthesize proteins from the information in their genome: they have no ribosomes or organelles such as mitochondria. For this reason they are strict intracellular parasites and can only replicate after infection of a living host cell. Viruses are resistant to antimicrobial agents used to treat bacterial and fungal infections but are very sensitive to interferon.

In addition to the nucleic acid and protein capsid, some viruses have an outer coat known as an envelope. This is a lipoprotein structure and is derived from either the plasma- or nuclear-membrane of the infected cells. In general, non-enveloped viruses are relatively resistant to environmental factors such as drying, gastric acidity, and bile, whilst enveloped viruses are more susceptible.

Symmetry of viruses

The complete unit of capsid and nucleic acid is termed the nucleocapsid. Viral nucleocapsids have a strict geometric structure and can be divided into two main symmetrical forms – icosahedral cubic or helical. The icosahedral viruses, for example the herpesviruses, comprise an outer icosahedral protein shell which houses the nucleic acid (Fig. 5.2). Others, for example influenza viruses, have a helical symmetry, in which the capsomeres are arranged intimately around the spiral of nucleic acid (Fig. 5.3). Most helical viruses are enveloped. A small number of viruses, for example poxviruses, have neither icosahedral nor helical symmetry and are described as complex.

Classification of viruses

Viruses may be classified into families on the basis of a number of features including symmetry, the presence or absence of an envelope, type of nucleic acid in the genome, the number of nucleic acid strands and their polarity. None of these methods permit an ideal classification, but a useful 'supergrouping' of viruses has been proposed which is known as the Baltimore classification (Fig. 5.4). This classification is based upon the type of genome, its polarity, and the route by which messenger RNA (mRNA) is produced within the infected cell.

Detection of viruses

The laboratory detection of viruses is important both for diagnostic and research purposes. The methods available are summarized in Fig. 5.5. More comprehensive details of methodology are given in Chapter 12.

Viral particles may be detected by electron microscopy following appropriate negative staining with phosphotungstic acid (Fig. 5.6). This may allow the rapid identification of viruses directly in clinical specimens, for example herpesvirus particles in vesicle fluid. The specificity of the method is poor, but in some cases may be improved by adding specific immune serum that agglutinates a particular virus.

Since viruses are strict intracellular parasites they must be provided with living cells if they are to be cultured in the laboratory.

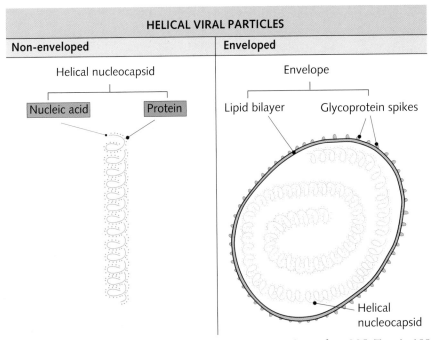

Fig. 5.3 Diagram illustrating the generalized structure of helical viral particles. (Redrawn from M.J. Taussig 1984; with permission from Blackwell Scientific Publications.)

THE BALTIMORE CLASSIFICATION OF VIRUSES

Class II **+DNA**

Class I **±DNA**

Class VI

Class IV

+RNA

+mRNA

– RNA
Class V

±RNA
Class III

Fig. 5.4 The Baltimore classification of viruses. Messenger (m) RNA and strands of the same polarity as mRNA are designated '+'. Viral DNA and RNA strands complementary to mRNA are designated '–'. Double-stranded nucleic acid is denoted '±'. Arrows indicate the route of arriving at mRNA. (Redrawn from M.J. Taussig 1984; with permission from Blackwell Scientific Publications.)

METHODS OF DETECTING VIRUSES

- Electron microscopy
- Culture in living cells
- Antigen detection
- Serology
- Molecular methods

Fig. 5.5 Summary of the methods available for diagnosing viral infections.

Most viral culture is now performed in tissue-culture systems (Figs 5.7(a), (b)); although for some viruses, such as hepatitis B, no cell lines are available which will permit viral culture in the laboratory. The specimen is collected into virus transport medium and inoculated into the cell-culture tube or flask. The cells are then incubated and observed for the development of a cytopathic effect. This appears within 48 hours for some viruses, but it may take as long as 14 days to develop. The changes in cell morphology which constitute a cytopathic effect may be characteristic of a particular virus. Some viruses induce no cytopathic effect and must be detected by other means.

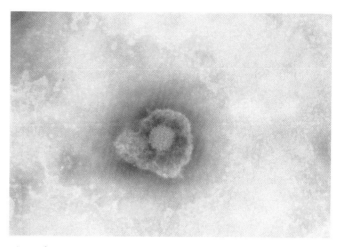

Fig. 5.6 Photomicrograph illustrating a herpes simplex virus particle negatively stained with phosphotungstic acid. The envelope is clearly visible. (Courtesy of Ian Miller.)

Detection of antiviral antibodies (serology) may be useful in diagnosis, although for common viral infections this requires the collection of two blood samples, 10–14 days apart, to permit detection of a rising titre of IgG antibodies. For some infections, such as rubella, a more rapid diagnosis can be made on the basis of detection of specific IgM class antibodies in a single specimen. In the case of certain viral infections for which the causative agent cannot be readily cultured, such as HIV, hepatitis B, and hepatitis C, serology is the main method of clinical diagnosis.

With the advent of specific antiviral drugs such as aciclovir there is now a need for the rapid diagnosis of viral infections. The use of direct antigen detection in tissues, for example by immuno-fluorescence, has become popular. These rapid antigen detection techniques have been greatly improved by the availability of highly specific monoclonal antibodies (see Chapter 7).

Methods for diagnosing viral infections by molecular biological techniques, such as DNA hybridization and the polymerase chain reaction (PCR), are now being developed. These tests are very sensitive and do not rely on the presence of viable virus. Confirmation of infection with hepatitis C virus is now routinely performed using PCR.

Viral replication

The processes involved in viral replication are summarized in Fig. 5.8. The initial stage of adsorption involves binding of the virus with the host cell. This is a specific interaction between a binding protein on the virus and a host cell-membrane receptor. The process has been well studied for influenza virus, where a viral protein known as haemagglutinin interacts with a host cell receptor, N-acetyl neuraminic acid.

Following binding, the virus penetrates the host cell. Enveloped viruses commonly enter the cell via fusion of the lipid membrane with the envelope, while non-enveloped viruses enter

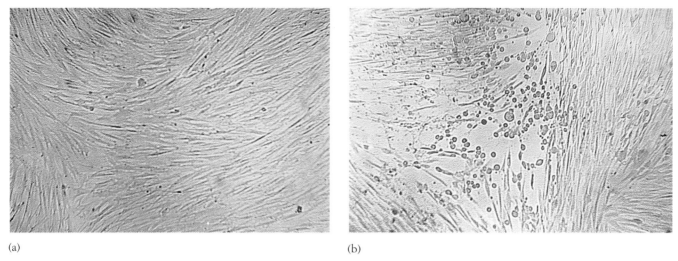

(a)   (b)

Fig. 5.7 The cytopathic effect of herpes simplex virus. (a) Photomicrograph illustrates the morphology of uninfected fibroblasts; (b) shows the cytopathic effect of the virus on the fibroblasts, which 'round up' and die. (Courtesy of Ian Miller.)

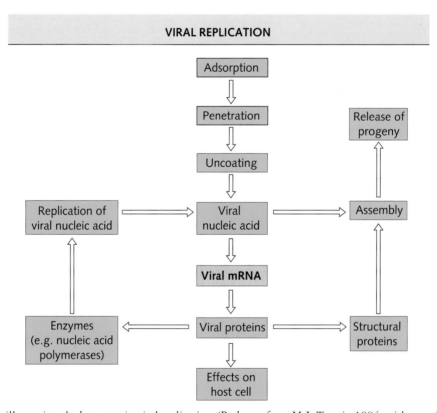

Fig. 5.8 Flow diagram illustrating the key steps in viral replication. (Redrawn from M.J. Taussig 1984; with permission from Blackwell Scientific Publications.)

by a process known as viropexis, which is similar to phagocytosis.

Once inside the host cell, the process of uncoating occurs, whereby the capsid proteins are removed to release naked viral nucleic acid within the host cell. The subsequent process of the production of viral messenger RNA (mRNA) may occur in several ways depending on the nature of the viral genome. These pathways are defined in the Baltimore classification (see Fig. 5.4). In viruses which contain DNA, mRNA can be formed using the host cell RNA polymerase to transcribe directly from the viral DNA (Baltimore Classes I and II).

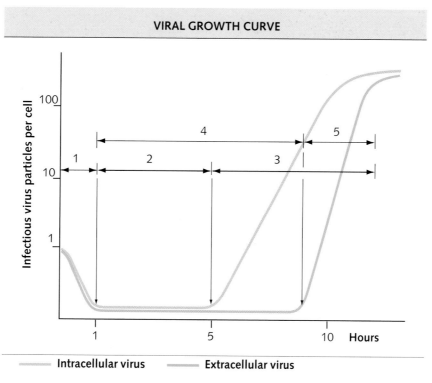

Fig. 5.9 Growth curve for an animal virus which matures intracellularly and is released by lysis. 1, adsorption and penetration; 2, eclipse period; 3, maturation; 4, latent period; 5, lytic release. (Redrawn from M.J. Taussig 1984; with permission from Blackwell Scientific Publications.)

For RNA-containing viruses, direct transcription is not possible, since host cell polymerases do not work from RNA molecules. If transcription is necessary, the virus must provide its own polymerases, either by carrying them in the nucleocapsid or coding for their synthesis after infection. RNA viruses produce mRNA via several routes. In double-stranded RNA viruses (Baltimore Class III), one strand is first transcribed by viral polymerase into mRNA.

For single-stranded RNA viruses there are three pathways to mRNA formation:

1. If the single strand is of the positive-sense configuration (Baltimore Class IV) it can be used directly as mRNA.

2. If it is negative-sense RNA (Baltimore Class V) then it must first be transcribed, using viral polymerase, into a positive-sense strand which can then act as mRNA.

3. Finally, retroviruses (Baltimore Class VI) convert their positive-sense RNA into negative-sense, single-stranded DNA under the influence of reverse transcriptase. Double-stranded DNA is then formed, which enters the host cell nucleus and becomes integrated into the host genome. The integrated viral DNA is then transcribed by host cell polymerase into mRNA (Chapter 19).

Following the production of viral mRNA the host cell produces viral proteins. Some of these proteins may have direct effects on the host cell but the remainder are of two main types. Some are enzymes (mainly nucleic acid polymerases) which allow the replication of more viral nucleic acid. The other group are the structural proteins which form the viral capsid. These separate elements are assembled within the host cell to form new progeny viral particles.

The viral particles may be released from the cell either by lytic release when the cell dies, or by a process known as budding in which the nucleocapsid becomes associated with that part of the host cell membrane which subsequently forms the viral envelope.

These processes result in the kinetics of viral replication illustrated in Fig. 5.9. The first phase represents adsorption and penetration of the virus. No viral particles are detectable during the subsequent eclipse period (phase 2) when the virus has been uncoated and new viral nucleic acid and structural proteins are being produced. The third phase, maturation, represents the period of time when new viral particles are being assembled within the cell. Phase 4 is the latent period during which no extracellular virus is detectable. The final phase (5), lytic release, represents the release of the newly packaged progeny viral particles into the surrounding environment.

Effects of viruses on host cells

The possible outcomes of viral infection at the individual host cell level are summarized in Fig. 5.10. The most common effect of

---

EFFECTS OF VIRUSES ON HOST CELLS

- Cytocidal (lytic) infection
- Persistent (steady state) infection
- Latent (integrated) infection
- Transforming infection
- Abortive infection

Fig. 5.10 Summary of the possible outcomes of viral infection on a host cell.

viruses on host cells is a cytocidal or lytic infection. In such infections there is death of the host cell with release of progeny virions (single, complete virus particles).

In persistent or steady-state infections, host cells may multiply and continue to produce the virus through several generations. Examples include the paramyxoviruses, such as mumps virus, and the continuous production and release of tumour viruses by neoplastic cells.

A third possible outcome is a latent or integrated infection in which viral nucleic acid persists in the cell but mature viral particles are undetectable. The herpesviruses are a good example.

Viruses may also transform susceptible cells. These transformed cells proliferate free from the normal restraints on divi-sion, with the resultant formation of tumours. Tumour viruses integrate their genome into host cell DNA.

Finally, it should be noted that some interactions between viruses and host cells do not continue to completion. This may be, for example, because of the lack of a necessary enzyme within the host cell. Such infections are known as abortive infections.

Routes of viral infection

The possible routes of viral infection are similar to those for other micro-organisms and are summarized in Fig. 5.11.

Whilst intact skin is a good barrier against viral infection, damage to or perforation of the skin may permit viral infection. This is of particular relevance to blood-borne viruses in health-care workers who have suffered needlestick or sharps injuries.

The respiratory tract represents a major route for infection with viruses. These include local respiratory tract infections, such as the common cold, and also generalized infections, for example chickenpox. Infection is established following the inhalation of infected droplets.

Some viruses infect via the alimentary tract and others are spread via the oropharynx, typically in saliva. This is a particularly important route for some of the herpes group viruses and is again relevant to cross-infection risks in the dental surgery.

Finally, transmission of viruses may occur in the genital tract, either during sexual contact or by transplacental spread. Trans-

---

ROUTES OF VIRAL INFECTION

Route	Examples
Skin	
Mechanical trauma	Cowpox virus
Injection	Hepatitis B virus; HIV
Bite	Rabies virus
Respiratory tract	
Droplet infection	
Localized respiratory infections	Common cold virus; influenza virus
Generalized infections	Chickenpox virus
Alimentary tract/oropharynx	
Faecal – oral	Hepatitis A virus
Saliva	Mumps virus
	Herpes simplex virus
	Epstein – Barr virus
Genital tract	
Sexual intercourse	HIV; hepatitis B virus
Transplacental	Rubella virus
	Cytomegalovirus

Fig. 5.11 Summary of the important routes of infection with viruses.

PATTERNS OF VIRAL INFECTION	
Pattern	**Examples**
Acute Infections	
Many febrile diseases	Influenza
Short incubation period	
Recovery or death of host in 2–3 weeks	
Many are asymptomatic or subclinical	
Persistent Infections	
Virus persists for months or years	
Four categories	
1. **Latent**	
Acute infection with apparent recovery	Herpetic gingivostomatitis
Minute amount of virus sequestered	
Later recurrence of acute symptoms	Herpes labialis
2. **Chronic**	
Virus persists in large quantity over long period; virus continuously detectable	Hepatitis B
3. **Slow**	
Rare, but often affect central nervous system; long incubation period; gradual, inexorable progression to death	Subacute sclerosing panencephalitis (secondary to measles)
4. **Oncogenic**	
Integration of viral genetic information into host cell chromosome; results in tumour production	Burkitt's lymphoma (Epstein – Barr virus)

Fig. 5.12 Main patterns of infection with viruses in the human host.

mission of cytomegalovirus via the transplacental route is now the commonest infective cause of congenital abnormalities.

Patterns of viral infection

The various patterns of viral infection observed at the level of the host are summarized in Fig. 5.12. Many are short-lived acute infections, such as influenza or the common cold. However, viruses are also renowned for establishing persistent infections, of which there are four types. The herpesviruses, which are of great importance in relation to oral disease, are an important cause of latent infections. Chronic infections, such as the carriage of hepatitis B virus, are very relevant to cross-infection control in dentistry. The role of viruses in causing tumours (oncogenic infections) is also of interest to the dental surgeon. Some benign tumours of the mouth, such as squamous papillomas, have a viral aetiology; the Epstein–Barr virus plays a role in the pathogenesis of Burkitt's lymphoma, a lymphoblastic lymphoma endemic in Africa that frequently affects the jaws.

Host response to viral infection

The host responses to viral infection can be divided into non-specific and specific responses.

Non-specific defence mechanisms (see Chapter 7) include intact skin and the mucus and cilia which protect the lower respiratory tract. The gastrointestinal tract is protected by virtue of the acidity of the stomach, lysis of enveloped viruses by bile, and viral uptake by gut-associated lymphoid tissue. Both the urinary tract and the conjunctiva are protected by the physical flushing effect of body fluids. Phagocytosis, which may be enhanced by antibody, is also an important non-specific defence mechanism.

The interferons play an important antiviral role. This family of protein molecules includes the three types alpha, beta, and gamma. The first two types of interferon are produced principally by virus-infected cells and are host-specific, but they do have a wide antiviral spectrum. The antiviral activities of interferon are summarized in Fig. 5.13. Interferon binds to cell-surface receptors and induces intracellular enzymes. These inhibit viral

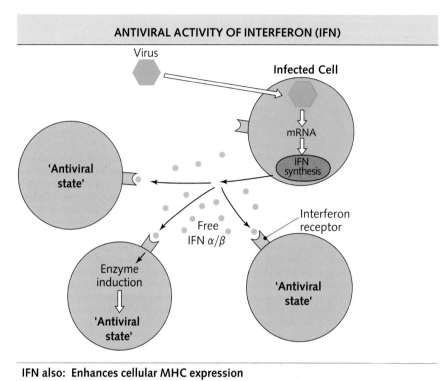

Fig. 5.13 Diagram illustrating the antiviral activities of interferon.

replication and render the cells treated with interferon resistant to virus infection.

In relation to the specific immune response (see Chapter 7) to viral infection, the roles of both humoral and cell-mediated immunity are summarized in Fig. 5.14. The humoral response is important in the prevention of reinfection with a previously encountered virus, but since antibody cannot interact with intracellular virus particles and the process takes too long to develop, it does not play an important role in recovery from primary infections. However, the cell-mediated immune response, which can identify and attack host cells containing intracellular parasites, plays a key role in recovery from primary viral infection.

SPECIFIC IMMUNE RESPONSE TO VIRAL INFECTION
Humoral (Antibody) Response
Neutralizes virus in body fluids
Reacts with viral adhesins
IgA important at mucosal surfaces
Encourages phagocytosis of viral particles
Main role is PREVENTION OF RE-INFECTION
Cell-mediated Immune Response
Required for RECOVERY FROM PRIMARY INFECTIONS
Production of lymphokines
Macrophage recruitment and activation
T-cells seek out and destroy virus-infected cells
Role in protective immunity

Fig. 5.14 Summary of the roles of humoral and cell-mediated immunity in the defence against viral infection.

Key facts

- Viruses are strict intracellular parasites and can only replicate inside living cells.

- Viruses have a strict geometric structure, which may be icosahedral or helical.

- The genome is protected by a protein coat (capsid) and some viruses also possess a lipid envelope.

- The genome may be DNA or RNA, but *never* both.

- Viral infection may be diagnosed by electron microscopy, culture in living cells, and detection of cytopathic effect, serology, direct antigen detection, or nucleic acid detection.

- Viruses gain access to the host via skin and mucous membranes and through the gastrointestinal, respiratory, and genital tracts.

- The stages of viral infection of cells are adsorption, penetration, uncoating, genome transcription to form mRNA, translation of mRNA to allow formation of viral proteins, genome replication, assembly and release.

- Infection of a host cell may result in cytocidal, persistent, latent, transforming, or abortive infection.

- Both non-specific and specific immune defences provide protection against viral infection.

- Interferons help to suppress viral replication, especially in the early stages of infection.

- In general, antibodies protect against reinfection with viruses, while cell-mediated immunity plays the main role in recovery from primary infections.

References and further reading

Collier, L and Oxford, J (1993). *Human virology: a text for students of medicine, dentistry, and microbiology*. Oxford University Press, Oxford.

Evans, AS and Kaslow, RA (ed.). (1997). Epidemiologic concepts and methods. In *Viral infections of humans. Epidemiology and control* (4th edn), Chapter 1. Plenum, New York.

Murray, PR, Rosenthal, KS, Kobayashi, GS, and Pfaller, MA (1998). Viral classification, structure and replication. In *Medical microbiology* (3rd edn), Chapter 6. Mosby Year Book, St Louis.

Taussig, MJ (1984). Infection: viruses. In *Processes in pathology and microbiology* (2nd edn), Section 3. Blackwell, Oxford.

6

Bacterial genetics and molecular biology

- Genes and DNA

- Genetic-transfer mechanisms in bacteria

- Manipulation of DNA and recombinant DNA technology

- Techniques for the molecular 'typing' of micro-organisms

- Clinical applications of molecular biology

Bacterial genetics and molecular biology

Genes and DNA

Genes are the elements of the hereditary material of living cells that carry the information to code for all the necessary components and reactions of life. At cell division the genes are replicated and a copy goes to each daughter cell. It was not until the 1950s that deoxyribonucleic acid (DNA) was recognized as being the substance of genes. During the past half century the subject of molecular biology has developed into a major discipline, underpinning many of the other fields of biology and medicine. Molecular biology had its roots in bacteriology, and many of the continuing advances in the subject still depend on bacteria. Molecular biology is a vast and rapidly developing subject, much of which is beyond the scope of this book. This chapter will give a brief introduction to the basics of the subject, describe some of the important aspects of bacterial molecular genetics, and demonstrate some of the uses to which molecular biological techniques are being directed.

The structure of DNA

DNA consists of the famous 'double helix', two antiparallel strands (3′ to 5′ and 5′ to 3′) of a sugar–phosphate backbone substituted with purine and pyrimidine bases. Complementary base pairs are cross-linked through hydrogen bonds, guanine (G) pairing with cytosine (C) and adenine (A) with thymine (T) (Fig. 6.1). The four bases represent the letters in a four-letter alphabet that are read linearly in three-lettered 'words'.

DNA replication

During cell growth the DNA replicates by a process known as semi-conservative replication (Fig. 6.2 (a)). This takes place at a replication fork, where the separate helices of the DNA act as templates for the new, daughter strands. Deoxyribonucleotides are added sequentially, a phosphodiester bond forming between the deoxyriboses while a guanine pairs through hydrogen bonds with a cytosine, and an adenine with a thymine, and so on. However, as the DNA polymerase enzyme can only add bases to the 3′ end of a growing strand, and the two parent strands are antiparallel, the replication processes at the division fork are asymmetrical (Fig. 6.2 (b)). The initiation of a replication fork and the subsequent DNA replication is performed by a series of enzymes co-ordinated with the DNA polymerase. These include a topoisomerase (DNA gyrase) to relieve helical winding and tangling problems, a DNA ligase to join together newly synthesized fragments, and initiator proteins which bind to specific DNA sequences and initiate a replication fork.

Mutation

Although the process of DNA replication is highly efficient and accurate, with built-in repair mechanisms, mistakes can occur. For example, one or more nucleotides can be omitted, or extra ones can be inserted, a G can be added instead of an A, or a T instead of a C. These mistakes occur in fewer than 1 in 10^9 nucleotides added. Such mispairings are one of the methods by which mutations occur. Other methods by which mutations occur include direct damage to the DNA by radiation or chemicals. These errors in the DNA can be passed on to future generations.

The result of a mutation can vary, depending on the site and its extent. The transcription and subsequent translation (see later) of the mutant genes produces variations in the amino acid sequence in the proteins, which may have properties so different that they do not function as well, or they may be inactive and result in cell death. Some transcription errors of DNA may be silent because the change in the resultant protein is insignificant. Some mutations can even be better than the original – this is the basis of 'natural selection', where beneficial mutations can be selected for better survival of the organism.

The genetic code and protein synthesis

The processes by which the base sequence of the DNA is converted to proteins are termed transcription (Fig. 6.3) and translation (Fig. 6.4). The DNA sequence must first be transcribed to a complementary messenger ribonucleic acid (mRNA), which is then read as a three-letter code – the genetic code. RNA polymerase makes a complementary copy of one of the strands of DNA from the 5′ end to the 3′ end. There is only one type of RNA polymerase in bacteria, but three in eukaryotes. Note that the mRNA has uridine (U) in place of the thymine (T) of DNA. The RNA polymerase binds to the DNA at a starting point termed the promoter. A length of mRNA is transcribed for a specific protein, the transcription stopping when the polymerase reaches a stop or termination signal, which in bacteria (*E. coli*) is when a series of U's

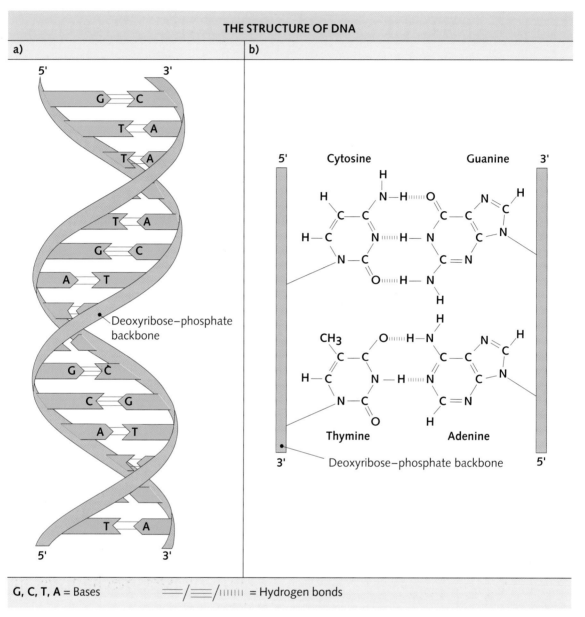

Fig. 6.1 The structure of DNA. (a) The double helix: two antiparallel strands of deoxyribose nucleotides, linked along their length with phosphodiester bonds, and cross-linked through hydrogen bonding between complementary bases. (b) Detailed diagram demonstrating base pairing.

is added from a complementary series of A's on the transcribed DNA.

In the cell, each amino acid has one or more of its own transfer RNA (tRNA) molecules which are specific short chains of folded RNA. One end of the tRNA binds an amino acid, while the other end has a three-base recognition sequence (anticodon) which binds to a complementary three-base sequence in the mRNA – the codon. The genetic code is a series of codons (three-base sequences) that determines the sequence of the amino acids in the primary structure of the protein. Protein synthesis takes place by a ribosome moving step-wise along the mRNA chain (Fig. 6.4). Each ribosome has two binding sites, one which holds the tRNA attached to the growing peptide, the P site, and the other the incoming tRNA with the amino acid attached, the A site. Peptide bond formation occurs here. Special codons code for the start and stop of the peptide. In bacteria, formyl methionine, coded for by the sequence AUG, is the initiator tRNA which always starts the peptide chain.

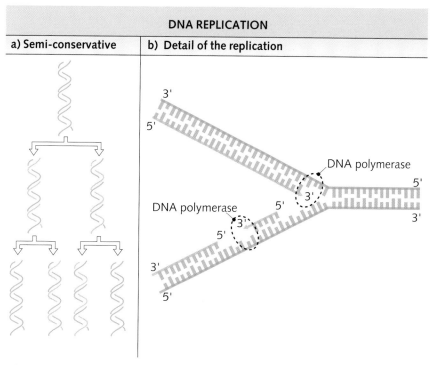

Fig. 6.2 The replication of DNA. (a) Semi-conservative replication: on replication each daughter cell receives an original strand plus a newly synthesized strand. (b) Detailed diagram showing the asymmetrical synthesis of DNA at the replication fork. Both strands are synthesized from the 5′ end to the 3′ end by the DNA polymerase. The lower strand is replicated in short sections which are subsequently joined.

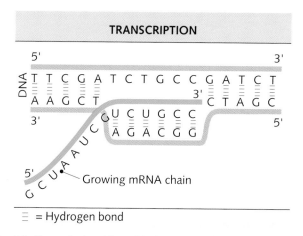

Fig. 6.3 Transcription. The mRNA is transcribed from the DNA template, producing a complementary copy of the DNA strand from which it is being synthesized.

Genetic recombination

This is a basic mechanism by which genetic variation can occur, and is an important phenomenon in survival and evolution. In simple terms, recombination is the rearrangement of DNA that involves the breaking and rejoining of two homologous DNA

double helices and is guided by base-pairing interactions between complementary strands. This is shown simply in Fig. 6.5.

So far, the basic synthesis of nucleic acids and proteins has been described, and this forms much of the basic knowledge required for understanding the mechanisms of genetic transfer and genetic techniques that are the subject of the remainder of this chapter.

Genetic-transfer mechanisms in bacteria

One of the earliest observations in bacterial genetics was that bacteria could easily transfer genes from one organism to another. This was most dramatic when it was realized that resistance to antibiotics was readily transferred from one bacterium to another.

There are three general methods for genetic exchange in bacteria: transformation, transduction, and conjugation. The key points of each are summarized below, and the latter two mechanisms are represented diagrammatically in Figs 6.6 and 6.7.

Transformation

- DNA is released from a bacterium on lysis.
- DNA is 'naked' – it is sensitive to the action of DNA-degrading enzymes (DNase).
- The recipient bacterium must be competent.

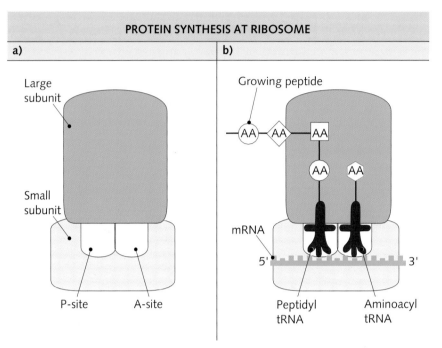

Fig. 6.4 Translation of mRNA at the ribosome leading to protein synthesis. (a) The 'empty' ribosome showing binding sites for transfer RNAs. (b) The incoming tRNA carrying an amino acid enters the A-site, the anticodon matching to the three-base codon of the mRNA. A peptide bond is formed and the ribosome moves along the mRNA so that the aminoacyl-tRNA moves to the P-site where it becomes the peptidyl tRNA.

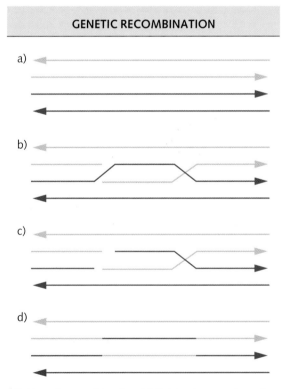

Fig. 6.5 Genetic recombination. (a) Pairing between homologous lengths of DNA. (b) The upper strand is nicked which permits partial exchange of strands. (c) The lower strand is nicked. (d) The recombinant molecules are resolved by further nicking and joining.

- Transferred genes are inserted into the genome of the recipient cell by recombination.

Transduction (Fig. 6.6)

- Bacterial viruses (bacteriophages), during their normal lytic cycle, package a short length of DNA from the bacterial chromosome into a virus 'shell'.

- DNA is transferred by the bacteriophage to a recipient bacterium.

- Only short lengths of DNA (a few genes) can be transferred in each virus particle.

Conjugation (Fig. 6.7)

- This is only possible between closely related species.

- A sex pilus produces a bridge between conjugating cells in Gram-negative bacteria (in Gram-positives, mating cells lie side by side with no visible connecting pilus).

- Long lengths of DNA can be transferred.

- Conjugative plasmids are most commonly transferred.

- A whole chromosome can be transferred if it contains an integrated F plasmid (Hfr donor: high-frequency recombination).

- Genes can be mapped (in minutes) on the chromosome by performing interrupted mating at set times and observing the genes that have been transferred up to that time.

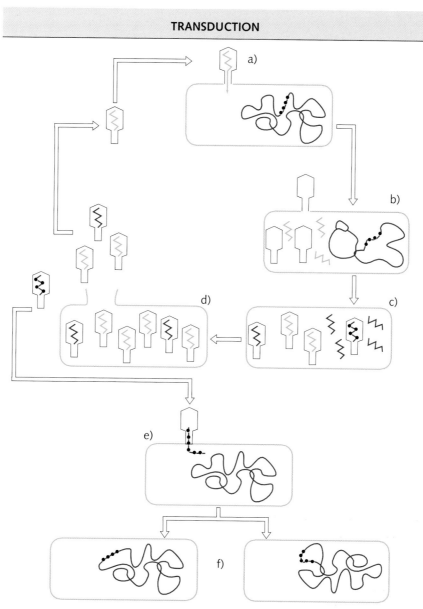

TRANSDUCTION

Fig. 6.6 Transduction. (a) A lytic bacteriophage attaches to a susceptible bacterium and injects its DNA. (b) The bacteriophage DNA codes for new bacteriophage coats and DNA. (c) The bacterial DNA is disrupted and, during assembly of new bacteriophage particles, some of the bacterial DNA is packaged inside bacteriophage coats. (d) The bacterium lyses, releasing both normal bacteriophage and those carrying some bacterial DNA. (e) A bacteriophage carrying bacterial DNA can infect a new bacterium, carrying into it genes from the donor bacterium. (f) This DNA can integrate into the chromosome of the recipient bacterium by recombination and then be transferred to daughter cells on cell division.

Resistance transfer

This is the term given to the genetic transfer of antibiotic-resistance genes from one bacterium to another. The resistance genes are carried on plasmids known as R-plasmids and are transferred by conjugation to other, usually closely related, bacteria. R-plasmids of *E. coli* can be transferred to such species as *Salmonella*, *Shigella*, *Proteus*, and *Haemophilus*. R-plasmids often carry several different genes coding for resistance to different antibiotics.

Transposons and insertion sequences

The fact that several different resistance genes could be carried on the same R-plasmid has been recognized for many years.

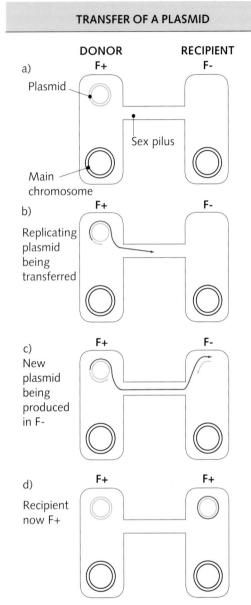

TRANSFER OF A PLASMID

DONOR — F+ RECIPIENT — F-

a)
Plasmid
Sex pilus
Main chromosome

b)
Replicating plasmid being transferred — F+ / F-

c)
New plasmid being produced in F- — F+ / F-

d)
Recipient now F+ — F+ / F+

Fig. 6.7 Bacterial conjugation. Demonstration of plasmid transfer. (a) The donor (F⁺) cell is carrying a plasmid which carries a motility or F factor. It also codes for a specialized pilus, the F or sex pilus, which is used to bind this cell to a recipient (F⁻) cell. (b) The phage replicates, and one strand of DNA moves through the sex pilus to the recipient cell. (c) The incoming DNA is copied in the recipient cell to form a new double-stranded DNA plasmid. (d) The recipient cell now carries the plasmid with the F factor and has become an F⁺ cell.

However, the reasons why this was so common were not understood until the existence of mobile genetic elements was discovered. Transposons are a type of mobile DNA of 2000–20 000 base pairs. They do not exist independently but have the characteristic of jumping from one part of a chromosome to another or to a plasmid, or from one plasmid to another, or back to the chromosome. If they are plasmid-located they can easily transfer from one bacterium to another. Characteristically they carry several different antibiotic-resistance genes. They are identified by having palindromic sequences of bases (inverted repeats) at their ends (Fig. 6.8). Shorter lengths of mobile DNA are termed insertion sequences which, by moving from one site to another, can create genetic variation and are also believed to control various cellular processes.

Manipulation of DNA and recombinant DNA technology

DNA denaturation (melting)

On heating DNA the strands separate. On cooling, the strands renature by complementary base pairing. The slower the rate of cooling, the more accurate is the process of renaturation (Fig. 6.9 (a)). The melting temperature gives an indication of the proportion of G/C and A/T in a sample of DNA.

Restriction endonucleases

These enzymes (commonly, simply termed restriction enzymes), occur naturally and cut DNA at specific sites. They recognize a short sequence of base pairs (bp), usually 4–6 in number, and cut at that site. The enzyme recognizes a palindromic sequence of bases and cuts in a straight or staggered manner, resulting in blunt or sticky ends, respectively (Fig. 6.9 (b)). Sticky ends are perhaps more common, and are certainly more useful in DNA technology where they can be used for grafting other pieces of DNA cut by the same restriction enzyme. Pieces of DNA with sticky ends are also able to circularize readily, a sort of event which may be how plasmids originate.

Gene cloning

Gene cloning is simply the artificial introduction of a gene, or a series of genes, from one source into a new host cell where they are incorporated by genetic recombination into that cell's genome. Here they can be expressed and passed to daughter cells on cell division, resulting in millions of cells producing the same product. Multiple copies of the gene can be made which can then be transferred, allowing hyperproduction of the gene product. Many biotechnological processes now depend on gene cloning, for example genetic engineering and the promised revolution in gene therapy. Thus, one insulin preparation used to treat humans with diabetes mellitus is produced by bacteria which have been cloned with human insulin genes. Also the hepatitis B virus vaccine is produced in yeasts cloned with genes encoding part of the coat of the hepatitis B virus.

A generalized scheme for DNA cloning is shown in Fig. 6.10. The DNA to be cloned is usually extracted from the cells and purified. It is then cut into short fragments by means of a restriction enzyme – leaving sticky ends. These can then be

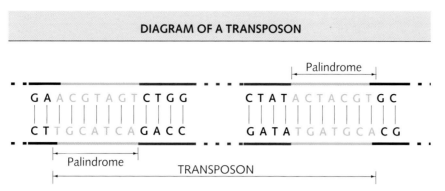

Fig. 6.8 Diagrammatic representation of a transposon, demonstrating palindromic sequences of base pairs (inverted repeats) characteristic of insertion sequences and other mobile genetic elements.

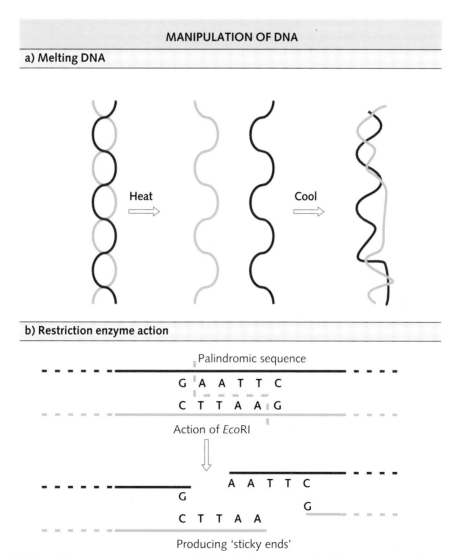

Fig. 6.9 Manipulation of DNA. (a) Melting and renaturation of DNA. (b) The action of *Eco*RI, a restriction endonuclease producing sticky ends.

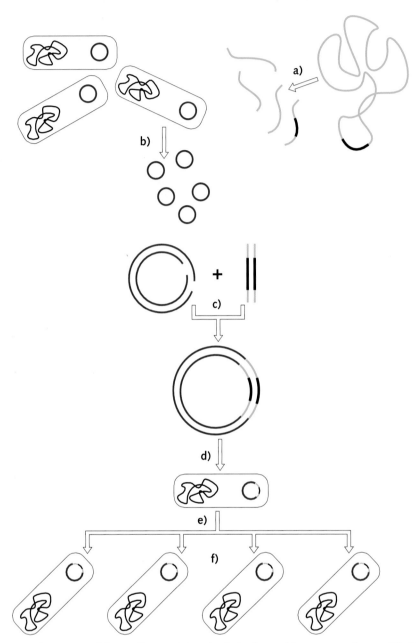

GENE CLONING

Fig 6.10 Gene cloning. (a) DNA is extracted from cells containing the desired gene (the gene may be amplified by PCR – see later), and cut into fragments by a restriction endonuclease. (b) A suitable vector is prepared, in this case a plasmid. (c) The plasmid DNA is cut by the same restriction enzyme as the DNA containing the gene to be cloned. The two DNA preparations are then mixed and treated with DNA ligase to produce recombinant DNA molecules. At this stage there will be many different recombinant plasmids, most not containing the particular DNA to be cloned, as well as normal plasmids not containing extra DNA. (d) The recombined DNA is inserted into a population of the recipient bacteria, and again the bacteria will contain many different lengths of DNA. These recombinant bacteria are the gene library. (e) Bacteria expressing the particular gene(s) must be selected (see text for methods). (f) Once selected, all progeny of the cloned bacteria will express the selected gene.

inserted into vector DNA by first cutting the vector with the same restriction enzyme, and then allowing complementary sticky ends to pair up, treating finally with a DNA ligase which joins the breaks.

Specific genes can be amplified from minute amounts of DNA by the polymerase chain reaction (PCR) (see below). Also, RNA can be the source of specific genes by using reverse transcription: complementary DNA is produced from an RNA template when the enzyme reverse transcriptase and DNA bases are incubated together.

The vector used for the transfer is usually a plasmid or a virus. When on a plasmid, the gene does not need to integrate into the host genome as the plasmid will self-replicate at cell division. If it is an R-plasmid it can move into other bacteria and be selected by antibiotic resistance. A virus vector can carry more genes than a plasmid, and a lysogenic bacteriophage – which has the property of being integrated into the host chromosome as part of its normal life cycle – is usually used. For example, bacteriophage lambda (λ) is often used when *E. coli* is being cloned.

The vector containing the DNA has to be inserted into a cell by one of several means:

- *Transformation* – the easiest, if cells can be made competent, but may need treatment, e.g. *E. coli* is treated with weak calcium chloride solution.

- *Electroporation* – uses an electric current to make pores in the cell membrane.

- *Gene gun* – minute tungsten or gold particles are coated with the DNA to be inserted, and are propelled into cells by a burst of helium; particularly useful for plant cells.

- *Microinjection* – the vector can be injected directly into an animal cell by means of a glass micropipette.

As in all genetic experiments, selection of the clone with the required gene(s) is the final crucial step. Antibiotic resistance is one of the main methods. For example, the plasmid vector might carry the genes for resistance to two antibiotics A and B. The restriction site into which the foreign DNA is inserted is chosen to be in the middle of the gene for resistance to antibiotic B. Therefore bacteria containing a plasmid into which foreign DNA has been inserted will be resistant to A, but sensitive to B, since the gene for resistance to B will be inactivated by insertion of the DNA. This permits bacteria with cloned foreign DNA to be selected – these are termed a gene library.

Identification and selection must then be made from this library for clones producing specific genes. This may be done by probing for the gene using specific gene probes (see below) if available, or the gene product (protein) may be detected by a specific antibody using a method similar to Western blotting (Chapter 7).

Gene probes

DNA or gene probes are simply pieces of labelled, single-stranded DNA or RNA from a known source that can be mixed with an unknown single-stranded (melted/denatured) DNA. If complementary base sequences are recognized the probe will hybridize, thus labelling the unknown DNA. The label can be radioactive or fluorescent. The technique is summarized in Fig. 6.11. DNA probes are highly sensitive and are a powerful method for diagnostic microbiology. Probes may be made from whole genomic DNA, or more specifically by cloning, direct chemical synthesis (if the base sequence is known), or PCR. The method can be used to probe DNA purified from whole cells in a test tube, DNA applied directly to a nitrocellulose or nylon support (dot blotting), or DNA restriction fragments separated on an electrophoresis gel (Southern blotting). 'Blots' of bacterial colonies can be made directly on to nitrocellulose membranes, and following lysis of the bacteria and denaturation of the DNA, can be probed for identification purposes.

Polymerase chain reaction (PCR)

In recent years this extremely powerful technique has revolutionized many nucleic acid-based procedures. In simple terms, the

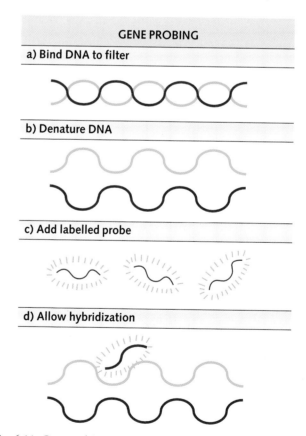

Fig. 6.11 Gene probing. (a) The DNA is bound to a nitrocellulose or nylon membrane filter. (b) The DNA is denatured (melted). (c) The labelled probe is added. (d) The reaction mixture is cooled to allow hybridization of the probe with complementary sequences. Any unhybridized probe is removed and the radioactivity or fluorescence is measured.

technique allows the amplification of DNA sequences over a million-fold in a matter of 2–3 hours by repeating a cyclic procedure of DNA denaturation, annealing of short primers (specific short sequences of DNA at either side of the required section to be amplified – one for each strand), followed by DNA synthesis. The technique is summarized in Fig. 6.12. The major discovery that made the technique possible was the isolation of a heat-stable DNA polymerase, the most widely used being the *Taq* poly-

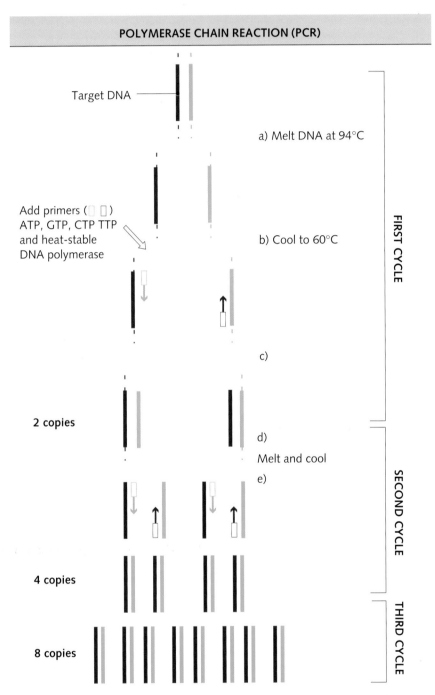

Fig. 6.12 The polymerase chain reaction (PCR). (a) The DNA containing the target sequence to be amplified is heated to 94°C to melt the DNA. (b) This is then cooled to 60°C and the reaction mixture added. This mixture contains the heat-stable DNA polymerase, the four nucleotides ATP, GTP, CTP, and TTP, and a pair of short primer sequences which are known to be complementary with base sequences on each strand at either side of the target DNA. (c) The mixture is incubated for a few minutes at 60°C to allow the synthesis of complementary strands. (d) This produces two copies of the target sequence. (e) The temperature cycle of heating to 94°C for a few minutes followed by cooling to 60°C is repeated 30–40 times, giving rise to over a million copies of the target DNA in 2–3 hours.

merase, isolated from *Thermus aquaticus*, a thermophilic bacterium isolated from hot springs. This polymerase is stable at the denaturation temperature of the DNA (which repeatedly reaches 92–94 °C), so that the enzyme and nucleotides need only be added to the reaction mixture once at the beginning. Theoretically, if a single target molecule of DNA is amplified through 30 cycles, typically in 2–3 hours, it will be amplified 2^{30} times, i.e. 10^9-fold. However, in practice, the procedure is not 100% efficient, but 10^6–10^7-fold amplification is typical. Purpose-made pieces of apparatus known as thermal cyclers are available which can be programmed to run the whole series of cycles at the required temperatures and times. The product of the PCR is detected by electrophoresis on agarose gels, stained with ethidium bromide, and visualized in ultraviolet light or by Southern blotting, or it can be done without the electrophoresis step by dot-blot hybridization using a standard DNA probe.

The standard PCR method described here is constantly being modified and made more sophisticated to increase specificity and to extend its uses. For example, reverse-transcription (RT)-PCR can be used to detect RNA in RNA viruses, or it can detect mRNA to indicate transcription of a specific gene, i.e. gene activity.

The extreme sensitivity of PCR is also its main drawback. To prevent amplification of contaminating DNA – giving rise to false-positives – it is essential that all PCR equipment and reagents, and the environment in which they are used is kept free from any extraneous DNA. This is crucially important in laboratories where the organisms from which the DNA is being detected are being worked on.

Techniques for the molecular 'typing' of micro-organisms

These techniques are used primarily for taxonomic, diagnostic, and epidemiological purposes in microbiology. Some of the basic principles have been described earlier in this chapter, while some of the uses in taxonomy have been described in Chapter 3.

Restriction enzyme analysis

This simply utilizes restriction enzymes to cut the DNA into small fragments (see Fig. 6.9 (b)). The fragments are run on an agarose electrophoresis gel, and the fragments viewed under ultraviolet illumination after staining with ethidium bromide. The banding patterns ('fingerprints') produced tend to be extremely complex – they resemble massive bar codes – but similarities and differences can be seen between different strains.

Restriction fragment length polymorphism analysis (RFLP)

This technique is very similar to the above method; in fact the first stages are identical. However, after the restricted DNA is separated on the agarose gel, it is transferred by blotting onto a nitrocellulose or nylon membrane, and probed with DNA probes which react with specific DNA sequences (Southern blotting). Restriction length polymorphisms are commonly occurring short deletions or insertions in the DNA which will change the size of restriction fragments between different organisms but will be identical in clones from the same organism, or in different tissues from the same organism. This forms the basis of DNA fingerprinting in forensic science. A commonly used probe is for genes coding for ribosomal RNA. These genes are highly conserved, and in bacteria the sequences can be readily detected by probes produced to *E. coli* rRNA genes. This technique is known as ribotyping.

PCR–RFLP

If the source of DNA to be probed is present in extremely small amounts, e.g. viral DNA in tissue from an infected individual, or in minute amounts of tissue or body fluid collected at a crime scene, it would be insufficient for the above sort of fingerprinting. In such situations the DNA can be amplified by PCR, and then analysed as above.

Pulsed-field gel electrophoresis

This technique is similar to restriction enzyme analysis. However, the restriction enzymes used are selected to cut the chromosomal DNA into large fragments. By conventional agarose gel electrophoresis these fragments would be too large to be resolved in the gel. The large molecules become stretched out and work their way snake-like through the gel, and are not well separated. However, with the advent of a special electrophoresis power supply, where the polarity of the current is regularly reversed, these large fragments are sufficiently distorted so that they can be resolved by the system.

Clinical applications of molecular biology

Clinical applications of recombinant DNA technology range from the relatively simple detection and identification of an infecting organism – especially those that cannot be cultured, e.g. the hepatitis viruses – to the techniques which are verging on science fiction, such as gene therapy (using genetic techniques to replace defective mutant genes) or cloning animals. Most of the applications are still in their infancy and many are still at the research laboratory stage. However, this is an extremely rapidly developing field and commercial kits for a variety of applications, based on molecular biology, are becoming increasingly available. Figure 6.13 is an attempt to summarize some of these applications.

SOME CLINICAL APPLICATIONS OF MOLECULAR BIOLOGY	
Detection/diagnosis of:	• Many bacteria and viruses including those that are difficult, slow, or impossible to culture, for example hepatitis B and C viruses, HIV • Genomic typing of any micro-organisms, RFLP, ribotyping
Recombinant therapeutic products:	• Hepatitis B virus vaccine • Insulin • Factor VIII • Monoclonal antibodies (chimaeric and class switching) • Various cytokines, for example TNF, interleukins, and interferons

Fig. 6.13 Examples of some clinical applications of molecular biology.

Key facts

- DNA consists of two antiparallel strands of deoxyribose phosphates cross-linked through purine and pyrimidine bases.

- The bases of DNA are guanine (G), cytosine (C), adenine (A), and thymine (T). G pairs with C, A with T.

- DNA replicates by a process known as semi-conservative replication. New bases are added asymmetrically at the replication fork.

- Mutations are faults in the DNA that are the result of errors in DNA replication or damage caused by chemicals or radiation. Consequences can be malfunction of cellular processes, lethality, or sometimes even beneficial changes. They can be passed on to future generations and are the basis of natural selection.

- DNA is transcribed to messenger RNA which is translated to protein. The sequence of the amino acids in the protein is determined by a three-base code – the genetic code – which is organized linearly on the mRNA. Transfer RNAs carry the amino acids and recognize specific three-base sequences – the codon – by part of their structure termed the anticodon at ribosomes – the site of protein synthesis.

- Gene cloning, the introduction of foreign DNA into another cell where it can replicate and be expressed, is the basis of biotechnology.

- Gene probes, or DNA probes, are small pieces of labelled DNA that can be used to detect specific sequences of DNA by pairing with complementary bases following melting of the target DNA into single strands.

Key facts – (cont.)

- Genetic transfer in bacteria occurs by one of three methods: transformation (naked DNA), transduction (via bacteriophage), and conjugation (directly from one bacterium to another – transferring a plasmid or part of, or the whole, chromosome).

- Resistance transfer is when antibiotic resistance is transferred by a plasmid.

- Transposons and insertion sequences are mobile lengths of DNA able to jump from one site in the chromosome or plasmid to another. They are characterized by having palindromic base sequences (inverted repeats) at their ends. Transposons commonly carry several different antibiotic-resistance genes.

- DNA strands separate on heating – DNA melting – and reassemble on cooling.

- Restriction endonucleases cut double-stranded DNA at specific sites leaving blunt or sticky ends.

- Polymerase chain reaction (PCR) is a system for amplifying the number of copies of a sequence of DNA over a million-fold in a few hours by repeating a cycle of denaturation (melting), primer binding, and DNA synthesis. It was made possible by the discovery of a heat-stable DNA polymerase that is stable to the high temperature used for the denaturation step.

- Restriction analysis can be used to fingerprint organisms. It can be made easier to analyse by combining it with Southern blotting and hybridization.

- The clinical application of recombinant DNA technology is in its infancy.

Further reading

Alberts, B, Bray, D, Lewis, J, Raff, M, Roberts, K, and Watson, JD (1994). *The molecular biology of the cell* (3rd edn). Garland, New York.

Murray, PR, Rosenthal, KS, Kobayashi, GS, and Pfaller, MA (1998). Bacterial genetics. In *Medical microbiology* (3rd edn), Chapter 5. Mosby Year Book, St Louis.

Smith, AJ and Riggio, M (1996). Current developments in microbiological diagnostic tests for oral diseases. *Dental Update*, 7, 296–302.

7

Host defences

Host defences

Introduction

The study of the natural defences of the host against foreign materials or infectious agents is known as 'immunology'. It is a large subject of increasing complexity but a good knowledge of the principles of immunology is crucial to the study of how micro-organisms cause disease (pathogenesis). The aim of this chapter is to give an overview of the immune system and to describe, as clearly as possible, the various immunological mechanisms which operate during any association between the pathogenic micro-organism and the defence systems of the host. While the main function of the immune system is to protect the host, the complex processes involved not infrequently result in varying degrees of damage to the host. Thus, a question often posed is: is the immune system friend or foe?

All immune responses must begin with the recognition by the host of a pathogenic micro-organism or other foreign substance. The body's defence system can conveniently be divided into innate (natural) immunity and acquired (adaptive) immunity. Innate immunity is non-specific and includes natural mechanical, chemical, and biological barriers to infection, which have no degree of specificity or memory. Acquired immunity is specific for a particular foreign agent, but has the advantage that if the host is re-exposed to the same agent the response is massively increased. Study of the immune system soon reveals that there is a great deal of interaction and communication between all the components, many of which are common to more than one pathway. Even between the main divisions of innate and acquired immunity there are several common features.

Innate immunity

The innate defences are summarized in Fig. 7.1. They have been subdivided into four broad groups but, as in any classification system, there is overlap in function between divisions. Some of the important biological processes relevant to innate immunity will now be described in more detail.

Phagocytosis and intracellular killing

Many cells are capable of engulfing micro-organisms, but the main phagocytic cells of the body are the so-called 'professional phagocytes' These comprise the neutrophils (polymorphonuclear leucocytes), the monocytes of the blood, and the macrophages of the tissues. The process of engulfment and killing is summarized in Fig. 7.2.

The intracellular killing of ingested micro-organisms can occur in two ways: oxidative or non-oxidative. The former involves the production by the phagocyte of reactive oxygen intermediates such as superoxide ions, hydrogen peroxide, and free hydroxyl radicals, all of which are toxic to micro-organisms. Non-oxidative mechanisms involve the products of the phagocyte granules which are delivered to the phagolysosome. These comprise a range of proteins which include lysozyme, myeloperoxidase, and acid hydrolases.

Complement

Complement (Figs 7.3 and 7.4) is a series of plasma proteins that have many functions in both the innate and acquired immune response. The innate functions include:

- lysing Gram-negative bacteria;

- enhancing the phagocytosis of foreign particles (opsonization);

- contributing to several aspects of the inflammatory response, including promoting chemotaxis of lymphoid cells.

Many of the complement proteins are produced as proenzymes, which require proteolytic cleavage to become active. In health, most of the complement components exist in the plasma in their inactive form. Once activated, the product of one reaction is the trigger for the next reaction, and hence the overall process can be thought of as a cascade (Fig. 7.4). This cascade can be activated by micro-organisms, immunoglobulins, and a variety of polysaccharides. Initial activation can occur in two ways – either via the classical or the alternative pathways (Fig. 7.3). The components of the classical pathway and the membrane-attack complex are termed C1–C9, while those of the alternative pathway are designated as Factor B, Factor D, or more often as simply 'B', 'D', and so on. The overall scheme is summarized in Fig. 7.4 and the consequences of the activation of complement are illustrated in Fig. 7.5.

Complement plays an important role in discriminating between self and non-self. The key step in the recognition process is the binding of C3b to cell surfaces or immune complexes. The surfaces of the cells and tissues belonging to an individual (self)

THE INNATE IMMUNE SYSTEM		
General category	**Component**	**Comment**
Barrier	Skin	The largest organ of the body, waterproof, highly resistant to penetration by micro-organisms. Chemical antimicrobial properties
	Mucous membranes	Often colonized with micro-organisms but mucus is an effective barrier. Mucus is constantly moving, and is swallowed or expelled
	Connective tissue	Prevents spread through tissues
Flushing action	Peristalsis	Flow rate through gastrointestinal tract important. The greater the flow rate the less chance of colonisation
	Cilia	Aid flow of mucus
	Flow of body fluids	Of great importance in preventing urinary tract infections
	Saliva	Important as a flushing agent in mouth and around teeth. Also important as a vehicle for chemicals (buffers and enzymes) and immunoglobulins
	Cough/sneeze reflex	Expels micro-organisms and contaminated secretions
(Bio)chemical	Enzymes	Proteases, lipases, polysaccharidases, nucleases, lysozyme: damage pathogens
	Gastric acid	Low pH destructive to most micro-organisms
	Bile	Detergent action disrupts membranes
	Sweat	High osmolarity
	Fatty acids	Antibacterial
Biological	Inflammation	Localization of cells of the immune system and their products at the site of infection
	Complement	A group of serum proteins involved in activation of phagocytes, the control of inflammation and lysis of some cells, including some bacteria (Gram-negative)
	Phagocytosis	Ingestion of foreign materials, mainly by macrophages/monocytes and neutrophils
	Natural Killer (NK) cells	A type of lymphocyte which can intrinsically kill cells infected with virus, and some tumour cells
	Acute-phase response	Production of certain serum proteins during inflammation
	Cytokines	Soluble molecules which mediate interactions between cells, for example during inflammation
	Competition with normal flora	Colonization resistance. Prevents occupation of colonized sites by pathogens

Fig. 7.1 Summary of key components of the innate immune system.

possess molecules which limit C3b deposition. This is in contrast to non-self surfaces which allow the rapid deposition of many C3b molecules and actually amplify C3b production through generation of a C3 convertase.

Interferons

Interferons (IFN) are a group of cytokines (see later) produced very early in the immune response, and are often referred to as acute-phase proteins. Alpha-interferon (IFN-α) and beta-interferon (IFN-β) are very important in the response to viral infections. They are produced by virally infected cells and act on other cells, rendering them resistant to viral infection (Chapter 5). Gamma-interferon (IFN-γ) is produced by a type of T lymphocyte (TH1 cells) following activation by antigen (see later). This interferon is involved in the activation of macrophages and has much less antiviral activity than IFN-α and IFN-β.

PHAGOCYTOSIS

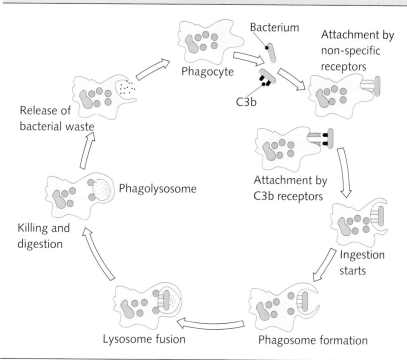

A foreign particle such as a bacterium first adheres to a phagocytic cell. This attachment can be through a non-specific receptor or a receptor for an opsonin on the surface of the particle, such as the C3b complement component, or an antibody. The particle is engulfed by the extending pseudopodia, and becomes enclosed within a phagosome. Lysosomes fuse with the phagosome resulting in a phagolysosome, in which the bacterium is killed and digested by the lysosomal enzymes and reactive oxygen intermediates

Fig. 7.2 Flow diagram illustrating the essential stages in phagocytosis.

Inflammation

The process by which cells of the immune system and their active products are concentrated at a site of infection or tissue damage is termed inflammation. The major purpose of the inflammatory response is to aid in eradicating the infection and in repairing damaged tissue. Three major events occur:

- The blood supply to the site is increased.
- Capillary permeability is increased to allow soluble mediators of the immune system (complement and antibodies) to reach the site.
- White blood cells migrate from the capillaries into the affected tissues.

Neutrophils are the earliest cells to arrive, followed by monocytes/macrophages and lymphocytes. The inflammatory reaction is controlled by a number of factors. The first are the cytokines. These are soluble proteins, usually glycoproteins, with molecular weights between 8 and 50 kilodaltons (kDa) which mediate interactions between cells. Vasoactive mediators released from mast cells, basophils, and platelets, together with by-products of plasma enzyme systems are also involved. The initial inflammation is a result of the fast-acting vasoactive amines histamine and 5-hydroxytryptamine (5-HT; serotonin), and products of the kinin system such as bradykinin. These are followed by the leukotrienes produced by the lipo-oxygenase pathway and mediators released from leucocytes once they accumulate.

The migration of leucocytes to the site of inflammation commences with their initial adherence to the inflamed endothelium through adhesion molecules. This is followed by movement up gradients of chemotactic peptides, the most important of which is C5a. Other important chemotactic molecules are f–Met–Leu–Phe, the initiator of protein translation in bacteria; interleukin (IL)-8, a small cytokine produced by activated mononuclear cells which can induce neutrophil and basophil chemo-

COMPLEMENT ACTIVATION	
Activators of classical pathway	
Immunoglobulins	Complexes containing IgG1, IgG2, or IgG3
Bacteria	None (but see below for lipid A from LPS)
Viruses	Some, for example murine retroviruses
Other micro-organisms	Mycoplasmas
Macromolecules	Polyanions DNA, Lipid A, cardiolipin (all contain PO_4^{3-}) Dextran sulphate, chondroitin sulphate and heparin (all contain SO_4^{2-}) Mannan proteins
Activators of alternative pathway	
Immunoglobulins	Complexes containing IgG, IgA, or IgE (less efficient than classical pathway)
Bacteria	Many Gram-positive and Gram-negative bacteria
Viruses	Some virus-infected cells, for example Epstein–Barr virus
Other micro-organisms	Many fungi, *Leishmania* spp., trypanosomes
Macromolecules	Dextran sulphate, erythrocytes from heterologous species Carbohydrates, for example agarose

Fig. 7.3 Activators of the classical and alternative pathways of complement.

taxis; and leukotriene B4, which is a metabolite of arachidonic acid produced by activated macrophages. The accumulated leucocytes release other cytokines which enhance the inflammatory response. These proinflammatory cytokines such as IL-1, IL-4, IL-6, tumour necrosis factor (TNF), and gamma-interferon (IFN-γ) further enhance cellular migration by their action on the local epithelium. Figure 7.6 summarizes the most important cytokines involved in inflammation.

Other mediators of inflammation include platelet-activating factor (increases vascular permeability and neutrophil activation), C3a (mast cell degranulation), fibrin breakdown products (increase vascular permeability and neutrophil and macrophage chemotaxis), and prostaglandin E2 (vasodilation, potentiates vascular permeability produced by histamines and bradykinin).

Acquired immunity

Acquired immunity differs from innate immunity in two key respects. First, acquired immune responses are specific for individual antigens and, second, immunological memory is produced. This means that a subsequent exposure to the same antigen results in a rapid and more intense response. The most important cells involved in acquired immunity are the lymphocytes, and the responses can be divided into humoral – also known as antibody-mediated immunity – and the cell-mediated response. The various components of the acquired immune system will now be discussed.

Antigens

The strict definition of an antigen is 'a substance which induces the production of antibody'. Antigens are large molecules (>10 kDa) that are foreign to the host and which bind antibody. They are usually proteins or carbohydrates, or both, and are recognized as being 'not self'. The antibody produced in response to an antigen binds only to a very small site on the antigen known as an antigenic determinant or epitope. The form of an epitope is due to the three-dimensional arrangement of the amino acid or sugar components. The term 'immunogenicity' means eliciting an antibody response. An antigen is, therefore, by definition an immunogen.

Many small molecules are capable of reacting with antibodies, but are too small themselves to elicit an antibody response. These are termed haptens, and can be made immunogenic by chemically conjugating the molecule to a larger carrier molecule, usually a protein.

Cells of the immune system

The two main categories of cells, the lymphocytes and the myeloid cells, originate from a common haemopoietic precursor

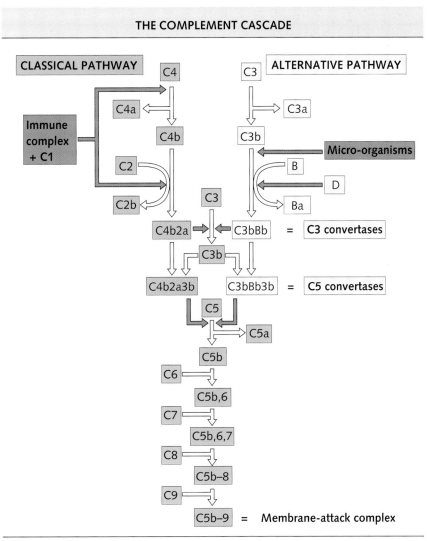

THE COMPLEMENT CASCADE

The classical and alternative pathways join at the point of the conversion of C3 to C3b by the C3 convertases. Either of the two C5 convertases, which are subsequently assembled, act on C5 to produce C5b (and C5a) to which C6 to C9 are added to form the membrane-attack complex

Fig. 7.4 Flow diagram illustrating the complement cascade.

stem cell (Fig. 7.7). Some of these cells, notably the professional phagocytes and natural killer (NK) cells, also participate in innate immunity. The myeloid cells have roles in phagocytosis, antigen presentation, and the production of pharmacologically active agents.

Lymphocytes

The lymphocytes are the main cells involved in acquired immunity. They are found throughout the body in the tissues, blood, and lymph and in specialized, organized lymphoid tissues. They recognize and react with antigens. There are three main types of lymphocytes: the B lymphocytes (B cells), the T lymphocytes

(T cells), and the large granular lymphocytes (LGL) or natural killer (NK) cells.

Lymphocytes originate in the bone marrow from stem cells which migrated from the liver during fetal development. The path of development from stem cell to either mature B or T cell is dependent on stimulation by particular cytokines and whether or not the cells are processed in the thymus.

T CELLS

Those cells destined to be T cells leave the bone marrow via the bloodstream and move to the thymus. There the T cells become able to differentiate between self and non-self antigens. This

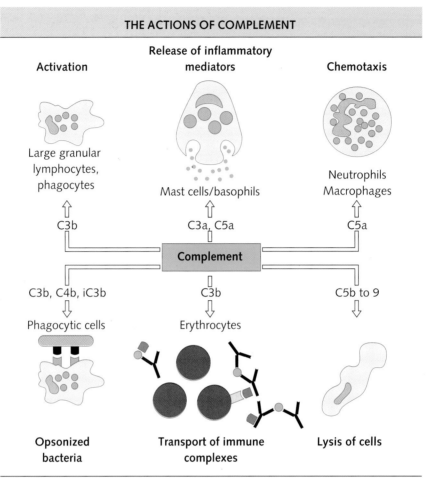

THE ACTIONS OF COMPLEMENT

The major complement components with biological activity are summarized here. C3 is a central component which is cleaved into C3a and C3b. C5 is acted on by C3 convertase and C3b to produce C5a and C5b. C3b has several different activities, the major one being as an opsonin. C3a and C5a are anaphylotoxins which trigger mast cells to release inflammatory mediators. C5a is a chemotactic agent which recruits professional phagocytes to a site of inflammation. C5b to C9 interact to form the membrane-attack complex (MAC) which inserts into membranes and results in cell lysis

Fig. 7.5 The major biological activities of the complement system.

process involves the immature T cell being presented with cell-surface self molecules termed major histocompatibility complex (MHC) molecules, of which there are two types termed class I and class II.

In the thymus, those T cells which react very strongly or very weakly with self MHC molecules are destroyed by a process known as apoptosis. The remaining T cells then mature and are able to recognize foreign antigens in conjunction with MHC molecules. Also in the thymus, fragments of self antigens are presented with MHC molecules to immature T cells, and these are also destroyed thereby preventing any T cells reacting with self.

The T cells recognize antigen through a surface molecule termed the T-cell receptor (TCR) (see Fig. 7.14). Each T cell possesses a different TCR to allow it to recognize a different antigen. After leaving the thymus, T cells locate in the lymph nodes and spleen.

B CELLS

B cells are derived from immature lymphocytes which have not passed through the thymus. These cells go directly to the lymph nodes and spleen after they have matured in the bone marrow, but they are not selected as highly as the T cells. They recognize antigen through the expression of antibody molecules on their

CYTOKINES AND INFLAMMATION			
Cytokine	Source	Target cell(s)	Main action
IFN-γ	T cells, NK cells	Lymphocytes, monocytes, tissue cells	Immunoregulation, B-cell differentiation
IL-1	Monocytes, dendritic cells, fibroblasts, epithelium and endothelium, astrocytes, macrophages	Thymocytes, neutrophils, T and B cells, tissue cells	Immunoregulation, inflammation, fever
IL-2	T cells, NK cells	T and B cells, monocytes	Proliferation, activation
IL-4	T cells	T and B cells	Division and differentiation
IL-6	Macrophages, T cells, fibroblasts, some B cells	T and B cells, thymocytes, hepatocytes	Differentiation, acute-phase protein synthesis
IL-8	Macrophages, skin cells	Granulocytes, T cells	Chemotaxis
TNF	Macrophages, lymphocytes	Fibroblasts, endothelium	Inflammation, cachexia, fibrosis, production of other cytokines (IL-1, IL-6, GM-CSF, adhesion molecules)

Fig. 7.6 Summary of the most important cytokines involved in inflammation.

CELLS OF THE IMMUNE SYSTEM

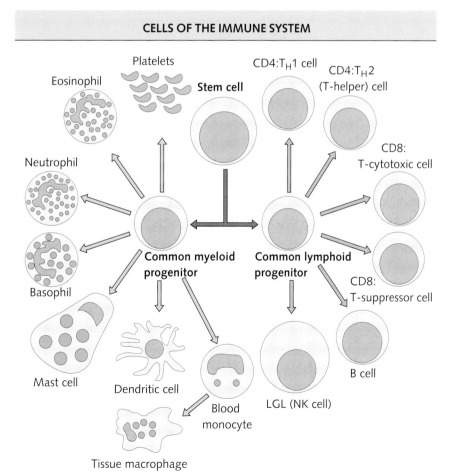

Fig. 7.7 The origin of the main cells of the immune system.

surface, each B cell being able to react with a different antigen. Antibody molecules expressed on B cells and TCR molecules on T cells both recognize antigen, but while they possess some common structural features, TCR molecules are not antibodies.

Myeloid cells

The main myeloid cells include the monocytes in the blood, which move into the tissues and become macrophages, the dendritic cells which are involved in antigen presentation (see later), and the neutrophils, basophils, and eosinophils. The major functions of these cells are summarized in Fig. 7.8.

Antigen presentation

Before an antigen can activate B and T cells, it must first be processed and then presented to these lymphocytes. This is undertaken by antigen-presenting cells (APC); these are mainly dendritic cells and macrophages, although activated B cells can also perform this function. The process is summarized diagrammatically in Fig. 7.9. The antigen is enzymatically degraded into small peptides which can then become anchored to MHC class I or II molecules. Peptides consisting of 8–9 amino acids bind to class I and those with 12 or more bind to class II molecules. Those antigens which have been taken up by the APCs via endocytosis or phagocytosis are degraded in the lysosomal vesicles and are linked to class II molecules before being presented at the cell surface. Those antigens which bind to class I have been synthesized within the cell itself (i.e. self or viral antigens), and are linked to class I in the Golgi body before being transported to the cell surface.

The activation of B and T lymphocytes is described later, but it should be noted here that the class II pathway activates CD4+ T cells (TH2 (helper) and TH1 cells), while the class I pathway activates CD8+ (cytotoxic) T cells. This process ensures that the correct T cells are activated for the right antigen in the right place and at the appropriate time.

Humoral immunity

Antibodies

The terms antibody and immunoglobulin are synonymous. There are five different classes of immunoglobulin (Ig). All are produced by activated B cells (plasma cells) and react specifically with antigens. Structurally, antibodies are made up of one or more units (monomers) comprising four polypeptides: two identical heavy (H) chains and two identical light (L) chains. These chains are connected to form Y-shaped molecules. IgM is a pentamer of the basic structure, IgA is usually a dimer, and IgG, IgD, and IgE are monomeric (Fig. 7.10). The arms of the molecule together comprise the Fab part of the immunoglobulin. The ends of the 'arms' have a variable structure (the V region) which recognizes the antigen. The generation of antibody V-region diversity is a result of the original B cell which recognized the antigen. Gene segments in the DNA of B cells are randomly recombined to produce an infinite number of different V regions. The Fc part is the 'tail' of the molecule, which is a constant region and is associated with effector functions of the antibody (Fig. 7.11).

FUNCTIONS OF THE MYELOID CELLS		
Myeloid cell	**Main sites of action**	**Properties**
Macrophage	Tissues (Kuppfer cells of liver)	Phagocytic; antigen presentation; when activated produces proinflammatory cytokines
Monocyte	Blood	After brief period in blood it migrates into tissue and becomes a macrophage
Dendritic cell	Lymph nodes, spleen, and low levels in blood (Langerhans cells are dendritic cells of the skin)	Antigen presentation
Neutrophil (polymorphonuclear leucocyte)	In blood and migrates into tissues	The most numerous of the professional phagocytic cells; has receptors for Fc region of immunoglobulins
Mast cell and basophil	Mucosal surfaces	Have IgE on their surface which, on binding antigen, brings about degranulation resulting in local inflammation. Important in allergic (type I) reactions
Eosinophil	Blood	Important in controlling parasitic infections when parasite is coated with IgG or IgE, and in type I hypersensitivity (allergic) reactions. May modulate inflammatory reactions

Fig. 7.8 The major groups of myeloid cells and their functions.

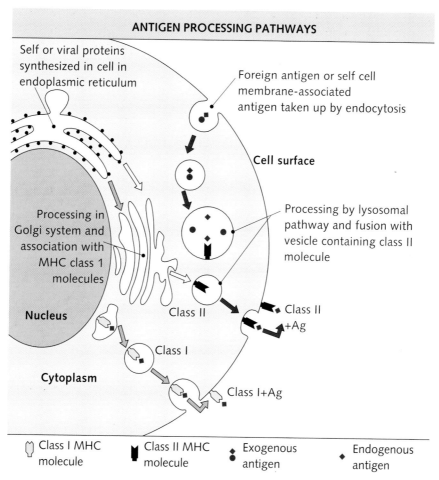

ANTIGEN PROCESSING PATHWAYS

Self or viral proteins synthesized in cell in endoplasmic reticulum

Foreign antigen or self cell membrane-associated antigen taken up by endocytosis

Cell surface

Processing in Golgi system and association with MHC class 1 molecules

Processing by lysosomal pathway and fusion with vesicle containing class II molecule

Nucleus

Class II

Class II +Ag

Cytoplasm

Class I

Class I+Ag

Class I MHC molecule   Class II MHC molecule   Exogenous antigen   Endogenous antigen

Fig. 7.9 Diagrammatic summary of antigen presentation, showing delivery of processed antigen to MHC class I and II molecules.

Activation of B cells: antibody production

Once a B cell recognizes an antigen, it is clonally expanded to produce antibody-secreting plasma cells (Fig. 7.12). On initial exposure to an antigen, antibody is slowly produced as a consequence of the B cells growing and differentiating into plasma cells. The level of antibody reaches a peak, and then declines as the plasma cells die. This pattern of antibody secretion is the primary response. Some of the antigen-activated B cells do not become plasma cells, but survive as memory cells. On subsequent exposure to the same antigen the antibody secretion is rapid, much more intense, and longer lasting, because of clonal expansion of the memory cells. This is the secondary response.

The primary response is characterized by the B cells producing predominantly IgM antibody, the pentameric immunoglobulin which is very effective at binding bacteria in the bloodstream. On repeated B-cell stimulation, class switching occurs, whereby IgG is produced which acts in the blood and tissues, or IgA which acts at mucosal surfaces (Fig 7.12).

Antibody–antigen reactions

The Fab region binds to the specific antigenic determinant or epitope to produce an antibody–antigen complex (immune complex). As there are at least two Fab regions per antibody molecule (they are divalent), the antibody can bind two antigen molecules and large immune complexes, or precipitates can form.

Antibodies function in various ways. By simply binding to an antigen they can block the properties of that antigen. Thus, a toxin can be neutralized, a histolytic enzyme may be inactivated, bacterial surface-attachment sites may be masked, and nutrient uptake by bacteria may be impaired. Viruses or bacterial cells may be aggregated, thus facilitating phagocytosis, and viruses can be prevented from binding to their receptors. The antigen is not directly damaged by the binding of an antibody. The Fc part of the molecule is the effector region. Various cells possess Fc receptors, perhaps the most important being the phagocytic cells, which are able to phagocytose antibody-coated micro-organisms or immune complexes much more efficiently. Mast cells and

CLASSES OF IMMUNOGLOBULINS

Class	Basic structure	Principal functions
IgG	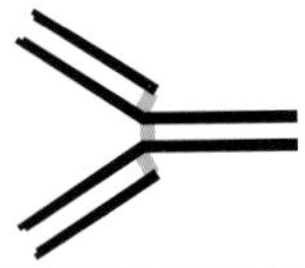	Protects extravascular compartment from micro-organisms and their toxins
IgM	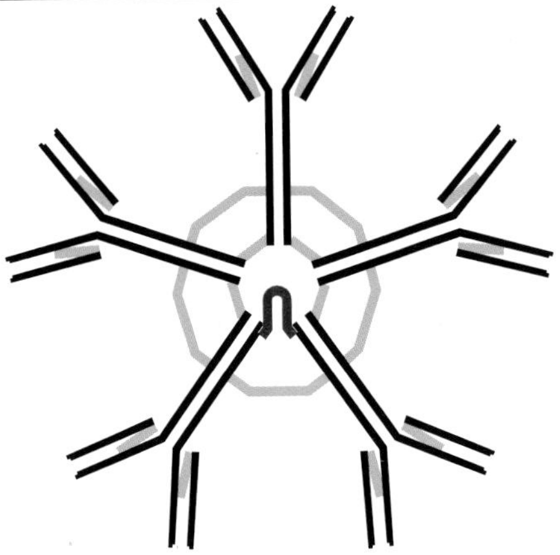	**Pentameric:** effective first line of defence against micro-organisms in the bloodstream. Produced in the primary response
IgA	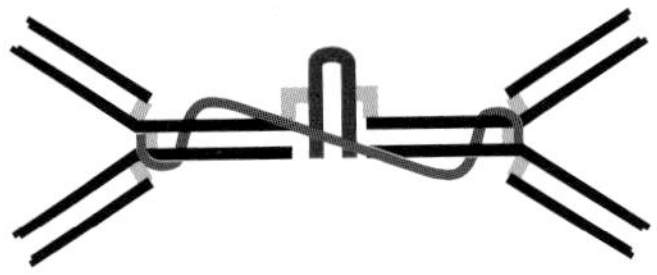	**Dimeric:** protects mucosal surfaces
IgD	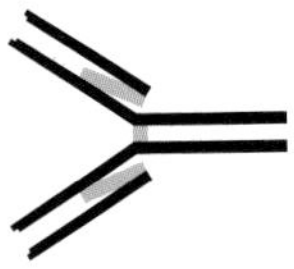	Influences lymphocyte functions
IgE	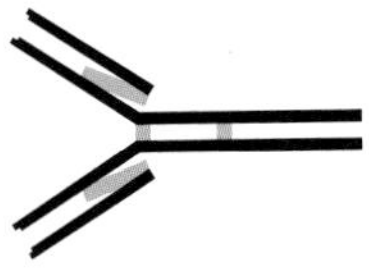	Protects against intestinal parasites. Responsible for many of the symptoms of allergy

Secretory component   J chain   Disulphide bridge

Fig. 7.10 The five classes of immunoglobulin.

basophils are activated by binding antigen through their Fc receptor.

Monoclonal antibodies

The Nobel Prize-winning procedure, developed by Köhler and Milstein for the immortalization of an antibody-secreting plasma cell by fusing it to a myeloma cell, results in a clone of a monoclonal antibody-secreting hybridoma. The procedure is summarized in Fig. 7.13. Monoclonal antibodies (mAb) are by definition standardized and have numerous uses in a huge range of immunoassays. They have largely obviated the use of animals for the production of standard antisera for diagnostic and research use.

Cell-mediated immunity

Activation of T cells

In contrast to B cells, T cells do not make antibodies or secrete special forms of their antigen-receptor molecules. They react

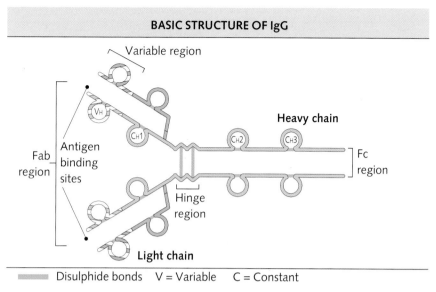

Fig. 7.11 The structure of immunoglobulin G.

to antigen by going through stages of activation: growing, differentiating, and secreting a range of cytokines which regulate the functions of other lymphocytes. T cells are divided into several subsets with different functions:

- T-helper cells or TH2 cells: express CD4 molecules on their surface and function by secreting cytokines (IL-4, IL-5, IL-6, and IL-10) that promote B cells to produce antibody by stimulating their growth and differentiation.

- T-suppressor (TS) cells are thought to control the action of TH2 cells by producing cytokines that suppress the immune response.

- CD8+ T cells function as cytotoxic T (TC) cells and can kill other cells, primarily those infected by viruses.

- Some CD4+ T cells, which produce different cytokines (IL-2, IFN-γ) from the TH2 cells, are involved in hypersensitivity reactions (see later) and are known as TH1 (formerly TDTH: delayed-type hypersensitivity) cells.

T cells are activated by antigens to produce cytokines following presentation of the antigen by the MHC complex to the T cell receptor (TCR). The TCR is a heterodimer of two transmembrane peptide chains on the surface of the T cell (Fig. 7.14). It is always associated with the CD3 transmembrane molecule which transmits the signal to produce cytokines when the receptor binds an antigen. The majority of T cells have heterodimers consisting of an α and a β chain, with the distal end having a variable (V) region, reminiscent of immunoglobulins, which recognizes the antigen located in the binding groove of the MHC molecule (Fig. 7.14). The binding of antigen-presenting cells (APCs) to the TCR also involves other cell-adhesion molecules such as the intercellular adhesion molecule-1 (ICAM-1) of the antigen-presenting cell which binds to the lymphocyte functional antigen-1 (LFA-1) on

the T cell, and the LFA-3 molecule on all antigen-presenting cells which binds to CD2 surface molecules on the T cell. A very simplified diagram of how antigen is presented to T cells is shown in Fig. 7.15.

Superantigens

Some bacterial antigens, such as the staphylococcal enterotoxins and Toxic Shock Syndrome Toxin (TSST-1), are able to stimulate cytokine production from T cells without the processing and presentation required by conventional antigens. These have been termed superantigens. They bind directly to MHC class II molecules and activate a distinct set of Vβ-expressing T cells (Fig. 7.16).

Activated macrophages, cytokines, and systemic inflammation/shock

Another important source of cytokine release, which is independent of T cells or antigen, are macrophages that have been activated by microbial components, especially the lipopolysaccharide (LPS) of Gram-negative bacteria (endotoxin). The most important cytokine produced by this route is tumour necrosis factor alpha (TNF-α) which enhances the antimicrobial activity of macrophages and neutrophils. It increases the adhesion of phagocytes to vascular endothelium allowing increased entry by phagocytes to sites of inflammation, and induces other cytokines, especially IL-1 and IL-6, to be produced by macrophages. Although normally a beneficial activity within the host, overstimulation of macrophages by excessive amounts of endotoxin can result in the dramatic symptoms of endotoxic shock (or SIRS: systemic inflammatory response syndrome), which is a major cause of death in severely ill patients (Chapter 17). The excessive activation of the coagulation and complement cascades by LPS, together with the

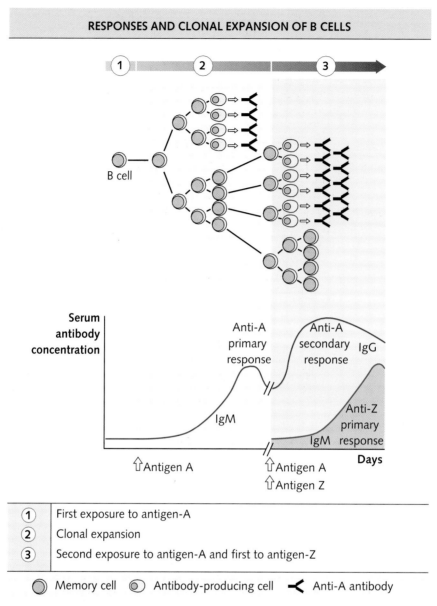

RESPONSES AND CLONAL EXPANSION OF B CELLS

B cell

Serum antibody concentration

Anti-A primary response

Anti-A secondary response

IgG

IgM

Anti-Z primary response

IgM

Days

⬆Antigen A

⬆Antigen A
⬆Antigen Z

① First exposure to antigen-A

② Clonal expansion

③ Second exposure to antigen-A and first to antigen-Z

⊙ Memory cell   ⊙ Antibody-producing cell   ◄ Anti-A antibody

Fig. 7.12 Diagram to show primary and secondary antibody responses and clonal expansion of B cells.

cytokines produced by the macrophages, result in the characteristic symptoms of fever, hypotension, disseminated intravascular coagulation and multi-organ failure typical of SIRS. The source of the LPS which brings about these symptoms can be from a systemic Gram-negative sepsis as typified by meningococcal disease or typhoid fever. However, the LPS may be more commonly derived from the normal bacterial flora of the gastrointestinal tract, which is released into the portal circulation following translocation across an ischaemic bowel wall, as a consequence of fluid loss following major trauma, surgery, or severe burns.

Lymph nodes and the lymphatic system

The lymphatic system of the body consists of the main lymphoid organs (spleen, thymus, and bone marrow), together with a network of smaller concentrations of lymphoid tissue called lymph nodes. These lymph nodes are found at branches of the lymphatic vessels and are present in clusters in the neck, groin, axillae, mediastinum, and the abdominal cavity. Typically, a lymph node consists of three main regions – the cortex (B cell area), the paracortex (T cell area), and the medulla which contains cords of lymphoid tissue (T and B cell area rich in plasma cells).

MONOCLONAL ANTIBODY PRODUCTION

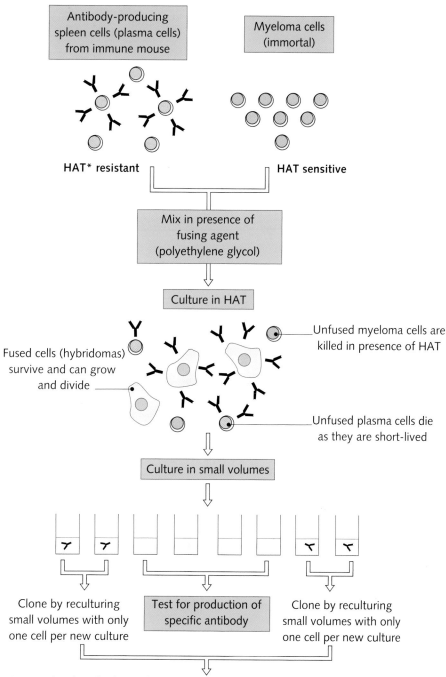

*HAT = Hypoxanthine aminopterin and thymidine

Fig. 7.13 Flow diagram illustrating the steps involved in the production of a monoclonal antibody.

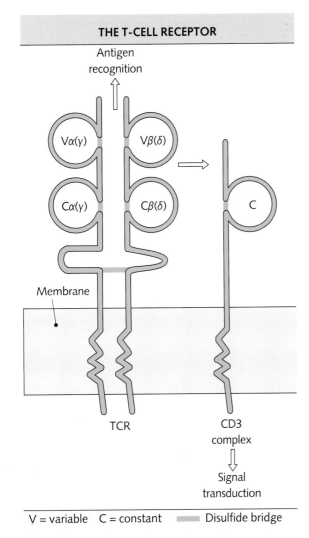

THE T-CELL RECEPTOR

Antigen recognition

Vα(γ)   Vβ(δ)

Cα(γ)   Cβ(δ)   C

Membrane

TCR   CD3 complex

↓

Signal transduction

V = variable   C = constant   ▬▬ Disulfide bridge

Fig. 7.14 Diagram of the T cell receptor.

PRESENTATION OF ANTIGEN

Antigen (peptide) in peptide groove of APC

T Cell

LFA-1   TCR   CD2

ICAM-1   MHC II   LFA-3

APC

Fig. 7.15 Simplified diagram showing the presentation of antigen by an MHC class II molecule to a T cell. Some of the accessory adhesion molecules are shown.

Lymph nodes function by filtering antigen from the lymphatic ducts and presenting it to the lymphoid cells.

Protection at mucosal surfaces and the MALT

The mucosal surfaces of the body are secretory in nature and have their own immune system, the mucosa-associated lymphoid tissue, or MALT. The main mucosal surfaces are the gastrointestinal tract (including oral mucosa and the salivary glands), the genitourinary tract, and the respiratory tract. The secretion of the mammary glands (colostrum) is also part of the MALT. This branch of the

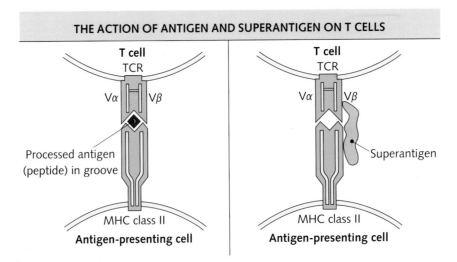

THE ACTION OF ANTIGEN AND SUPERANTIGEN ON T CELLS

T cell
TCR

Vα   Vβ

Processed antigen (peptide) in groove

MHC class II
Antigen-presenting cell

T cell
TCR

Vα   Vβ

Superantigen

MHC class II
Antigen-presenting cell

Fig. 7.16 Diagram demonstrating the difference between activation of T cells by conventional processed antigen and superantigen.

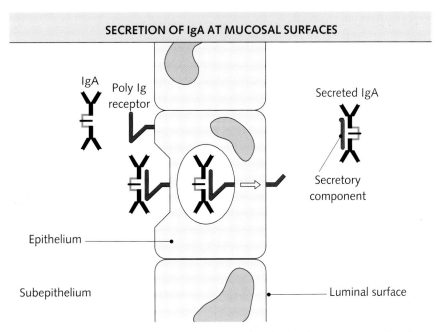

Fig. 7.17 Diagram illustrating the mechanism by which IgA crosses mucosal surfaces.

immune system is stimulated through mucosa-associated lymphoid tissue which is organized into discrete areas in the gut known as Peyer's patches, just below the epithelial cells in the lamina propria. Antigen travels through specialized epithelium (M cells) to the subepithelial lymphoid tissue. The main antibody produced at these sites is secretory IgA, a dimeric immunoglobulin which acquires its secretory component during transport across the epithelium (Fig. 7.17).

Hypersensitivity

Classically, hypersensitivity is thought of as being an allergic reaction, in which the normal acquired immune response is exaggerated or inappropriate and causes damage to the host. Hypersensitivity reactions are divided into four types. Types I–III are predominantly antibody-mediated, while type IV is mediated through T cells and macrophages and is antibody-independent.

Type 1 hypersensitivity: atopy and anaphylaxis

These reactions include atopic allergies such as asthma, hay fever, and eczema. They result from exposure to environmental allergens, for example pollen and dust, that react with specific IgE antibody present on the surface of mast cells and basophils. These cells degranulate, releasing inflammatory mediators as described earlier in this chapter. Since many of these cells are found in the tissues beneath the skin and mucous membranes of the airways, eye, nose, and throat, it is these sites which are particularly affected.

Anaphylaxis is an acute, immediate, and intense form of the type I reaction which results in vasodilation and contraction of smooth muscle. The body becomes shocked, and the response may be fatal. It can be caused by food allergy (for example peanuts), drug allergy (for example penicillin), and wasp or bee stings.

Type II hypersensitivity: cytotoxic hypersensitivity

This occurs when antibodies, either IgG or IgM, are directed against the cells of the host or against foreign antigens such as transfused red blood cells, and brings about the destruction of the cells in the same way that an invading micro-organism would be destroyed. This can be through phagocytosis (antibody acting as an opsonin), by complement-dependent lysis, or by the cytotoxic reaction of killer (K) cells. Lysis of blood cells following an incompatible blood transfusion is an example of type II hypersensitivity.

Type III hypersensitivity: immune-complex disease

Immune complexes (antigen–antibody complexes) are usually eliminated by macrophages/monocytes. However, sometimes when complexes are deposited in tissues a damaging inflammatory response may develop through complement activation and attraction of polymorphs to the site. This is sometimes referred to as the Arthus Reaction. Antigens can be of microbial, animal, or plant origin, and the glomeruli of the kidneys are the most susceptible tissues, for example glomerulonephritis following a streptococcal infection. Immune-complex disease is a frequent complication of autoimmune disease where the kidneys, joints, arteries, and skin can be damaged. Repeated inhalation of moulds and plant or animal material can cause type III reactions in the lung, for example Farmers' lung and Pigeon fanciers' lung.

Type IV hypersensitivity: delayed-type hypersensitivity (DTH)

Following a second exposure to the appropriate antigen, antigen-sensitized T cells (TH1 CD4+ cells) release lymphokines which activate macrophages and induce an inflammatory response. The reaction is slow to develop, taking days or sometimes weeks. The three main types of DTH are:

- *Allergic contact dermatitis* or eczema which develops on the skin within 48–72 h following contact with certain chemicals, e.g. nickel, chromate, or poison ivy.
- The *Tuberculin-type reaction* also occurs in 48–72 h, typically after the injection of soluble mycobacterial antigens into the skin of an individual immune to, or infected with, *Mycobacterium tuberculosis*.
- *Granulomatous hypersensitivity* occurs in tuberculosis or leprosy. It results from the persistence of the bacteria within macrophages which are unable to destroy the micro-organism. Granulomas develop which consist of a central zone of macrophages, epithelioid cells, and giant cells, sometimes with an area of necrosis. The whole is surrounded by lymphocytes, often with considerable fibrosis.

Much immunopathology is the result of an exaggerated immune response to invading micro-organisms or other foreign antigens, and hypersensitivity states, as described above, also contribute to damage to the host. However, damage can also be caused if the immune system reacts to self tissues (autoimmunity), or if a component of the immune system fails (immunodeficiency), or is suppressed as a consequence of disease or therapy. The following section of this chapter will briefly deal with these points.

Deficiencies in the immune system

The immune system must function normally if the host is to survive the constant assaults by micro-organisms and other foreign agents. It is not surprising that defects in the immune system can result in disease, while some diseases themselves are the cause of immune deficiencies. Some of the more common states and causes of immunodeficiency are summarized in Fig. 7.18.

Autoimmunity

Normally the immune system 'sees' its own tissues as 'self' and does not react to them. Rarely, however, there is a breakdown in this recognition and the immune system destroys its own tissue, a phenomenon termed autoimmunity. As the specificity repertoires that are expressed by both B and T cells are random, it is perhaps not surprising that antiself specificities occur. There are mechanisms which kill these self-reactive cells, as described earlier, but some escape this surveillance. Many autoimmune diseases have a poorly understood aetiology. However, some are triggered by microbial antigens which mimic or cross-react with self components. The best known of these is rheumatic fever (Chapter 16), in which carbohydrate antigens in the cell wall of *Streptococcus pyogenes* cross-react with antigens of the heart sarcolemma, and bypass T cell self-tolerance.

Other known autoimmune diseases include pernicious anaemia, insulin-dependent diabetes mellitus, and rheumatoid arthritis. Some diseases of unknown cause, such as multiple sclerosis, are also suspected as having an autoimmune aetiology.

Immunosuppression

When patients are undergoing organ transplantation it is essential that the recipient is immunosuppressed to prevent rejection. Various immunosuppressive agents are available, including purine analogues which inhibit nucleic acid synthesis, corticosteroids, and cyclosporin – a fungal peptide which preferentially affects dividing T cells and inhibits cytokine production.

Immunosuppression occurs during many eukaryotic parasitic infections. Most are thought to be caused by overloading of the macrophages as a result of a massive production of soluble antigen by the parasite. In malaria, the *Plasmodium falciparum* is thought to mop up circulating antibody by producing soluble antigen – a process termed immune distraction.

Immunosuppression can also be a result of therapy. Chemo- and radiotherapy are used in the treatment of tumours in an attempt to kill the rapidly growing cancer cells. A side-effect is that the host's rapidly dividing leucocytes are also killed, resulting in immunosuppression.

The concept of the immunocompromised host

The term 'immunocompromised host' refers to patients who are susceptible to infection as a result of an underlying defect or illness which results in a less than perfect immune system. This defect can be in either the innate or acquired branches of the immune system, and virtually any aspect of the immune response can be involved. Patients include those undergoing organ transplants and those being treated for cancer, patients with haematological malignancies, burns patients, those with specific immunodeficiencies, and malnourished individuals. This group of patients is becoming increasingly significant and their numbers will continue to increase in the future. The micro-organisms infecting such patients are commonly members of the normal bacterial flora of the host, often referred to as opportunistic pathogens.

Immunological techniques

The final part of this chapter will briefly describe a few of the most commonly used immunological techniques. Over the past few decades many different techniques that employ immunological components, especially antibodies, have been developed for use in the study of biological reactions relevant to the pathogenesis of disease, epidemiology, and diagnosis. Serology, the measurement of specific antibodies in serum to diagnose indirectly a specific infection, still has a major role in clinical microbiology. Some of the most commonly used techniques involve the use of tagged, or labelled antibodies, where the label can be a fluorescent dye, an enzyme, or a radioactive isotope. Two of the most commonly used techniques are enzyme-linked immunosorbent assay (ELISA), and immunoblotting (Western blotting). Both techniques involve the ultimate detection of antibody–antigen complexes, where either the antigen or the antibody is being assayed. The third technique, latex agglutination (or a variation called coagglutination) is used as an extremely rapid technique for the detection of antigen or

IMMUNODEFICIENCIES	
Deficiency	**Cause/consequence**
B cell deficiencies X-linked agammaglobulinaemia	Affected males have no B cells, no IgA, M, D, or E and only small amounts of IgG. Protection from maternal antibody exists for 6–12 months and then severe pyogenic infections develop. Can be treated with large doses of gammaglobulin
IgA deficiency with IgG subclass deficiency	Tend to develop immune-complex disease. Those which also lack IgG2 and 4 also develop pyogenic infections
T cell deficiency Severe combined immunodeficiency (SCID)	Infants develop prolonged diarrhoeal disease (viral and bacterial), pneumonia as in AIDS patients (see below), and candidal infections. A lethal disease unless rescued by bone marrow transplant
MHC class II deficiency	Failure to express MHC II on antigen-presenting cells. Affected infants have recurrent infections, especially of the gastrointestinal tract
Acquired immunodeficiency syndrome (AIDS)	Infection with HIV. Affects CD4+ T cells, and monocyte/macrophages, dendritic cells and microglia of the central nervous system. Fall in CD4+ T cells results in opportunistic infections such as *Pneumocystis carinii* pneumonia, mycobacterial infections, toxoplasmosis, cryptosporidiosis, and severe candidal and herpes infections. Kaposi's sarcoma and Burkitt's lymphoma are common malignancies
Defects in the complement system	Defects in C1, C4, or C2 result in immune-complex diseases. Deficiencies in C3, Factor H or I result in poor opsonization and an increased susceptibility to pyogenic infections. Deficiencies in the C5-C8, Factor D, and the alternative pathway results in susceptibility to neisserial infections because of failure to lyse these bacteria
Defects in phagocytosis Chronic granulomatous disease (CGD)	Patients are unable to form oxygen radicals (O_2^-) and hydrogen peroxide in their phagocytes and therefore cannot kill ingested bacteria. Bacteria remain alive intracellularly and granulomas form to which there is a cell-mediated response. Children with CGD develop pneumonia, infections of the lymph nodes, and abscesses in the skin, liver, and other viscera
Neutropenia	A general deficiency of neutrophils brought about by immunosuppressive therapy, for example cancer chemotherapy and radiotherapy Great susceptibility to bacterial infections

Fig. 7.18 Summary table of the major types of immunodeficiency.

toxin in clinical specimens. It is gaining popularity as a technique that can be performed in a surgery or side-room by semi-skilled operators, a development which some see as a cause for concern.

ELISA

The simplest form of this technique is summarized in Fig. 7.19. It can be used to detect antibodies in serum or other body fluids, by binding them to an antigen coated to a solid phase (a well in a polystyrene, multiwell microtitre plate). The bound antibody can then be detected by adding a tagged second antibody, which recognizes the first as an antigen. For example, if the assay is being used to detect a specific human IgG, then the second antibody might be antibody to human IgG (which has been produced by immunizing another species, commonly a goat, with human IgG). This second antibody is covalently labelled with an enzyme. The complex of antigen, first antibody, and second antibody–enzyme conjugate is detected by adding a chromogenic substrate for the enzyme, i.e. the product of the enzyme is coloured, or a different colour from the substrate. The intensity of the colour produced, which is proportional to the amount of antibody bound by the antigen, can be read quantitatively in a purpose-designed microplate spectrophotometer.

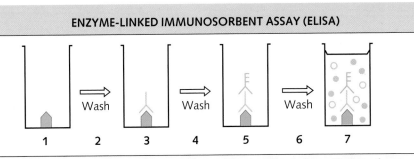

ENZYME-LINKED IMMUNOSORBENT ASSAY (ELISA)

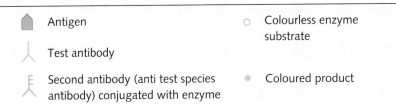

Steps: 1 Coat wells with antigen; 2 wash; 3 add test antibody (e.g. dilution of serum); 4 wash; 5 add enzyme conjugate (antibody to first antibody conjugated with enzyme); 6 wash; 7 add chromogenic enzyme substrate and read colour change

Antigen

Colourless enzyme substrate

Test antibody

Second antibody (anti test species antibody) conjugated with enzyme

Coloured product

Fig. 7.19 Diagrammatic representation of the simple ELISA technique to detect antibody.

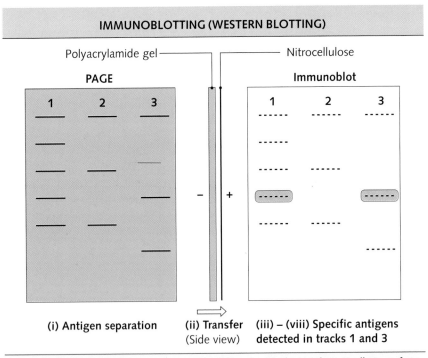

IMMUNOBLOTTING (WESTERN BLOTTING)

Polyacrylamide gel — Nitrocellulose

PAGE

Immunoblot

(i) Antigen separation

(ii) Transfer
(Side view)

(iii) – (viii) Specific antigens detected in tracks 1 and 3

Steps: (i) Separate antigens on polyacrylamide gels; (ii) electrophoretically transfer to a sheet of nitrocellulose; (iii) block unbound sites with an irrelevant protein (e.g. gelatin or serum albumin); (iv) add specific (first) antibody; (v) wash; (vi) add tagged second (anti-first) antibody, which is enzyme- or radiolabelled; (vii) wash; (viii) detect antibody–antigen reactions by addition of chromogenic substrate or by autoradiography

Fig. 7.20 Diagram of the immunoblotting technique (Western blotting) for the detection of specific antigens.

A converse assay for the detection and quantitation of antigen can be performed by a capture or sandwich ELISA where the capture antibody is bound to the plastic. After capture of the antigen, it can be detected either directly with an enzyme-labelled antibody, or indirectly with a second antibody raised in a different species from the capture antibody. This second antibody can be detected as described above for the antibody-detection ELISA.

In diagnostic procedures, ELISA is now one of the standard assays used to detect antibody to a vast range of microbial pathogens, particularly in virus serology. Detection of antigen is less frequently used but it has a role in the rapid detection of micro-organisms or toxins from normally sterile sites, such as antigens of meningitis-causing micro-organisms in cerebrospinal fluid.

Immunoblotting or Western blotting

This is an immunoassay employed for observing antibody–antigen reactions in a (sometimes) complex antigen mixture (Fig. 7.20). Antigens are first separated by polyacrylamide gel electrophoresis (PAGE). The separated antigens are transferred electrophoretically (blotted) to a nitrocellulose membrane to which they bind. After the blot is treated with antibody, the antigen–antibody complexes are detected with either an enzyme-labelled second antibody as for ELISA or a radioactively labelled second antibody. The enzyme is located with a chromogenic substrate – but a different one from the ELISA, as here the product must be insoluble as well as coloured. Radioactivity is located by exposing the nitrocellulose membrane to X-ray film (autoradiography).

Latex agglutination

This is performed with microscopic latex (really polystyrene) beads which have been coated with a specific antibody. When these beads are mixed with a fluid containing the specific antigen they bind to the antigen and agglutinate, forming a visible precipitate (Fig. 7.21). A variation of this technique employs killed *Staphylococcus aureus* cells in place of the latex beads. *Staph. aureus* contains Protein A molecules on its surface which bind to the Fc region of many IgG molecules. These bacterial cells bind antibodies so that their antigen-binding sites are free to bind antigen. The resultant agglutination reaction is referred to as coagglutination.

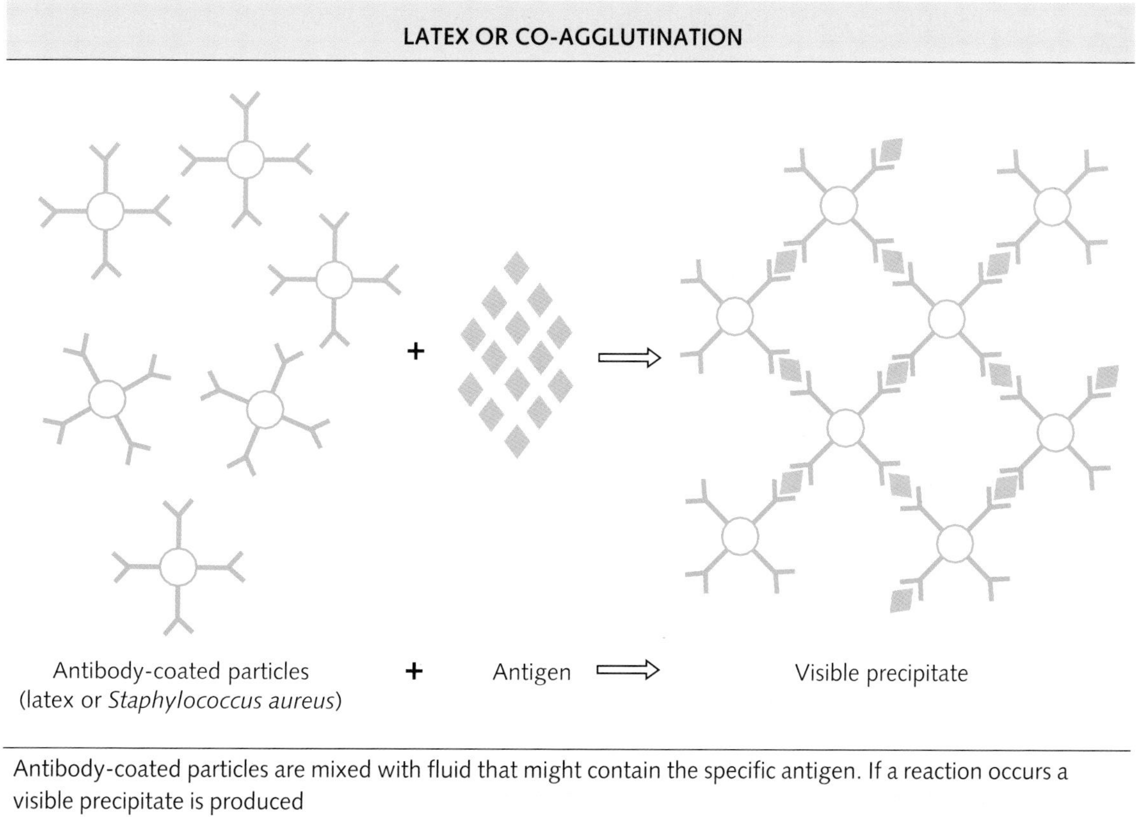

LATEX OR CO-AGGLUTINATION

Antibody-coated particles (latex or *Staphylococcus aureus*) + Antigen ⟹ Visible precipitate

Antibody-coated particles are mixed with fluid that might contain the specific antigen. If a reaction occurs a visible precipitate is produced

Fig. 7.21 The latex or co-agglutination test for the detection of specific antigens.

Key facts

- Host defence, or the immune response, consists of innate (or natural) immunity and acquired (or adaptive) immunity. The latter is specific for a particular antigen, and on re-exposure to that antigen, produces an increased response due to immunological memory.

- There is a great deal of interaction and communication between all aspects of the immune system, performed largely by cytokines.

- Innate defences include: phagocytosis and intracellular killing; the complement system; interferons; and inflammation.

- Acquired immunity: important cells include B and T cells. It can be divided into humoral (antibody-mediated) and cell-mediated.

- Antibodies are produced by activated B cells. Antibodies or immunoglobulins (Ig) have a monomeric Y-shaped structure, with antigen-binding sites at the arms of the Y and an Fc tail part which is responsible for effector functions of the molecule. IgM is pentameric, IgA is usually dimeric, and IgG, IgD and IgE are monomeric.

- B-cell activation: antibody molecules are randomly expressed on B cells. When a B cell recognizes and binds an antigen it is clonally expanded to produce antibody-secreting plasma cells. The primary response produces largely IgM, and some B cells survive as memory cells. The secondary response is much more pronounced and is due to clonal expansion of the memory cells with IgG being the predominant antibody.

- Monoclonal antibodies are artificially created by fusing an antibody-producing plasma cell with a myeloma cell line to produce immortalized clones secreting a specific antibody.

- T cell, or cell-mediated immunity, is primarily the activation of T cells to grow, differentiate, and produce a range of cytokines which regulate the functions of other lymphocytes.

- T cells are activated to produce cytokines following the presentation of antigen by the MHC complex to the T cell receptor.

Key facts – (cont.)

- T cells include: T-helper or TH2 cells which express CD4 molecules and promote B cells to produce antibody; T-suppressor (TS) cells; cytotoxic CD8+ (TC) cells; TH1 cells which are also CD4+ but produce different cytokines than the TH2 cells.

- Superantigens stimulate T cells to produce cytokines by binding directly to the MHC class molecule without the need for antigen processing and presentation.

- Systemic inflammation or shock is a response to bacterial endotoxin (LPS), whereby the macrophages overproduce tumour necrosis factor (TNF) and other cytokines such as interleukin (IL)-1 and IL-6 which result in the symptoms of shock.

- The main lymphoid organs of the body are the spleen, thymus, and bone marrow together with lymph nodes at branches in the lymphatic system.

- The mucosae have their own immune system – which is primarily secretory – and dimeric, secretory IgA is the principal immunoglobulin.

- Hypersensitivity, an allergic or an exaggerated or inappropriate immune response is divided into four types: I, atopy and anaphylaxis; II, cytotoxic; III, immune-complex disease; and IV, delayed-type hypersensitivity.

- Other deficiencies in the immune system include autoimmunity and immunosuppression.

References and further reading

Mims, CA, Playfair, JHL, Roitt, IM, Wakelin, D, Williams, R, and Anderson, RM (1993). *Medical microbiology*, Mosby, London.

Murray, PR, Rosenthal, KS, Kobayashi, GS, and Pfaller, MA (1998). Basic concepts in the immune response. In *Medical microbiology* (3rd edn), Section II. Mosby Year Book, St Louis.

Playfair, J (1995). *Infection and immunity*. Oxford University Press.

Roitt, I, Brostoff, J, and Male, D (1997). *Immunology* (5th edn). Mosby, London.

Staines, N, Brostoff, J, and James, K (1994). *Introducing immunology* (2nd edn). Mosby, London.

8

Immunization

- Introduction
- Types of immunization
- Current vaccine practice

Immunization

Introduction

The introduction of immunization against infectious disease has been one of the most successful developments in medicine. It was pioneered at the end of the eighteenth century by Edward Jenner to prevent smallpox and due to the remarkable success of worldwide vaccine programmes in the latter half of this century, the disease has been totally eradicated from the planet.

The aim of immunization is to produce resistance in the population to natural clinical infection with microbial agents by means of a range of artificial and safe procedures.

Prophylactic immunization is only one of the measures available to control infectious disease, but its efficacy and cost must be assessed against other forms of protection, for example safe water supply and sewage disposal, a high standard of food hygiene, good socioeconomic living conditions, as well as organized surveillance of infectious disease with early detection and prompt treatment and prevention. The mortality and morbidity of a number of infectious diseases have been dramatically reduced by immunization, while many others are currently not amenable to control by specific vaccines.

At present, vaccines do not form part of the armamentarium employed by dentists to control and treat oral and dental infections, although research has demonstrated that this is possible for dental caries and perhaps, in the future, for certain forms of periodontal disease. However, immunization of dental staff and, in some cases, patients, against a number of common infections plays an important role in preventing cross-infection during dental treatment.

Types of immunization

A summary of the different types of immunization available is presented in Fig. 8.1. Active immunization is associated with the production of antibody and often cell-mediated immunity, while passive immunization depends on a supply of antibodies from outside the host.

Passive immunization

Immunoglobulins used in passive immunization are usually derived from human serum but horse serum is also sometimes used. The indications for using artificial passive immunization are

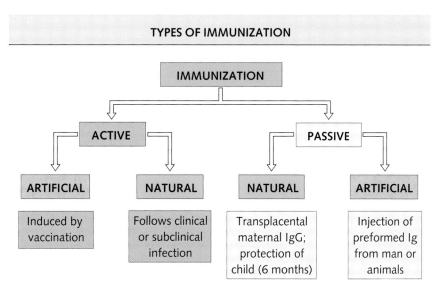

Fig. 8.1 Summary of the different types of immunization.

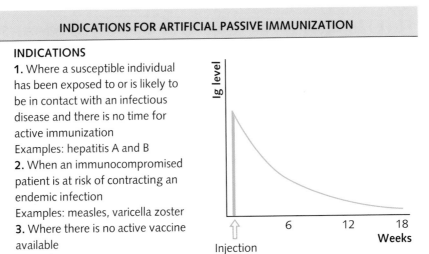

INDICATIONS FOR ARTIFICIAL PASSIVE IMMUNIZATION

INDICATIONS

1. Where a susceptible individual has been exposed to or is likely to be in contact with an infectious disease and there is no time for active immunization
Examples: hepatitis A and B

2. When an immunocompromised patient is at risk of contracting an endemic infection
Examples: measles, varicella zoster

3. Where there is no active vaccine available
Example: gas gangrene

Fig. 8.2 Indications for artificial passive immunization and the resultant pattern of immunoglobulin level with time.

listed in Fig. 8.2, and the short-term nature of passive immunization is illustrated in the graph (Fig. 8.2) which shows the fate of immunoglobulin over a 3-month period. Generally, specific passive immunotherapy is becoming increasingly less common but can still save lives in certain circumstances. Some of the common examples of passive immunotherapy in infectious diseases are described in Fig. 8.3. In recent years it has become clear that there are a number of cytokines, for example IFN-α, which can assist in the treatment of certain chronic viral infections, for example hepatitis B (Fig. 8.4).

SPECIFIC PASSIVE IMMUNOTHERAPY WITH ANTIBODY

Infection	Source of antibody	Indication
Diphtheria	Human	Prophylaxis; treatment
Tetanus	Human	Prophylaxis; treatment
Varicella zoster	Human	Treatment in immunodeficiencies
Gas gangrene	Horse	Postexposure
Hepatitis B	Human	Postexposure plus vaccine
Hepatitis A	Pooled human immunoglobulin	Prophylaxis (travel)
Measles	Pooled human immunoglobulin	Postexposure

Fig. 8.3 Specific forms of passive immunotherapy with antibody.

POTENTIALLY THERAPEUTIC CYTOKINES

Interferons	Infective agents	General side effects
IFN - α (leucocyte) **IFN - β (fibroblast)**	Hepatitis B (chronic) Hepatitis C Herpes zoster Papillomavirus	Fever, malaise, muscle pains, toxicity to kidney, liver, and bone marrow

Fig. 8.4 Potentially therapeutic cytokines in the management of chronic viral infection.

Active immunization by vaccine

Since active immunization relies on the host's immune system it takes months before the individual becomes adequately protected against the infective agent concerned. It is important that the resultant immunity is long-lasting and persists for many years, so that natural infection in the future will still stimulate an accelerated antibody response.

There are three main types of vaccine against a range of bacteria and viruses (Fig. 8.5). Live vaccines consist of attenuated micro-organisms which multiply in the body and mimic natural infection as far as antibody production is concerned but without producing symptoms; reactions are mild and similar to the natural disease. A single dose can give long-lasting immunity which can be reinforced with later booster doses.

The reactions to killed vaccines do not resemble those of the natural disease and usually three doses are required before long-lasting immunity can be achieved. Additional doses are necessary because there is no multiplication of the infective agent in the body.

Vaccines containing toxoid are only possible with infections caused by a single exotoxin, for example tetanus. Toxins are rendered harmless by chemical means (usually formaldehyde treatment) but retain their antigenicity.

Live and killed vaccines each have their advantages and disadvantages (Fig. 8.6). Live vaccines are most effective in preventing infections which normally induce long-term immunity

VACCINES IN CURRENT USE		
	Bacterial vaccines	**Viral vaccines**
Live	BCG (tuberculosis)[a]	Poliomyelitis (Sabin) Measles, mumps, rubella (combined MMR vaccine) Rubella Varicella[b] (chickenpox)
Killed	Pertussis *Haemophilus influenzae* b *Streptococcus pneumoniae*	Influenza Poliomyelitis (Salk) Hepatitis A Hepatitis B
Toxoids	Diphtheria Tetanus	

Fig. 8.5 Summary of the types of vaccine currently in use. [a]BCG not used routinely in USA; [b]Live attenuated varicella vaccine has recently been licensed in some countries, including the USA, but currently no vaccine is licensed for use in the UK.

LIVE AND KILLED VACCINES		
	Live	**Killed**
Preparation	Attenuation (not always feasible)	Inactivation
Administration	May be natural route (e.g. oral) or injection May be single dose	Injection Usually multiple doses
Adjuvant	Not required	Usually required
Safety	May revert to virulence	Pain from injection
Cost	Low	High
Duration of immunity	Usually years	May be long or short
Immune response	IgG, IgA, cell-mediated	Mainly IgG; little or no cell-mediated

Fig. 8.6 Advantages and disadvantages of live and killed vaccines.

following recovery, such as the common childhood viruses, since they produce many of the features of the infection itself, in particular virus replication and a cell-mediated immune response. Many natural infections do not produce solid immunity, especially if the agent has marked antigenicity or evokes a response that protects the microbe. In these infections, the rationale for a living attenuated vaccine is relatively weak; whereas the use of non-viable subcellular components that induce strong immunity which attack the microbe at specific weak spots – possibly consisting of a mixture of the different antigenic types present in the population – is more likely to be effective. The patterns of antibody response to active immunization with a live attenuated compared to a killed vaccine are illustrated in Fig. 8.7, and show clearly why the latter requires a number of doses to achieve a satisfactory response.

Safety is one of the main problems with vaccines, and therefore each batch is subjected to stringent legal controls to ensure safety and potency. In fact, considering the enormous number of vaccine administrations (about 20 million per year in the USA alone) the safety record is extremely good. The main problems with vaccine safety are listed in Fig. 8.8.

PROBLEMS WITH VACCINE SAFETY	
Live attenuated vaccines	Insufficient attenuation
	Reversion to wild type
	Administration to immunodeficient patient
	Persistent infection
	Contamination by other viruses
	Fetal damage
Non-living vaccines	Contamination by live organisms
	Contamination by toxins
	Allergic reactions
	Autoimmunity
Genetically engineered vaccines	?Inclusion of oncogenes

Fig. 8.8 Problems associated with the safety of vaccines.

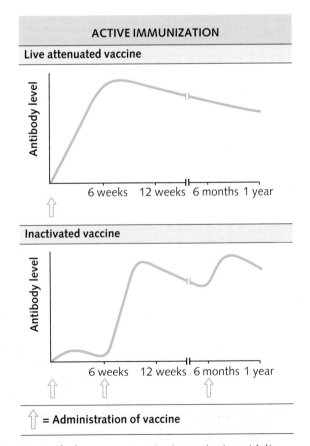

Fig. 8.7 Antibody response to active immunization with live attenuated and inactivated vaccines.

In recent years a number of new vaccines have been produced which consist of purified bacterial or viral proteins obtained by genetic engineering. For example, hepatitis B vaccines have been produced by gene cloning and peptide synthesis by a yeast. Another ingenious development has been the insertion of genes coding for antigens of one or more micro-organisms into a carrier virus or bacterium. Following injection of this vaccine into the patient, the carrier organism would proliferate sufficiently to release an immunizing amount of the foreign protein but without inducing the disease itself. Carrier viruses or bacteria need to be attenuated and able to grow inside the host – BCG (bacillus Calmette–Guérin) and *Salmonella typhi* have been suggested. This technology has resulted in the hypothesis that in future a 'one-shot' vaccine could be produced (Fig. 8.9).

Current vaccine practice

The provision of a programme of active immunization to a community should be linked to considerations of need, efficacy, safety, and ease of administration. Circumstances vary widely in different countries and priorities vary. The range of vaccines currently available in the UK and the USA and the recommended administration schedules are summarized in Figs 8.10 and 8.11.

It is important to try to achieve the status of herd immunity with immunization against an infection that is transmitted from individual to individual. If 90% of a community are immune to an infectious agent then the chances of the few non-immune individuals becoming infected is relatively small. However, if only 50% of the community are immune to the agent the chance of a

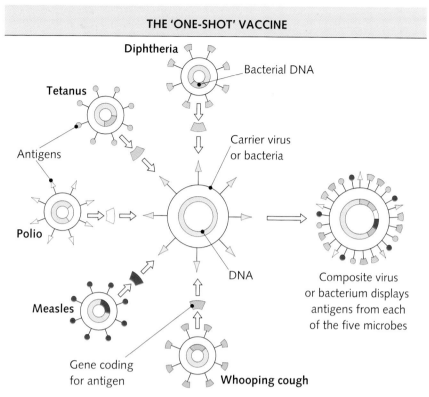

THE 'ONE-SHOT' VACCINE

Fig. 8.9 In the future, vaccines may consist of a single viral or bacterial vector containing genes for all required vaccines – the 'one-shot' vaccine.

susceptible individual becoming infected is much higher and the possibility of an epidemic is raised. Clearly, vaccines should be targeted at the age group at greatest risk of infection. Most vaccines are given to children because most of the diseases that can be prevented by vaccines are encountered in the early years of life. Ideally, vaccination should start soon after birth. However, it is usually delayed for about two months, since the immune system of the neonate is not fully developed and circulating maternal antibody from the placenta may inactivate a response from live virus vaccine and reduce it to that of some killed vaccines. It is common practice to give more than one vaccine at a time wherever possible, since this not only reduces the number of injections required but combined vaccines may enhance antibody production.

There are a number of potential contraindications to a vaccine. Live vaccine should never be given to immunocompromised patients because of the risk of a severe generalized infection. If a live vaccine is given to a pregnant woman there is a danger of transplacental spread to the fetus with the possible risk of abortion. Other contraindications include a previous history of severe local or generalized reaction to the vaccine or a history of hypersensitivity to some of its components.

Whilst it is government policy that all individuals in the UK should receive the triple (DTP; diphtheria, tetanus, pertussis)

vaccine, a polio vaccine, the 'MMR' (measles, mumps, rubella) vaccine, and BCG (Figs 8.10 and 8.11), the place of some of the other vaccines listed, for example those against pneumococcal disease and influenza, is less clear. The influenza virus has shifts and drifts in its antigenic pattern (Chapter 16) so that vaccines must be frequently updated. There is the additional problem of deciding which patients merit this special protection. In the USA, trivalent 'flu' shots are available to all, but are clearly recommended for the elderly and those with compromised respiratory defences.

There remains a long list of important infectious diseases for which vaccines, although desirable, are not yet available (Fig. 8.12). In some cases it is likely that successful vaccines will emerge in time, but in others there appear to be fundamental problems which will make the delivery of a vaccine very difficult. For example, problems associated with producing live herpes group vaccines include the danger of virus latency in the nervous system with reactivation and clinical disease, and also the difficulty of obtaining large amounts of virus from some members of the group such as Epstein–Barr virus. In the case of syphilis the lack of convincing immunity following natural infection is discouraging. Probably the most determined effort is being directed against HIV, where the production of a vaccine to limit the spread and progression of AIDS is a race against time. The

CURRENT VACCINE PRACTICE IN THE UNITED KINGDOM AND USA

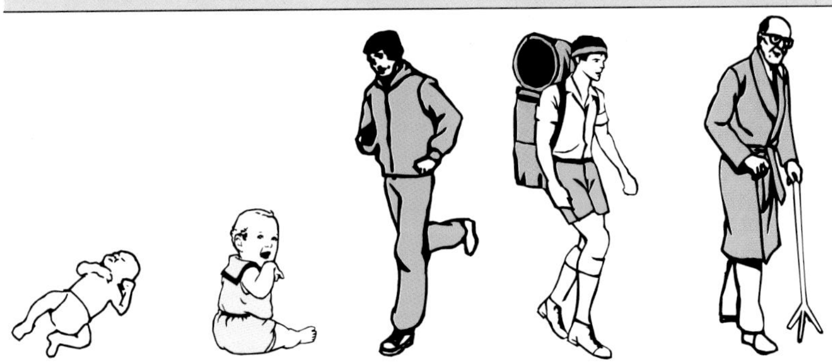

UK

2–6 months	12–18 months	Teenager	Traveller	Old age
Polio Diphtheria Pertussis Tetanus	Measles Mumps Rubella Hib*	Diphtheria Tetanus BCG	Hepatitis A and B Others e.g. cholera	Influenza *Streptococcus pneumoniae*

USA

Birth – 2 months	2–6 months	12–15 months	Teenager	Traveller	Old age
Hepatitis B	Polio Diphtheria Pertussis Tetanus Hib*	Measles Mumps Rubella	Diphtheria Tetanus Hepatitis B**	Hepatitis A and B Others e.g. cholera	Influenza *Streptococcus pneumoniae*

Fig. 8.10 Current vaccine practice in the UK and the USA. Administration of most vaccines is relatively standard world-wide, but there are important local differences due to variations in risk of infection or in government health policy. *Haemophilus influenzae* Type b; **recommended for 12-year-olds who were not vaccinated as infants.

ADMINISTRATION SCHEDULE		
Vaccine	**UK and USA**	**(a) Adverse reactions** **(b) Protection**
Triple (DTP) vaccine: **diphtheria, tetanus, pertussis**	**Primary:** given to all at 2–6 months (3 doses at 4-week intervals) **Booster:** 15 months (USA) and 4 years (UK and USA); DT every 10 years (USA)	**Diphtheria and tetanus:** (a) Rare and minor (b) Excellent **Pertussis:** (a) Local and trivial. Doubt about attributed brain damage (b) About 80% success
Polio vaccine: **Sabin (live, oral)** **Salk (killed)**	**Primary:** given to all concomitantly with DTP vaccine **Booster:** 4 and 16 years (UK), 15 months, 4 years, and high-risk adults (USA) Immunocompromised	(a) Unusual. Rare case of paralysis in adults with Sabin vaccine (b) Excellent for both vaccines. In UK, Sabin vaccine has been preferred to Salk, but this is under debate
'MMR' vaccine: **measles, mumps, rubella**	Introduced into UK in October 1984. Given to all at 12–18 months. In UK, second dose given before school entry and rubella given to seronegative girls at 10–14 years. In USA, second dose of MMR at 4–6 or 11–12 years	(a) Few. Transient rash, fever, mild parotitis (1%) (b) Good response and long-lasting
BCG: **tuberculosis**	UK: given to all at 10–14 years. USA: high-risk groups only	(a) Limited. Ulcer discharging pus at infection site possible and axillary lymphadenopathy (b) Good
Hepatitis B	High-risk groups (e.g. travellers, homosexuals, health workers). In USA, given to infants and unvaccinated 11–12 year olds	(a) Local pain and redness occasionally (b) Good
Hepatitis A	Travellers to endemic areas (for example Africa, India, Far East)	(a) Mild local reaction (b) Good
Streptococcus pneumoniae **pneumonia**	Aged, high-risk groups	(a) Local reaction in 50% (b) Apparently good
Haemophilus influenzae **serotype b (Hib)**	Recommended for all infants from 2 months of age in UK. Given at 2–6 months in USA with a booster at 12–15 months	(a) Safe (b) Apparently good
Influenza A and B	Aged, high-risk individuals	(a) Contraindicated in people allergic to egg protein (b) Shortlived (a few months). Only 60% respond
Varicella (chickenpox)	(USA only) 12–24 months. 2 doses at 11–12 years if not previously vaccinated and have no history of disease	(a) Contraindicated in pregnancy (b) Apparently good

Fig. 8.11 Recommended vaccine administration schedules in the UK and the USA.

MAJOR INFECTIOUS DISEASES FOR WHICH THERE IS NO SATISFACTORY VACCINE

Organism	Disease
HIV	AIDS
Herpes simplex virus	Oral/genital infection
Cytomegalovirus	Fetal damage
Epstein–Barr virus	Glandular fever
Rhinoviruses	Common cold
Neisseria gonorrhoeae	Gonorrhoea
Treponema pallidum	Syphilis
Chlamydia trachomatis	Urethritis

Fig. 8.12 Important infectious diseases for which satisfactory vaccines are not currently available.

ideal properties of a vaccine are listed in Fig. 8.13, but few if any vaccines meet these high requirements. The details of vaccine choice, route, dose, and risk have to be considered disease by disease and there is room for considerable improvement in producing safe, effective and affordable vaccines.

Further reading

Janeway, CA Jr, Travers, P, Hunt, S, and Walport, M (1997). Manipulating the immune response to fight infection. In *Immunobiology* (3rd edn), Chapter 13. Current Biology Ltd, Churchill Livingstone, Gorland Publishing Inc., London.

Mims, C, Playfair, J, Roitt, I, Wakelin, D, and Williams, R (1998). Vaccination. In *Medical microbiology* (2nd edn), Chapter 31. Mosby, London.

Murray, PR, Rosenthal, KS, Kobayashi, GS, and Pfaller, MA. (1998). Antimicrobial vaccines. In *Medical microbiology* (3rd edn), Chapter 15. Mosby Year Book, St Louis.

Powell, MF and Newman, HJ (ed.). (1995). *Vaccine design*. Plenum, New York.

Roitt, IM (1997). *Roitt's essential immunology* (9th edn). Blackwell, Oxford.

Roitt, I, Brostoff, J, and Male, D (1997). Vaccination. In *Immunology* (5th edn), Chapter 19. Mosby, London.

Salisbury, DM and Begg, NT (1996) *Immunisation against infectious disease*. HMSO, London.

PROPERTIES OF AN IDEAL VACCINE

- Promotes effective immunity
- Provides lifelong protection
- Safe (no side–effects)
- Stable
- Inexpensive
- Seen by the public to be good and effective

Fig. 8.13 The properties of a hypothetical, ideal vaccine.

Key facts

- Successful immunization programmes produce herd (population) immunity to a range of natural microbial infections.
- Not all microbial infections are amenable to control by vaccines.
- Artificial passive immunization is effective immediately after inoculation of serum and short lived (3 months).
- There are 3 main types of vaccine used in artificial active immunization: live, killed, and toxoid.
- Successful artificial active immunization results in long-term protection (from 1 year to a lifetime) against specific natural infection.
- Vaccines are generally safe, but constant vigilance is required, and there are certain recognized groups of individuals in which their use is contraindicated.
- Three or more different vaccines can be given at the same time.
- Current vaccine practice in the UK provides protection against poliomyelitis, diphtheria, whooping cough, tetanus, measles, mumps, rubella, and tuberculosis.
- An ideal vaccine should provide effective, lifelong-immunity, with no side-effects, and be stable and inexpensive.
- Genetic and molecular techniques are being employed to produce a range of new vaccines, which may result in a 'one-shot' vaccine to cover many infectious diseases.

9

Antimicrobial agents

Antimicrobial agents

The management of infection is an important element of clinical dentistry, and antimicrobial drugs frequently play a role in the treatment of both purulent and mucosal infections in the head and neck region. Antimicrobial agents may also be used prophylactically, for example in the prevention of infective endocarditis among susceptible patients receiving dental treatment. An understanding of the principles of antimicrobial chemotherapy is, therefore, essential for dental surgeons.

The ideal antimicrobial agent

A fundamental concept in antimicrobial chemotherapy, first proposed by Paul Ehrlich, is known as 'selective toxicity'. This implies that the antimicrobial drug can damage the micro-organism without injuring the host, an outcome that can be achieved by the use of agents which act at target sites present in the organism but absent from host cells. The various mechanisms of selective toxicity will be described during the course of this chapter for each of the antimicrobial drugs discussed.

Other properties of an ideal antimicrobial agent are summarized in Fig. 9.1. Unfortunately, none of the antimicrobial drugs currently available satisfy all these criteria. Clinicians must, therefore, be familiar with the pharmacokinetics and possible side-effects of the antimicrobial agents they prescribe.

Strictly speaking, antibiotics are natural products of bacteria and fungi which kill, or inhibit the growth of, other micro-organisms. However, most antimicrobial drugs in current use have been chemically modified to improve their properties, whilst

THE IDEAL ANTIMICROBIAL AGENT
• Selective toxicity against microbial target
• Minimal toxicity to the host
• Cidal activity (kills micro-organisms)
• Long plasma half-life
• Good tissue distribution
• Low binding to plasma proteins
• Oral and parenteral preparations
• No adverse interactions with other drugs

Fig. 9.1 Summary of the properties of a hypothetical, ideal antimicrobial agent.

others are totally synthetic. Some authorities, therefore, prefer the more general term antimicrobial agent to that of antibiotic.

Antibacterial agents

Classification

Antibacterial agents may be classified in several ways, as summarized in Fig. 9.2. Classification on the basis of target site is a convenient system, which helps with understanding the molecular basis of antibacterial action, including selective toxicity. It will, therefore, be used in the following sections of this chapter.

CLASSIFICATION OF ANTIBACTERIAL AGENTS	
Bactericidal or bacteriostatic	Bactericidal agents KILL bacteria
	Bacteriostatic agents INHIBIT GROWTH of bacteria
Chemical structure	Diverse and of limited practical use
Target site	Cell-wall synthesis
	Protein synthesis
	Nucleic acid synthesis
	Cell-membrane function

Fig. 9.2 Summary of the criteria for classifying antibacterial agents.

Classes of antibacterial agents

Inhibitors of cell-wall synthesis

Peptidoglycan is a vital component of bacterial cell walls (Chapter 2) but is not found in eukaryotic host cells. This makes it an ideal target for selective toxicity. The beta-lactams and the glycopeptides are the two important groups.

BETA-LACTAMS

This is a large family of compounds that includes the penicillins and cephalosporins. Structurally these agents all contain the beta-lactam ring (Fig. 9.3). As shown in Fig. 9.4, they prevent cell-wall synthesis by binding to enzymes known as 'penicillin binding proteins'. These are responsible for the final stages of cross-linking of the bacterial cell-wall structure during growth and division. As a result, precursor cell-wall units accumulate, which in turn activate the cell's autolytic system.

There are many beta-lactam antibiotics available for clinical use. Dental surgeons are most likely to prescribe the penicillins (Fig. 9.5) because of their activity against organisms implicated in purulent infections of the head and neck. Some can be administered orally but others must be given intramuscularly or intravenously. Though many are active mainly against Gram-positive bacteria, in recent years new beta-lactams have been developed with activity against Gram-negative rods such as *Pseudomonas aeruginosa*.

INHIBITORS OF CELL-WALL SYNTHESIS

Beta-lactams

Examples: penicillins, cephalosporins
Bind to 'penicillin binding proteins'
⇩
Inhibition of cross-linking of cell wall
⇩
Accumulation of precursor cell-wall units
⇩
Cell lysis

Glycopeptides

Examples: vancomycin, teicoplanin
Bind to terminal D-ala-D-ala residues
⇩
Prevent incorporation of subunit into growing peptidoglycan

Fig. 9.4 The mechanism of antimicrobial activity of the beta-lactam and glycopeptide groups of antibiotics, both of which inhibit bacterial cell-wall synthesis.

Some patients are allergic to beta-lactam antibiotics and will suffer an immediate hypersensitivity reaction if such drugs are administered. This information must be elicited when taking a medical history.

It is also important not to prescribe ampicillin or amoxycillin for an oral or pharyngeal infection which may prove to be infec-

---

THE BETA-LACTAM RING

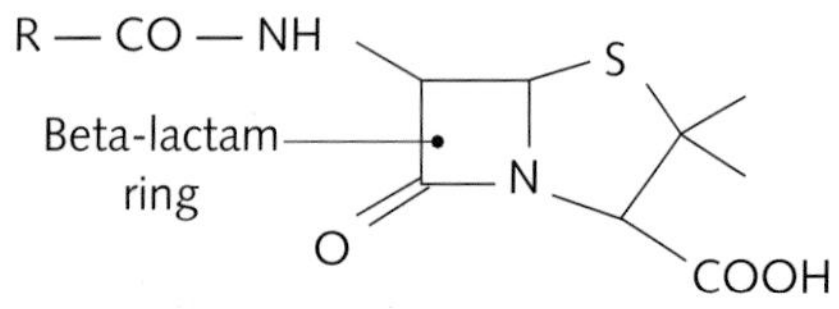

Examples of beta-lactam antibiotics

Benzylpenicillin

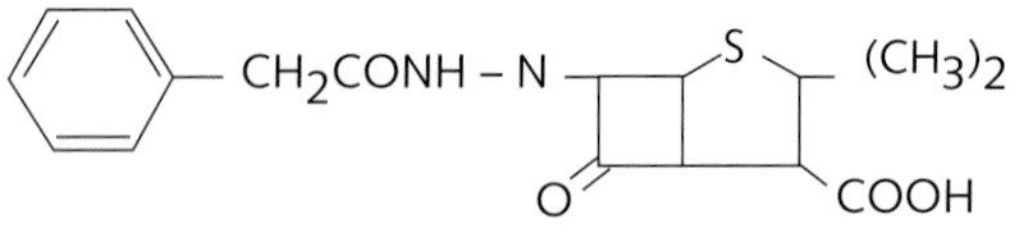

Cephalexin

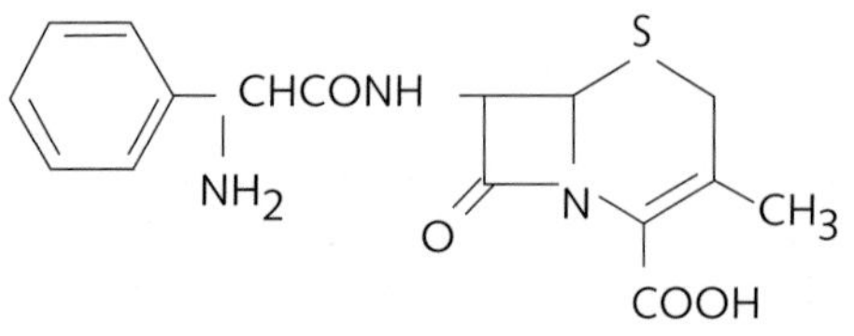

Fig. 9.3 The beta-lactam ring is common to the structure of all penicillins and cephalosporins.

TYPES OF PENICILLIN

Benzylpenicillin and its long-acting parenteral forms
Example: benzylpenicillin

Orally absorbed penicillins resembling benzylpenicillin
Example: phenoxymethyl penicillin

Penicillins resistant to staphylococcal *β*-lactamase
Example: flucloxacillin

Extended spectrum penicillins
Examples: ampicillin; amoxycillin

Penicillins active against *Pseudomonas aeruginosa*
Example: azlocillin

Fig. 9.5 Summary of the different types of penicillin. Dentists are likely to prescribe all these drugs, except for the antipseudomonal agents.

tious mononucleosis. Under such circumstances, over 95% of patients develop a persistent, itchy, macular rash due to a specific toxic reaction to the drug, which is a non-allergic reaction.

GLYCOPEPTIDES

These agents interfere with cell-wall synthesis by binding to terminal D-ala – D-ala residues at the end of pentapeptide chains that are part of the growing bacterial cell-wall structure (see Fig. 9.4). This prevents the subsequent incorporation of new subunits into the growing cell wall.

Vancomycin and teicoplanin are only active against Gram-positive organisms, and both must be given by injection. Whilst neither drug is clinically indicated for the management of oral infections, vancomycin is one of the antimicrobial agents used under certain circumstances for prophylaxis against infective endocarditis in special-risk patients (Chapter 17).

Inhibitors of protein synthesis

Whilst the mechanisms of protein synthesis are similar in prokaryotic and eukaryotic cells, there are certain differences which can be exploited to permit selective toxicity. The target sites for the more common groups are summarized in Fig. 9.6.

AMINOGLYCOSIDES

This is a large family of antimicrobial agents. The mode of action is still not completely understood, but an important element is the binding of drug to the 30S ribosomal subunit of the 70S bacterial ribosome (Fig. 9.6).

Aminoglycosides are not absorbed after oral administration and must be given intravenously or intramuscularly. Their main clinical indication is for the treatment of serious Gram-negative infections, including those caused by *Pseudomonas aeruginosa*. They may also be used in combination with a penicillin for the treatment of infective endocarditis (Chapter 17). Streptomycin is still sometimes prescribed as part of the treatment for mycobacterial infections.

The aminoglycosides are potentially nephrotoxic and ototoxic, which can lead to renal failure and deafness, respectively. Patients undergoing treatment, therefore, require regular monitoring of blood levels of the drug. In view of their antimicrobial spectrum, route of administration and toxicity, aminoglycosides are not indicated for the treatment of oral or dental infections.

TETRACYCLINES

There are several members of this group of antibacterial drugs, but the differences between them lie in their pharmacological properties rather than their antibacterial spectra. The mode of action is the same for all members of the group. The drug is actively transported into bacterial cells where it binds to 30S ribosomal subunits, preventing attachment of aminoacyl–tRNA to the acceptor sites and halting chain elongation (Fig. 9.6).

Tetracyclines are usually administered orally. Compared with earlier tetracyclines, absorption is more complete for the newer agents doxycycline and minocycline, resulting in higher serum concentrations and less gastrointestinal upset. Tetracyclines are active against a broad range of bacterial species, but their clinical

INHIBITORS OF PROTEIN SYNTHESIS
Aminoglycosides
Examples: streptomycin, gentamicin Interfere with binding of formylmethionyl-tRNA and subsequent formation of initiation complex on 70S ribosome
Tetracyclines
Examples: oxytetracycline, doxycycline Bind to 30S ribosomal subunits Prevents aminoacyl-tRNA from entering the acceptor sites on the ribosome
Macrolides
Examples: erythromycin, azithromycin Bind to 23S rRNA in 50S subunit of ribosome Blocks translocation step in protein synthesis
Lincosamides
Example: clindamycin Bind to 50S ribosomal subunit Inhibit peptide bond formation
Chloramphenicol
Blocks action of peptidyl transferase Prevents peptide bond synthesis
Fusidic acid
Forms complex with elongation factor EF-G and with GTP Blocks chain elongation

Fig. 9.6 The mechanisms of action of the antibiotics which function by inhibiting protein synthesis.

usefulness has been restricted because of the widespread development of resistance. Their ability to penetrate host cells has proved valuable in the treatment of infections with intracellular bacteria such as chlamydiae. Tetracycline mouthwashes are sometimes prescribed in dentistry for the treatment of herpetiform and other types of oral ulceration.

Suppression of the normal gut flora frequently results in gastrointestinal upset and overgrowth of resistant microorganisms such as *Candida* spp. The latter may result in oral candidosis. It should also be noted that tetracyclines are deposited in developing bones and teeth, which can result in unsightly staining of the teeth. This normally precludes their use in children under the age of 12 years and in women during late pregnancy.

MACROLIDES

Although the macrolides constitute a family of antimicrobial agents, erythromycin is the best known and most widely used, with useful activity against a number of the more recently described pathogens including *Campylobacter* and *Legionella* species. Some of the newer macrolides, for example azithromycin, also look very promising. Erythromycin acts through binding to the 50S bacterial ribosome and blocks the first translocation step in protein synthesis (Fig. 9.6). Erythromycin is usually given orally. Absorption can be irregular, but the drug is generally well distributed in the body and penetrates mammalian cells. Erythromycin is active against Gram-positive cocci and is a useful alternative to penicillin for the treatment of dental infections and other forms of streptococcal disease in patients who are penicillin-allergic. Its spectrum also includes *Neisseria* and *Haemophilus* species, mycoplasmas, chlamydiae, and rickettsiae.

Although erythromycin is a relatively non-toxic drug, nausea, vomiting, and epigastric pain are fairly common after oral administration, though they usually follow higher dosages. Rashes may also occur. Hepatic disturbance is associated with certain formulations, notably the esters of erythromycin.

LINCOSAMIDES

The important drug in this group is clindamycin. The mechanism of action is not fully understood but, like the macrolides, the lincosamides bind to the 50S ribosomal subunit. Ultimately they inhibit protein synthesis by preventing peptide bond formation (Fig. 9.6).

Clindamycin is usually administered orally and penetrates well into bone. It is active against only Gram-positive aerobes, but has potent activity against both Gram-positive and Gram-negative anaerobes. It is especially valuable in the management of staphylococcal infections of bones and joints. More recently, in the UK, it has been recommended as one of the drugs for the prophylaxis of infective endocarditis in patients who are allergic to penicillin (Chapter 17).

Rashes and diarrhoea are recognized side-effects. The association between clindamycin and pseudomembranous colitis has been well publicized, although it is now clear that this complication may follow the administration of many antibiotics.

CHLORAMPHENICOL

This was the first broad-spectrum antibiotic to be discovered. It acts by blocking peptidyl transferase and thus prevents peptide bond synthesis. The selective toxicity arises because chloramphenicol has a much higher affinity for the transferase in the 50S subunit of the bacterial ribosome than it has for the transferase in the 60S subunit of the mammalian ribosome.

Chloramphenicol is well absorbed after oral administration, but it can also be given intravenously or topically. It is active against a wide range of both Gram-positive and Gram-negative bacteria, aerobes and anaerobes, and intracellular organisms such as chlamydiae.

Unfortunately, these very favourable antimicrobial and pharmacokinetic properties have been marred by toxic, and occasionally fatal, effects on the bone marrow. Glossitis, associated with overgrowth of *Candida* species, is fairly common if treatment is continued for more than one week.

Chloramphenicol should never be prescribed for minor infections. It remains a drug of choice for typhoid fever and other severe infections due, for example, to *Salmonella* and *Rickettsia* spp. It may also be indicated in the management of meningitis, since it can penetrate cerebrospinal fluid (CSF) and for the treatment of severe respiratory infections caused by *Haemophilus influenzae*. Topical preparations are used commonly for eye infections. There is no place for chloramphenicol in the treatment of oral infections.

FUSIDIC ACID

This steroid-like compound is different from the other inhibitors of protein synthesis, because it does not bind directly to the ribosome. Instead, it forms a stable complex with elongation factor-G (EF-G), guanosine diphosphate (which provides energy for the translocation process), and the ribosome (Fig. 9.6).

Fusidic acid can be given orally or intravenously and is well absorbed, with good penetration into soft tissues and bone but not into the CSF. Topical preparations are also available, including an ointment for the treatment of angular cheilitis when *Staphylococcus aureus* has been isolated, but their use results in rapid emergence of resistance.

Fusidic acid is active against most Gram-positive bacteria. Its main use is in the treatment of staphylococcal infections resistant to beta-lactams, or in penicillin-allergic patients. In view of the rapid emergence of resistance to this drug, it should always be administered in combination with another antistaphylococcal agent.

Inhibitors of nucleic acid synthesis

Many compounds are known which interact with DNA. However, since the structure of DNA is shared by both eukaryotic and prokaryotic cells, compounds that bind directly to DNA are usually highly toxic to mammalian cells. However, there are a few compounds that interfere with DNA-associated enzymatic processes and which exhibit sufficient selective toxicity for use as antibacterial agents.

SULPHONAMIDES

The sulphonamides were the earliest of the modern antimicrobial agents used clinically and are all structural analogues of para-amino benzoic acid (PABA). The mode of action is shown in Fig. 9.7. Selective toxicity depends on the fact that most bacteria synthesize tetrahydrofolic acid and cannot utilize exogenous sources of the vitamin. Mammalian cells, by contrast, rely on an outside source of folic acid.

INHIBITORS OF NUCLEIC ACID SYNTHESIS

Inhibitors of synthesis of precursors:

Sulphonamides

Example: sulphamethoxazole

Structural analogues of para-amino benzoic acid (PABA)

Compete with PABA for active site of dihydropteroate synthetase

Inhibits synthesis of tetrahydrofolic acid

Inhibits synthesis of purines and pyrimidines

Trimethoprim

Example: may be given in combination with sulphamethoxazole (co-trimoxazole)

Pyrimidine-like structure

Inhibits dihydrofolate reductase

Inhibits synthesis of tetrahydrofolic acid

Inhibitors of DNA replication:

Quinolones

Examples: nalidixic acid, ciprofloxacin

Inhibit DNA gyrase

Prevents supercoiling of bacterial chromosome

Prevents 'packing' of DNA into bacterial cell

Inhibitors of RNA polymerase

Rifamycins

Example: rifampicin

Bind to RNA polymerase

Blocks synthesis of messenger RNA

Fig. 9.7 The mechanisms of action of the antibiotics which function by inhibiting nucleic acid synthesis.

Most sulphonamides are well absorbed orally. They exhibit a broad spectrum of activity, but resistance is widespread. There are few absolute indications for their use and their principal role, often in conjunction with trimethoprim (see below) has been in the treatment of urinary tract infections. Toxicity and side-effects, though rare, include skin rashes, bone marrow suppression, and hepatotoxicity. Stevens–Johnson syndrome is a rare but sometimes fatal complication.

TRIMETHOPRIM AND CO-TRIMOXAZOLE

Trimethoprim is a pyrimidine-like structure which is an analogue of part of the folic acid molecule. Like the sulphonamides it also prevents the synthesis of tetrahydrofolic acid, but by inhibiting dihydrofolate reductase, i.e. later in the pathway. This enzyme is also found in mammalian cells, but there is selective toxicity because trimethoprim has a far greater affinity for the bacterial enzyme.

Trimethoprim is often given in combination with sulphamethoxazole, as co-trimoxazole, since the two agents act synergistically against some bacteria. However, the clinical benefit of the combination is disputed and there have been a number of reports of adverse reactions. The indications for the use of co-trimoxazole have been restricted accordingly, but still include the treatment of *Pneumocystis carinii* pneumonia, toxoplasmosis and, in certain clinical situations, urinary tract, respiratory, and ear infections. Trimethoprim alone is used mainly in the management of urinary tract infections.

QUINOLONES

This large family of synthetic agents acts by inhibiting an enzyme called DNA gyrase, thus preventing supercoiling of the bacterial chromosome. The bacterial chromosome, which is more than 1 millimetre long, cannot then be packed into the cell.

The modern fluoroquinolones, such as ciprofloxacin, are generally well absorbed by mouth and well distributed throughout the body compartments. They are used not only to treat urinary tract infections, but also systemic Gram-negative infections including those caused by *Pseudomonas aeruginosa*. The commonest side-effects are gastrointestinal, but neurotoxicity and photosensitivity reactions occur in 1–2% of patients.

RIFAMYCINS

The important drug in this group is rifampicin, which acts by binding to RNA polymerase and preventing the synthesis of messenger RNA. The drug has little affinity for the equivalent human enzymes. Rifampicin is well absorbed orally, crosses the blood–brain barrier and reaches high concentrations in saliva.

The main use of rifampicin is in the treatment of mycobacterial infections, but it is also the drug of choice for the prophylaxis of close contacts of meningococcal and haemophilus meningitis. Rifampicin is of generally low toxicity but jaundice and rashes may occur.

METRONIDAZOLE

This antimicrobial drug is widely used by dentists because of its activity against anaerobic bacteria. After entry into the host cell, the drug is activated by a reduction process. Only obligate anaerobic bacteria can produce the low redox potential needed for activation, therefore this drug has no activity against facultative anaerobes or strict aerobes. The active intermediates of the drug probably interact with and break the bacterial DNA.

Metronidazole is well absorbed orally and well distributed in tissues. It is used for the treatment of certain parasitic infections and is very valuable for the management of anaerobic bacterial infections. Development of resistance is extremely rare. Serious side-effects are rare, but complaints of nausea, a metallic taste, and furred tongue are fairly common. Alcohol should be avoided by those taking metronidazole, to prevent disulfiram-like flushing and hypotension.

Antifungal agents

Only a small number of antifungal drugs are currently available, because of difficulties in achieving selective toxicity. However, these drugs are prescribed widely by dentists.

Most act on synthesis or function of the fungal cell membrane.

POLYENES

This group includes nystatin and amphotericin B. Polyenes bind avidly to sterols in eukaryotic cell membranes resulting in impairment of barrier function (Fig. 9.8).

Amphotericin B has a wide spectrum of antifungal activity. It is poorly absorbed by mouth and is administered by the intravenous route for the treatment of systemic fungal infections. Intravenous amphotericin B is still the drug of choice in most systemic mycoses, but it is very toxic. A liposomal formulation of amphotericin B (AmBisome) is better tolerated but expensive. Since the drug is not absorbed orally, topical preparations, including mouthwashes and lozenges, are widely used for the treatment of oral candidosis without toxic effects.

Nystatin is too toxic for parenteral use but, like amphotericin B, is commonly prescribed for topical use.

AZOLES

This large group of synthetic agents includes fluconazole, itraconazole, and miconazole. These drugs act by blocking the 14 (alpha)-demethylation step in the biosynthesis of ergosterol, thus interfering with fungal membrane functions.

Both fluconazole and itraconazole are triazole antifungals, effective in the treatment of oral or vaginal candidosis. Although the physicochemical properties of these two drugs are very different, both can be safely administered systemically. Fluconazole has been used widely for both the treatment and prophylaxis of oropharyngeal candidosis, particularly among immunocompromised patients, though more recently there have been concerns about the development of resistance.

Itraconazole also has potent anticandidal activity. Overall, it has a broader spectrum of activity than fluconazole and is of potential value in the treatment of other fungal infections such as aspergillosis. A promising liquid preparation has recently been developed, which has both topical and systemic activity.

IMPORTANT ANTIFUNGAL AGENTS
Disruption of cell-membrane function
Polyenes
Example: nystatin, amphotericin B

Bind to sterols in cell membrane

⇩

Impairment of barrier function

⇩

Leakage of cellular components and metabolic disruption

⇩

Cell death

Disruption of cell-membrane synthesis
Azoles
Examples: miconazole, fluconazole, itraconazole

Bind to cytochrome P450

⇩

Inhibition of lanosterol C14-demethylase

⇩

Inhibition of ergosterol synthesis

Disruption of nucleic acid synthesis
Pyrimidines
Example: 5-fluorocyyosine
Benzofurans
Example: griseofulvin

Fig. 9.8 The mechanisms of action of currently available antifungal drugs. The polyenes and azoles are prescribed widely by dentists in the management of oral candidosis.

Antiviral agents

Compared with the vast array of available antibacterial drugs, there are very few specific antivirals. This is largely due to the difficulty in devising mechanisms of selective toxicity for viruses, because of their replication within host cells. The long incubation periods of many viral infections and the ability of some viruses to establish latent infections add to the problems of specific antiviral therapy.

Some of the currently available antiviral drugs are listed in Fig. 9.9. Most are nucleoside analogues. Of these drugs, aciclovir is the only one likely to be prescribed by dental surgeons.

IMPORTANT ANTIVIRAL AGENTS

Nucleoside analogues

Interfere with DNA/RNA synthesis
Examples:

Aciclovir	–	herpes simplex virus
Ganciclovir	–	cytomegalovirus
Zidovudine	–	human immunodeficiency virus
Ribavirin	–	respiratory syncytial virus

Adamantanes

Interfere with virus uncoating within cell
Example:

Amantadine	–	influenza type A virus

Interferons

Example:

Interferon α	–	hepatitis B and C viruses

Fig. 9.9 Summary of the antiviral drugs currently in clinical usage. Aciclovir is prescribed by dentists in the management of oral herpes simplex virus infections.

ANTIVIRAL MECHANISM OF ACICLOVIR

ACICLOVIR

⇩

Addition of one phosphate group
by herpesvirus thymidine kinase

⇩

ACICLOVIR MONOPHOSPHATE

⇩

Addition of two further phosphate
groups by host cell kinases

⇩

ACICLOVIR TRIPHOSPHATE

⇩

Inhibition of herpesvirus DNA polymerase
Incorporation into viral DNA

⇩

DNA CHAIN TERMINATION

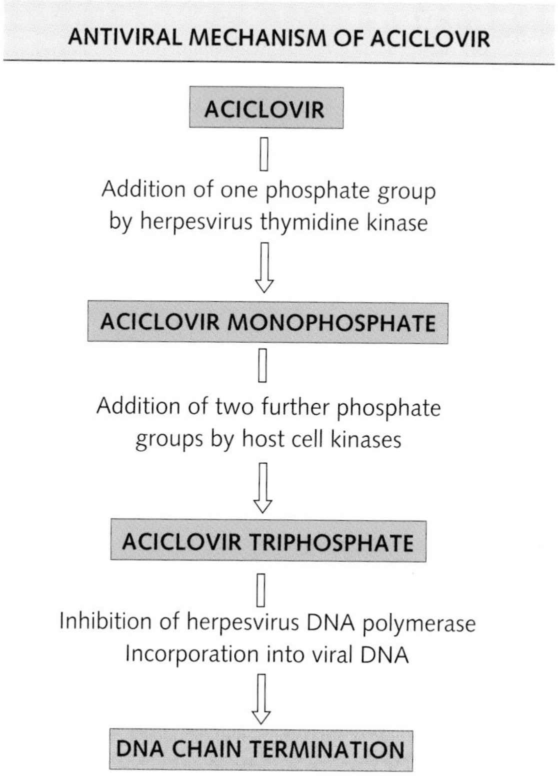

Fig. 9.10 Diagram outlining the antiviral mechanism of aciclovir. The drug is most active against herpes simplex virus, because of the efficiency of the viral thymidine kinase enzyme in phosphorylating aciclovir and trapping it within infected cells.

ACICLOVIR

This drug is valuable in the management of orofacial herpes simplex infections and is commonly prescribed by dentists. Its mode of action is illustrated in Fig. 9.10. Aciclovir is an analogue of guanosine and is very efficiently phosphorylated by the herpesvirus thymidine kinase enzyme which is present in infected host cells. This phosphorylation step traps the drug within infected cells only, and is the basis for its selective toxicity. Subsequently, two further phosphate groups are added under the influence of cellular kinases. The resultant triphosphate form is a potent and selective inhibitor of herpes simplex virus (HSV) DNA-polymerase and a DNA chain terminator.

Aciclovir may be administered orally, intravenously, or topically. Few adverse reactions have been reported, despite widespread clinical use. Systemic treatment for primary herpetic gingivostomatitis must be given early in the course of the disease if it is to be effective. Topical treatment is generally appropriate for herpes labialis. Aciclovir has revolutionized the treatment of herpes simplex virus infections in the immunocompromised, and has also been used prophylactically in that group.

INTERFERONS

Interferons (Chapter 5) are naturally produced proteins with potent antiviral activity, but their use in clinical practice has been disappointing. However, large doses of interferon, administered systemically, are currently the mainstay of active treatment for chronic hepatitis B and C infections. Many patients receiving interferons develop flu-like symptoms, whilst leucopenia, thrombocytopenia, and effects on the CNS have also been reported.

Resistance to antimicrobial agents

In the preceding sections of this chapter, frequent references have been made to the development of resistance to antimicrobial drugs. Some species of bacteria are innately resistant to certain families of antibiotics. This is usually because the bacteria either lack a susceptible target or because they are impermeable to the drug. However, strains of initially susceptible bacteria may develop or acquire resistance to particular antibiotics. For example, in recent years methicillin-resistant strains of *Staphylococcus aureus* (MRSA) have become far more common, greatly increasing the difficulty of treating infections caused by this important medical pathogen. Since the mid-1980s, resistance of enterococci to vancomycin (VRE) has also become an increasingly recognized problem. This is especially serious because of the very limited range of antibiotics to which these organisms are sensitive. There is also concern about the development of vancomycin resistance within strains of MRSA.

Acquired antimicrobial resistance is now a serious clinical problem, which can be limited by more responsible prescribing of these drugs by clinicians and by implementing scrupulous cross-infection control measures. Although this section will concentrate on resistance to antibacterial drugs, resistance to antifungals and antivirals can also develop under appropriate conditions of use, particularly with long-term prophylaxis.

Mechanisms of resistance

There are three main types of resistance mechanism, namely:

- *Altered target* – the target enzyme may change sufficiently, perhaps by mutation, to cause a lowered affinity for the antimicrobial drug. Normal bacterial metabolism and growth may then occur. Alternatively, an additional target enzyme that is resistant to the drug may be produced.

- *Alteration in access to the target site (altered uptake)* – the amount of drug reaching the target is reduced, either by altering entry, for example through changes in cell permeability, or by the bacterium actively pumping the drug out of the cell (efflux mechanism).

- *Drug inactivation* – enzymes may be produced that inactivate the antibacterial agent. Important examples of these enzymes include beta-lactamases, aminoglycoside-modifying enzymes, and chloramphenicol acetyl transferases.

The relevance of each of these mechanisms of resistance to the groups of antimicrobial agents already discussed is shown in Fig. 9.11.

Genetic aspects of resistance

Microbial genetics have already been discussed in Chapter 6. Antibiotic resistance may arise by a single, spontaneous chromosomal mutation in one bacterial cell, resulting in the synthesis of an altered protein. If this protein is, for example, a target site for a particular antibiotic, then the antimicrobial effectiveness of that drug will be severely compromised against the mutant cells. In the presence of that same antibiotic, such spontaneous mutants will have a selective advantage, surviving and outgrowing the susceptible population. These resistant organisms may then spread to other body sites and to other individuals.

In addition to spontaneous mutation, bacteria can acquire resistance genes via transmissible plasmids. An individual plasmid may code for resistance to several types of antibiotic, allowing bacteria to become resistant to as many as six different drugs simultaneously.

Finally, resistance genes may occur on transposons. These have also been termed 'jumping genes' and can be integrated into the chromosome or plasmids.

Laboratory control of antimicrobial drug treatment

Whilst clinical experience is helpful in determining which antimicrobial agents to prescribe for infections in specific sites and with particular organisms, susceptibility tests performed in the laboratory are a valuable aid to the antibiotic management of an infection. However, the conditions under which such tests are performed represent an artificial situation compared with use of the drug *in vivo*. The results require skilled interpretation and the final choice of agent must also take into account the clinical background.

Antibiotic susceptibility tests

There are two main types, diffusion tests and dilution tests.

DIFFUSION TESTS

The organism under test is inoculated onto an agar plate and filter paper discs containing the relevant antibiotics applied to the surface. After incubation, the plate is examined for zones of inhibition around each antibiotic disc (Fig. 9.12). By comparison with the zone sizes for reference strains, the organism can be categorized as susceptible, intermediate (may respond clinically to higher doses), or resistant.

DILUTION TESTS

These allow a more quantitative assessment of susceptibility, by determining the minimal inhibitory concentration (MIC) of the antibiotic for a particular organism. This is the lowest concentration that will inhibit visible growth *in vitro* (Fig. 9.13). The test can be extended to determining the minimal bactericidal concentration (MBC). This is the lowest concentration of an antibiotic that will actually kill the organism. For bactericidal antibiotics the MIC and MBC are very close to one another. Determining the MBC, together with measuring serum levels (see below), is important in the antibiotic management of patients with infective endocarditis (Chapter 17) to ensure that a bactericidal concentration of drug is maintained during treatment.

RESISTANCE TO ANTIBACTERIAL AGENTS

Antibacterial	Mechanism of resistance		
	Altered target	Altered uptake	Drug inactivation
Beta-lactams	-	+	++
Glycopeptides	-		
Aminoglycosides	-	+	++
Tetracyclines	-	+	
Chloramphenicol		-	+
Macrolides	++		
Lincosamides	++		
Fusidic acid	++		
Sulfonamides	++	-	
Trimethoprim	++	-	
Quinolones	-	+	
Rifampicin	++		
Metronidazole		-	

- rare   + common   ++ very common

Fig. 9.11 Table illustrating the common mechanisms of resistance of bacteria to antibacterial drugs.

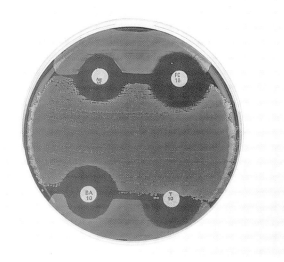

Fig. 9.12 An antibiotic susceptibility test. Growth of the organism (*Staph. aureus*) has been inhibited around the three filter paper discs containing antibiotics to which it is sensitive (neomycin, fucidin, and bacitracin) but not around the tetracycline disc, to which it is resistant. The control strain at the top and bottom of the plate is sensitive to all four antibiotics.

Special laboratory tests can be undertaken to determine synergistic activity between combinations of antibiotics, for example between aminoglycosides and penicillins.

Another important laboratory function is the measurement of drug levels in the serum of patients undergoing treatment with certain antibiotics, for example the aminoglycosides that are toxic at doses close to those required for successful treatment. It is also important to monitor blood levels in patients receiving prolonged therapy for serious infections such as endocarditis, to ensure that they remain above the MBC.

Responsible prescribing of antimicrobial agents

Although antimicrobial agents have revolutionized the treatment of infection, like most drugs their administration may be accompanied by unwanted effects. In addition to the necessary risk–benefit analysis which clinicians must undertake for the individual patient, one must also remember that the administration of antimicrobial agents carries the risk of selection and dissemination of resistant organisms. For this reason it is essential

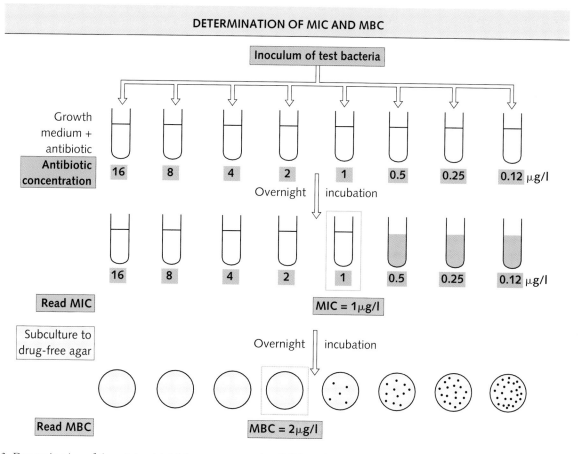

Fig. 9.13 Determination of the minimal inhibitory concentration (MIC) and minimal bactericidal concentration (MBC) of an antibiotic for a test strain.

that antimicrobial agents are administered appropriately; most hospitals have antibiotic control policies as a safeguard against indiscriminate prescribing.

In relation to common dentoalveolar infections, many will respond quickly and completely to appropriate surgical treatment, which usually involves drainage, with no need for recourse to antimicrobial treatment of any form.

If an antibiotic is deemed necessary then it should be chosen carefully in the light of a presumptive diagnosis. Where possible, clinical specimens should be collected for culture and sensitivity testing before antibiotic administration. The antibiotic regime can then be adjusted, if necessary, in the light of the laboratory results.

Further reading

House of Lords, Select Committee on Science and Technology. (1998). *Resistance to antibiotics and other antimicrobial agents*. HL Paper 81–1. HMSO, London.

Levy, SB (1992). *The antibiotic paradox. How miracle drugs are destroying the miracle*. Plenum, New York.

Mims, C, Playfair, J, Roitt, I, Wakelin, D, and Williams, R (1998). Antimicrobial agents and chemotherapy. In *Medical microbiology* (2nd edn), Chapter 30. Mosby, London.

Murray, PR, Rosenthal, KS, Kobayashi, GS, and Pfaller, MA (1998). Antibacterial agents; Antiviral agents; Antifungal agents. In *Medical microbiology* (3rd edn), Chapters 20, 47, and 67. Mosby Year Book, St Louis.

O'Grady, F, Lambert, HP, Finch, RG, and Greenwood, D (1997). *Antibiotics and chemotherapy (7th edn), their use in therapy*. Churchill Livingstone, Edinburgh.

Key facts

- 'Selective toxicity' implies that an antimicrobial drug can damage or kill a micro-organism without injuring the host.

- Antibacterial drugs may kill bacteria (bactericidal) or inhibit their growth (bacteriostatic).

- Major target sites for antibacterial drugs are cell-wall synthesis, protein synthesis, nucleic acid synthesis, and cell-membrane function.

- Beta-lactam antibiotics (penicillins and cephalosporins) inhibit bacterial cell-wall synthesis.

- Aminoglycosides, tetracyclines, macrolides, lincosamides, chloramphenicol, and fusidic acid all act by inhibiting protein synthesis.

- Sulfonamides, trimethoprim, quinolones, and rifamycins act by inhibiting nucleic acid synthesis.

- Metronidazole has potent activity against anaerobic bacteria.

- The two main groups of antifungal drugs, polyenes and azoles, act by interfering with cell-membrane functions.

- Most antiviral drugs are nucleoside analogues.

- Aciclovir, a structural analogue of guanosine, is very active against herpes simplex virus.

- Resistance to antibacterial, antifungal, and antiviral drugs is a major clinical problem.

- Resistance to antimicrobial drugs may be innate or acquired, the latter often through transfer of genetic material, for example via plasmids.

- Laboratory control provides important guidance in the use of antimicrobial agents.

10

Sterilization and disinfection

Sterilization and disinfection

Introduction

Prevention of cross-infection in the dental clinic is based upon the routine use of procedures that interfere with the spread of microbes between patients and the dental team. More specifically, disease prevention involves interfering with one or more of the steps involved in the development of an infectious disease as described in Chapter 11. Instrument processing and surface disinfection will be discussed here, while other infection-control procedures will be described in Chapter 28.

Sterilization and disinfection are the keystones of the control of infection in all clinical environments. Sterilization is an absolute term and refers to a process that kills or removes all types of micro-organisms. It is essential for any item that is to enter body tissues, for any fluids which are to be injected, and for instruments which contact mucosal surfaces. Disinfection is a lower grade process that kills or removes micro-organisms, excluding bacterial spores. It results in a reduction in the number of pathogenic organisms to a level that is unlikely to cause infection.

Instrument processing

The goal of instrument processing is to recycle contaminated instruments such that they are sterile for use on the next patient. Procedures must minimize the risk of exposure to the dental staff handling the instruments. Any item used in a patient's mouth should be cleaned, packaged, and sterilized before reuse on another patient, or alternatively it should be discarded. The steps for instrument processing and the rationale for each are presented in Fig. 10.1.

Cleaning

Large amounts of contaminated debris on instruments can insulate microbes from sterilizing agents. Cleaning is therefore an essential step prior to sterilization. Appropriate gloves, eyeglasses, mask, and protective clothing should be worn when processing instruments. The safest way to clean dental instruments is to use an ultrasonic bath or an instrument spray washer, following the manufacturer's instructions carefully. These methods effect-

STEPS AND RATIONALE FOR INSTRUMENT PROCESSING	
Cleaning	Cleaning instruments removes or reduces the bioburden so that the sterilization procedure will have the best chance to work
Packaging	Packaging items prior to sterilization protects them from re-contamination until they are opened at chairside
Sterilization	Sterilization will kill all remaining microbes on the instruments
Sterilization monitoring	Monitoring the sterilization process with either biological or chemical indicators helps assure that successful sterilization has occurred
Storage and distribution of sterile instruments	Storing sterile instrument packages and cassettes properly will maintain their sterility until they are opened at chairside for use on the next patient

Fig. 10.1 The steps involved in instrument processing.

ively clean the instruments and reduce the direct handling of contaminated items. Hand-scrubbing of contaminated instruments increases the chance of punctures and cuts from the sharp contaminated instruments. While ultrasonic units and instrument washers are effective in removing dried blood, saliva, and debris, occasionally an item may require additional hand-scrubbing to remove cement or other impacted material.

Instrument packaging

Packaging instruments before placing them in a sterilizer keeps them in functional groups and preserves the sterility of the instruments until the packs are opened at the chairside. Figure 10.2 describes various types of packaging materials and techniques. It is important to use materials designed as sterilization packaging, since many ordinary plastics or papers cannot withstand sterilizer conditions or will not allow penetration by the sterilant (e.g. steam). Instrument cassettes are becoming increasingly popular for housing dental instruments during use, cleaning, and sterilization. They are made of plastic, stainless steel, or aluminium, contain a varying number of instrument slots, and are perforated to facilitate cleaning and the entry of the sterilizing agent. The cassettes hold the instruments during chairside use and at all stages of the washing, packaging, and sterilization process. Since cassettes greatly reduce the direct handling of contaminated sharp instruments, staff safety during instrument processing is enhanced.

Carbon-steel items (for example many burs and the cutting edges of orthodontic pliers) will rust if processed through a steam sterilizer. A 'rust inhibitor' such as sodium nitrite may be added before instruments are packaged to retard this corrosion. Alternatively, a non-corrosive sterilization method like dry heat or unsaturated chemical vapour could be employed (see next section). Instruments should be dried before packaging. Internal chemical indicators and/or biological indicators (spore tests) are added during the packaging step.

It should be noted that currently in the United Kingdom there is debate about the efficacy of autoclaves without a vacuum phase for the sterilization of instruments placed in a sterilization bag or pouch. Although it has been suggested that effective sterilization

PACKAGING MATERIALS AND PROCEDURES	
Sterilizing method	**Packaging material**
Steam	Paper/plastic pouches, nylon type plastic tubing, sterilization paper, wrapped cassettes, thin cloth
Dry heat	Dry heat type nylon plastic tubing, some sterilization papers
Chemical vapour	Paper/plastic pouches, some sterilization papers

Use proper materials

- Use packaging materials designated for use in sterilizers to assure satisfactory performance
- Use the proper packaging material for the method of sterilization

Use proper wrapping procedure

- Make sure instruments do not protrude from package
- Do not cover tips of sharps with materials that will prevent contact with steam, dry heat or chemical vapour
- Instrument cassettes should be wrapped or packaged before sterilization
- Place biological and/or chemical indicators inside packages or cassettes
- Normally use no more than two layers of material when wrapping items

Use proper sealing procedures

- Some paper/plastic pouches are self-sealing
- Nylon type plastic tubing should be heat-sealed or double-folded and sealed with sterilization tape
- Paper-wrapped cassettes or packs should be sealed with sterilization tape
- Do not use metal fasteners of any kind, for example staples, paper clips
- Do not use aluminium foil or closed containers for steam or chemical vapour sterilization. Suitability of closed containers for dry heat sterilization should be confirmed by spore-testing

Fig. 10.2 Packaging materials and procedures for instrument sterilization. (Adapted from Miller 1996; with permission.)

can be achieved, the UK Department of Health maintains that wrapping instruments before sterilization in a non-vacuum autoclave (as used by many dentists) may result in inadequate air removal and a failure to sterilize. Routine use of a chemical monitor (see below and Fig. 28.5) is essential.

Instrument sterilization

Sterilization versus disinfection

Sterilization is defined as a process designed to kill all microbes, including spore-forming bacteria, viruses, fungi, and protozoa. The main exception here may be the Creutzfeldt–Jakob Disease (CJD) particle. Nevertheless, the killing of specific bacterial spores has been chosen as the test to determine whether sterilization in health-care settings has been achieved. Thus, the working definition of sterilization is 'a process that causes the death of a high level of specific bacterial spores'.

In contrast, disinfection is a process, usually involving liquid chemicals used at room temperature, which can kill many disease-producing microbes but is relatively ineffective against others, for example bacterial spores. When there is a choice between sterilization and disinfection, the former should be selected as it provides the best protection against the spread of disease-producing microbes.

Sterility is an absolute state indicating the absence of all living microbes, but in practice this cannot be confirmed for every item since this would require culturing them all before they were released for use. Thus, sterility assurance is best achieved by making a special effort to perform routinely all instrument processing procedures correctly and to monitor the sterilization process with biological and chemical indicators.

Heat sterilization

Microbes are killed soon after they come into direct contact with a heat-sterilizing agent such as steam, hot air, or hot chemical vapours that are at the proper temperature. The destruction of micro-organisms by heat is mainly a result of the thermal coagulation of proteins. Temperature, time, and exposure are the key

CAUSES OF STERILIZATION FAILURE	
Improper cleaning of the instruments	Bioburden left on items may insulate microbes from the steam, dry heat, or chemical vapour
Improper packaging	Slows down or prevents steam or chemical vapour from reaching items inside, or cloth absorbs excessive amount of moisture or chemical vapour • Wrong packaging material for the method of sterilization • Closed, solid container in steam or chemical vapour sterilization • More than two layers of wrapping material • Excessive cloth wrap
Improper loading of the sterilizer	Prevents items from being fully exposed to the steam, dry heat, or chemical vapour • Overloading with no separation between packages or cassettes • Layering (stacking up) of packages or cassettes rather than placing them on their edges
Improper timing of the sterilization cycle	Prevents sterilizing temperature from being held for sufficient time • Incorrect operation of the sterilizer • Timing started before the sterilizing temperature was reached on non-automatic units • Dry heat sterilizer door opened to add more items without re-starting sterilization cycle • Malfunction of the sterilizer
Improper temperature in the sterilizer	• Incorrect operation of the sterilizer • Malfunction of the sterilizer

Fig. 10.3 Causes of sterilization failure. (Adapted from Miller 1992; permission of ADA Publishing, Inc.)

factors that influence sterilization. The actual surface of the instruments to be sterilized must be exposed to an appropriate sterilizing agent at the correct temperature for the recommended time. Anything that interferes with these parameters may prevent sterilization. Specific causes of sterilization failure are listed in Fig. 10.3.

Figure 10.4 describes the various methods of sterilization commonly used in dentistry. Each method has its advantages and disadvantages, but all can achieve sterilization if recommended procedures are employed. The manufacturer's directions for loading, operation, and the maintenance of sterilizers must be followed. Of paramount importance is the correct loading of a sterilizer to ensure that each package or cassette will have access to the sterilizing agent. Items must not be packed tightly in the

sterilizer and a little space must be present between each item. This can be achieved by loading packages or cassettes on their edges rather than laying them flat in layers and by utilizing any loading racks supplied with the sterilizer.

STEAM STERILIZATION

The steam sterilizer (autoclave) is the most commonly used and efficient method of sterilization in dentistry. Its main advantage is its ability to achieve excellent heat penetration of the packages and cassettes being processed. Unfortunately, it causes corrosion of carbon-steel items, but stainless-steel instruments are not affected. Also, any paper packaging is wet at the end of the sterilizing cycle and should be allowed to dry before removal from the chamber.

HEAT STERILIZATION METHODS				
Method	**Temperature/Pressure**	**Exposure time** [a]	**Advantages**	**Concerns**
Steam autoclave [b]	121°C (250°F) 115 kPa 134°C (273°F) 216 kPa	15–30 minutes 3.5–12 minutes	Good penetration Non-toxic Time efficient	Non-stainless steel items corrode May damage rubber and plastics Do not use closed containers Unwrapped items quickly contaminated after cycle
Dry heat [c] **(oven type)**	160°C (320°F)	60–120 minutes	No corrosion Non-toxic Items are dry after cycle Can use closed container [d]	Long cycle time May damage rubber and plastics Door can be opened during cycle Unwrapped items quickly contaminated after cycle
Dry heat [c] **(rapid heat transfer)**	191°C (375°F)	12 minutes (wrapped) 6 minutes (unwrapped)	No corrosion Non-toxic Time efficient Items are dry after cycle	May damage rubber and plastics Door can be opened during cycle Unwrapped items quickly contaminated after cycle
Unsaturated chemical vapour [b]	134°C (273°F) 216 kPa	20 minutes	No corrosion Time efficient Items dry quickly	May damage rubber and plastics Do not use closed containers Must use special solution Uses hazardous chemical Unwrapped items quickly contaminated after cycle

Fig. 10.4 Heat sterilization methods. [a]These exposure times relate only to the sterilization portion of the total cycle and do not include any warm-up time, come-down time, or drying times. The exposure time may vary depending upon the load and should be verified during actual use by biological monitoring (spore-testing) and the use of chemical indicators. [b]Biologically monitor with spores of *Bacillus stearothermophilus*. [c]Biologically monitor with spores of *Bacillus subtilis*. [d]Confirm by using a biological indicator on the inside of the closed container. (Adapted from Miller 1993*a*; with permission.)

After filling the sterilizer reservoir with distilled or other good quality water the unit is activated, the water flows into the bottom of the chamber and electric coils heat the water under increased pressure. This cycle may last for several minutes until the predetermined sterilizing temperature (121°C at 115 kPa to 135°C at 216 kPa) is reached. At this time the temperature is held constant for the set time (usually 3.5 to 30 minutes) for what is referred to as the sterilizing cycle (time *at* the sterilizing temperature). The steam pressure is then released to zero, after which the door can be opened or the drying cycle activated.

Some sterilizers have a short-time, high-temperature cycle referred to as a 'flash' cycle, which can be used only with items that are not packaged, to avoid any interference with steam penetration during the shortened cycle time. The cycle should be reserved for emergency situations when an item is in short supply and needs to be sterilized quickly. When this cycle is used, a strict aseptic technique is required to protect the processed item from recontamination after removal from the sterilizer.

Dry heat sterilization

Dry heat kills micro-organisms by oxidizing the cell components. There are two forms of dry heat sterilizer, a standard oven type and a rapid heat-transfer model that involves the mechanical circulation of heated air around the items to be sterilized. The latter operates at a higher temperature but results in a shorter sterilization cycle. The advantages of dry heat over steam sterilization are that it does not corrode carbon-steel items and that packages are dry at the end of the cycle. Sterilization in a closed container is also better achieved in dry heat than in steam or unsaturated chemical vapour sterilizers. However, dry heat sterilization involves a long sterilization cycle and 'come-up' time (especially in the oven type sterilizer), together with a risk of damage to instruments due to the high temperature. A further disadvantage is that the doors of some units can be opened mid-cycle, thus interrupting the required constant high temperature needed during the entire sterilizing cycle.

Unsaturated chemical vapour sterilization

This method of sterilization is far more common in the USA than the UK. The unsaturated chemical vapour sterilizer is also called a chemiclave or a Harvey sterilizer. The sterilizing agent is a chemical solution containing 0.23% formaldehyde and 72.38% ethanol as the active ingredients along with a small amount of water. This sterilizer heats up to a sterilizing temperature of about 132°C, with a sterilizing cycle time of 20 minutes. Afterwards the pressure is released and the door can be opened. This method of sterilization has the advantages of corrosion-free sterilization and yielding dry packages after the sterilizing cycle. Some have concerns about handling formaldehyde and the repeated purchase of the special solution. A purging system (charcoal filter) that collects the vapours at the end of a cycle can be obtained with new units or can be retrofitted on old units.

Liquid chemical sterilization

The very few non-disposable plastic items used in a patient's mouth, that melt in heat sterilizers can be cleaned, dried, and sub-merged for 10 hours in a solution of 2.0% to 3.4% glutaraldehyde (1,5-pentanedial). Glutaraldehyde sterilants exist as acidic or neutral solutions, but the antimicrobial activity of glutaraldehyde is enhanced at alkaline pH, though this activity decays more quickly with time at the higher pH values. In use, glutaraldehyde is mixed with an 'activator' to bring the solution to about pH 8. Once activated, it has a shelf-life (activity when not in use) of no more than 28–30 days. However, using and reusing the solution may increase its decay so that its use-life (activity as it is being used) is shorter, perhaps 7–14 days depending upon its dilution with residual water on the items being processed, organic load, environmental contamination, and temperature.

A properly prepared and stored glutaraldehyde solution is considered to be a liquid sterilant if its contact time with the cleaned items is at least 10 hours. However, in use, the effectiveness of processing items through glutaraldehyde (in contrast to heat sterilizers) cannot be biologically monitored by spore testing. Thus, liquid chemical sterilization with a glutaraldehyde solution should be used only on items that are destroyed by heat sterilization and never as just a substitute for heat sterilization. Test kits are available that can estimate the remaining active glutaraldehyde concentration in a solution, and these should be used to estimate the quality of this liquid sterilant as it is being reused to process several batches of plastic items over a period of time. It should be noted that only antimicrobial solutions labelled as sterilants should be reused, and then only with strict controls and sterility assurance procedures. Reusing solutions that do not sterilize greatly enhances the risk of actually contaminating subsequent items with surviving microbes.

After 10 hours of complete submersion in a properly prepared solution of glutaraldehyde in a covered container, the processed items should be thoroughly rinsed to remove residual chemical, dried, and packaged to protect from recontamination until used on the next patient. Such items cannot be considered as sterile since they become exposed to the environment after processing, although they can be regarded as safe for clinical use. Glutaraldehydes sold for instrument sterilization should not be used to wipe down operatory surfaces for surface disinfection, since this creates an undesirably high level of glutaraldehyde vapour in the environment.

Skin and eye contact with glutaraldehyde or excessive inhalation of the vapour must also be avoided. The toxicity of glutaraldehyde has resulted in its withdrawal from use by many health authorities within the UK.

Other methods of sterilization

Although not used in dental clinics, sterilizers utilizing ethylene oxide gas can, if operated for several hours at temperatures below 140°C, achieve the sterilization of clean, dry, plastic, and rubber items that melt in heat sterilizers. Ethylene oxide sterilization plants are restricted to large hospitals. The gas is very toxic and must be handled with care, the processed items requiring aeration for a few hours to remove residual ethylene oxide. Ethylene oxide is an alkylating agent and kills by damaging proteins and nucleic acids.

Radiation sterilization, usually based on a ^{60}cobalt source (gamma irradiation), is used in industry for sterilizing pre-packaged items such as syringes, needles, catheters, and gloves. These are then purchased as sterile by the consumer. The killing of the organisms occurs through production of free radicals which break the bonds in DNA.

Sterilization monitoring

Biological monitoring

Biological monitoring involves the use of highly resistant bacterial spores, termed biological indicators (BI), to test the effectiveness of the sterilization process (Fig. 10.5). If these spores are killed during the normal sterilization cycles it is assumed that all other microbes present on instruments will also be killed. Spores of *Bacillus stearothermophilus* are used to monitor steam and unsaturated chemical vapour sterilization, whereas spores of *Bacillus subtilis* are used to monitor dry heat and ethylene oxide gas sterilization. The method is very sensitive, but because results are not available for several days it is not recommended for every load (see below).

There are two common forms of BI and each usually contains about 1 million spores. The spore strip consists of a small piece of filter paper impregnated with the spores and placed in a protective envelope. This indicator can be used to test any type of sterilizer as long as the correct type of spore is on the strip. After the sterilization cycle is complete, the envelope is collected from inside the instrument package or cassette. The spore strip is removed aseptically from the envelope, submerged in a growth medium and incubated aerobically at 55°C (for *B. stearothermophilus*) or 37°C (for *B. subtilis*). After 7 days the medium is observed for growth and, if positive, confirmed by microscopic observation of Gram-stained smears. Growth of the spores indicates sterilization failure, and steps must be initiated to identify and solve the sterilization problems (Fig. 10.6).

The other type of system is the self-contained BI which is used only with a steam sterilizer. It consists of a spore strip or disc inside a plastic vial that also contains an inner vial of growth medium. The inner vial of growth medium is mixed with the spores by a simple release mechanism and the whole item incubated.

	TYPES OF STERILIZATION MONITORING
Biological	Provides the main guarantee that sterilizing conditions have been achieved • Use biological indicator (BI) inside one package and/or cassette at least once a week • Use spore-strip BI for steam, chemical vapour, and dry heat or spore vial for steam • Use *B. stearothermophilus* for steam and chemical vapour and *B. subtilis* for dry heat • For analysis of BI, incubate *B. stearothermophilus* at 55°C and *B. subtilis* at 37°C or return the BI to a sterilization monitoring service for analysis. Always incubate a control BI (not processed through the sterilizer) with the test BI to validate results • If the spores are not killed, then the items in at least that load cannot be considered sterile
Chemical	**External indicator:** when a chemical indicator is on the outside of a package or cassette, it indicates that the item has been processed through a heat sterilizer to differentiate it from a non-processed item • Use a chemical indicator on the outside of every package or cassette • If an internal indicator (see below) is visible from the outside of the package or cassette, an external indicator is not needed • If the chemical indicator does not change properly, then the items in at least that load cannot be considered sterile **Internal indicator:** when a chemical indicator is on the inside of a package or cassette, it can indicate that the items inside the package or cassette have been exposed to heat • Use a chemical indicator or integrator* inside every package or cassette • If the chemical indicator does not change properly, then the items in at least that load cannot be considered sterile
Physical	Suggests that sterilizer may or may not be working properly • Visually observe the unit at times during a cycle and record (optional) readings from dials and gauges showing temperature, pressure, time • Observe and save print-outs of these time and temperature parameters on units having recording devices

Fig. 10.5 Types of sterilization monitoring. *Integrators are not available for the unsaturated chemical vapour or the rapid heat-transfer, dry heat sterilizers. (Adapted from Miller 1993*b*; with permission of ADA Publishing.)

STEPS TO TAKE AFTER A STERILIZATION FAILURE	
1. Take the sterilizer out of service	• After one positive spore test use any back-up sterilizer that has been routinely spore-tested • Resterilize all unused items processed through the sterilizer in question
2. Procedures to identify problems	• Review all records of all chemical monitoring since the date of the last negative spore test • Review with appropriate staff all packaging procedures, sterilizer loading, and operating procedures including procedures on how the biological indicator (BI) was handled and/or processed
3. Retest and observe the cycle	• Correct any procedural problems identified • Conduct a repeat spore test placing a chemical indicator next to the BI and operating the same cycle that failed previously • Observe the sterilizer during this retest cycle for any physical signs of a problem
4. Determine the fate of the sterilizer	• Observe the chemical indicator and obtain the results of the spore test • If the spores were killed and the chemical indicator changed colour, the sterilizer can be placed back into service. Test with a BI • If the spores were not killed, contact the appropriate person for repair or replacement of the sterilizer
5. Test the repaired or new sterilizer	• Spore test the repaired or new sterilizer and wait for the results before returning it to service

Fig. 10.6 Summary of the steps to take after a sterilization failure. (Adapted from Miller 1996; with permission.)

In the USA, the Centers for Disease Control and Prevention (CDC) and the American Dental Association (ADA) recommend at least weekly biological monitoring of all sterilizers used in dental facilities. It is important to keep records of spore testing so that, when necessary, sterility assurance can be documented after that fact.

Chemical monitoring

Chemical monitoring of the heat sterilization process is achieved by using heat-sensitive inks or other materials (e.g. markings on sterilization pouches and paper strips) that change colour or form when exposed to certain temperatures or other conditions. They produce an immediate result (in contrast to spore tests that require an incubation period of several days). Some types simply help to eliminate the accidental intermingling of 'sterilized' and 'non-sterilized' items (e.g. autoclave tape) and are not true indicators of successful sterilization. Others, called integrators, change colour more slowly because they are activated by a combination of temperature, time, and/or steam presence and can be employed to monitor the success of the sterilization cycle.

Physical monitoring

Physical monitoring is simply the occasional short-term visual observation of the sterilizer gauges indicating temperature, pressure, and time before, during, and after a cycle.

Distribution of sterile instruments

The sterility of processed instruments should be maintained until the packages or cassettes are opened at the chairside for care of the next patient. This can only be achieved if the packaging material is not compromised (Fig. 10.7).

Surface asepsis

Surface asepsis can be achieved either by cleaning and disinfecting the contaminated surfaces or by using surface covers (or disposable trays) to prevent underlying surfaces from becoming contaminated. Usually a combination of these is used. Surfaces should be divided into 'touch' and 'non-touch' surfaces. The former are those that are directly involved in clinical care and must be treated effectively between patients. These include surfaces touched with contaminated hands, such as light handles and switches, or those that come into contact with items used in the patient's mouth (e.g. instrument trays). 'Non-touch' surfaces are those that are not directly involved in the care of subsequent patients (e.g. some worktops, bracket table arms). While these surfaces may become contaminated by aerosols and spatter, they need be treated only at the end of each treatment session.

Cleaning and disinfecting surfaces

Cleaning

Cleaning surfaces prior to disinfection reduces the amount of bioburden (microbes and debris) and gives the antimicrobial substance the best chance to work. Sometimes the presence of organic material, for example blood and saliva, can interfere with the

MAINTAINING THE STERILITY OF INSTRUMENT PACKAGES AND CASSETTES	
Drying	Packages and cassettes processed through steam sterilizers should be dried before removal from the sterilizer • Either activate the automatic dry cycle or open sterilizer door slightly and allow to cool and dry for about 30 minutes • Packages from the unsaturated chemical vapour and dry heat sterilizers are dry after the sterilization cycle
Cooling	Hot or warm packages should be dried slowly to prevent the formation of condensation on the instruments inside • Do not place warm items on cold surfaces or under air-conditioning units • Do not use fans in the sterilizing area to cool items as this circulates potentially contaminated air over the sterile items
Storage	The sterility of a package or cassette is event-related, not time-related • Handle only dry packages and handle them as little and as gently as possible to avoid tearing or disrupting the packaging material • Store sterile packages or cassettes in a cool, dry, protected, low-traffic, raised low contamination area that does not touch walls, ceilings, sinks, overhead pipes or heat sources • Even though the sterility of a package or cassette is event-related, it is still a good idea to rotate stored items as first in, first out
Distribution and use	Maintain instrument sterility until just before use • Distribute the sterile packages or cassettes at chairside when needed at the next patient appointment • Open the sterile packages or cassettes at chairside

Fig. 10.7 Methods for maintaining the sterility of instrument packages or cassettes.

action of these chemicals and can protect microbes from direct contact with the killing agent.

Uncovered contaminated touch surfaces must be precleaned and then disinfected. Heavy duty gloves, eyeglasses, and a mask are recommended during these procedures. A liquid detergent is applied to the surface and wiped vigorously with towels or pads. These cleaned surfaces are then ready for disinfection.

Disinfection

PROCEDURES

Various aspects of surface disinfection are described in Fig. 10.8. A disinfectant is commonly applied to precleaned surfaces by spraying. This, along with the spray and wipe cleaning steps mentioned above, has been referred to as the 'spray–wipe–spray technique'. A pad saturated with the disinfectant may be used instead of spraying, but all the surfaces must become wet. Follow the manufacturer's directions on the disinfectant label, including those for use and contact time.

PROPERTIES OF DISINFECTANTS

The types and properties of various disinfecting chemicals are listed in Fig. 10.9.

Although there is no single best disinfectant, ideally the one selected should:

• have proper governmental approvals for safety and effectiveness;

• be tuberculocidal, in addition to killing other bacteria;

• kill hydrophilic viruses (e.g. polio, coxsackie), in addition to killing lipophilic viruses (e.g. HIV).

Selection of the two antimicrobial properties indicated above is based on relative microbial resistance to disinfecting chemicals (Fig. 10.10). Products that are tuberculocidal and can kill hydrophilic viruses are the 'strongest' surface disinfectants, and their use ensures the killing of all other disease-producing microbes except bacterial spores.

Surface covers

If contamination of a surface can be prevented by a barrier membrane, then the surface need not be cleaned and disinfected so frequently (see Fig. 10.8). The covers must be impervious to moisture and completely cover the underlying surface. They are carefully removed after each patient treatment and replaced with fresh covers before care of the next patient. The underlying surface is cleaned at the end of the day.

TIPS ON SURFACE PRECLEANING AND DISINFECTION

- Surfaces that are difficult to disinfect (e.g. chair buttons, control buttons on the air/water syringe, switches, light handles, hoses, handpiece and air/water syringe holders) should be covered with surface covers to prevent contamination. Replace the covers between patients. It may take less time to replace a cover than to clean and disinfect a surface

- Cleaning and disinfecting electrical switches on the chair, control unit, or X-ray viewing boxes may damage or short-circuit the switch. Cover them

- Use a disinfectant-cleaner rather than just a cleaner to preclean surfaces. Many of the water-based phenolic and iodophor agents sold as surface disinfectants can also be used in the precleaning step. This provides some protection during the precleaning step, helps sanitize any debris spattered by the precleaning procedure, and helps keep the number of products needed to a minimum

- Follow the disinfectant manufacturer's directions very carefully

- Water, rather than alcohol, should be used to dilute those agents requiring dilution before use

- Use heavy utility gloves during surface precleaning and disinfection to provide good protection to the hands

- Use a mask and protective eyewear to provide protection from the possible splashing of chemicals and contamination onto the mucous membranes of the eyes, nose, or mouth

- Frequently change the cleaning towels or pads when cleaning and disinfecting the operatory to reduce possible carry-over of contaminants from one surface to another

Fig. 10.8 Key elements of surface disinfection.

Disinfection of impressions and appliances

Every attempt must be made to clean and disinfect all contaminated items before they are sent to a dental technology laboratory, thus preventing contamination of the laboratory equipment and personnel (Fig. 10.11). It is important that the dentist communicates with the dental laboratory to agree on the procedures that each will use to ensure satisfactory infection control.

Management of contaminated dental instruments and surfaces

The overall procedures needed to manage contaminated instruments and surfaces in the dental environment are summarized in Fig. 10.12. Examples of these instruments and surfaces are given, together with their potential for involvement in spreading disease and the most appropriate microbial killing method for each item.

PROPERTIES OF DISINFECTANTS

Chemical class	Advantages	Concerns
Chlorines (e.g. sodium hypochlorite)	Rapid antimicrobial action Tuberculocidal Active against hydrophilic and other viruses Good activity in hard water	Should be prepared fresh daily Activity diminished by organic material Corrode metals May irritate skin and eyes Unpleasant odour Activity decreases as pH increases
Synthetic phenols [a] (e.g. o-phenylphenol, o-benzyl-p-chlorophenol, p-tertiary amylphenol)	Tuberculocidal Virucidal against lipophilic viruses Good activity in presence of organic material and hard water	Some may damage some plastics Some have lower activity against hydrophilic viruses May form film on surfaces May irritate skin and eyes
Iodophors (e.g. butoxypolypropoxy polyethoxyethanol-iodine)	Tuberculocidal Virucidal against lipophilic viruses May have residual activity	Should be prepared fresh daily Hard water reduces activity May discolour some surfaces Some may corrode metals
Quaternary ammonium compounds [b] (e.g. benzalkonium chloride, alkyldimethylethylbenzyl ammonium chloride, dioctyldimethyl ammonium bromide)	Non-irritating Detergent action Some bactericidal activity	Not tuberculocidal Reduced activity against hydrophilic viruses Weak activity against some Gram-negative bacteria Reduced activity in presence of organic material and soaps
Alcohols [c] (e.g. ethyl alcohol, isopropyl alcohol)	Tuberculocidal Virucidal mainly against lipophilic viruses Only slightly irritating	Evaporates quickly May damage some rubber and plastic materials

Fig. 10.9 Properties of disinfecting chemicals. [a]Water-based phenolics contain one or more of these phenolics in water. Alcohol-based phenolics contain o-phenylphenol or p-tertiary-amylphenol in ethyl alcohol or in isopropyl alcohol. [b]Some quaternary ammonium compounds are combined with an alcohol which gives the disinfectant tuberculocidal activity. [c]The antimicrobial activity of ethyl alcohol may vary from that of isopropyl alcohol with different microbes.

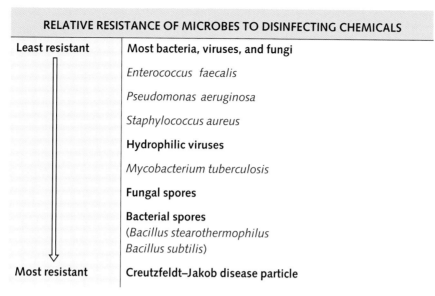

RELATIVE RESISTANCE OF MICROBES TO DISINFECTING CHEMICALS

Least resistant	Most bacteria, viruses, and fungi
	Enterococcus faecalis
	Pseudomonas aeruginosa
	Staphylococcus aureus
	Hydrophilic viruses
	Mycobacterium tuberculosis
	Fungal spores
	Bacterial spores (*Bacillus stearothermophilus* *Bacillus subtilis*)
Most resistant	**Creutzfeldt–Jakob disease particle**

Fig. 10.10 The relative resistances of microbes to disinfecting chemicals.

DISINFECTION OF IMPRESSIONS AND APPLIANCES

	Iodophor	0.5% Sodium hypochlorite	Synthetic phenolic (water-based)
Impressions			
Alginate	Yes	Yes	No
Polysulfide	Yes	Yes	Yes
Silicones	Yes	Yes	Yes
Polyether	Yes*	Yes*	Yes*
Hydrocolloid	Yes	Yes	No
Compound	Yes	Yes	No
Appliances			
Complete denture (acrylic/porcelain)	Yes	Yes	No
Removable partial (metal/acrylic)	Yes	No	No
Fixed prostheses (metal/porcelain)	Yes	No	No

Fig. 10.11 Disinfection of dental impressions and appliances. Rinse impression or prosthetic device under running tap water, immerse in disinfectant for 15 to 30 minutes, then thoroughly rinse with water. Because materials vary, contact the manufacturer for current recommendations. *Polyethers are sensitive to immersion. Spraying with disinfectant, then wrapping in disinfectant-soaked towel is least likely to damage an impression. (Adapted from Miller and Palenik 1994, pp. 198 and 201; with permission.)

CLASSIFICATION AND MANAGEMENT OF CONTAMINATED DENTAL INSTRUMENTS AND SURFACES			
Classification (*Risk in disease spread*)	**Examples**	**Involvement in patient care**	**Microbial killing method**
Critical (*High*)	Penetrates tissue Contacts open tissue	Hand instruments Cutting instruments Burs, files, needles Handpieces Scaler tips	Heat sterilization Sterile, single-use disposables
Semi-critical (*Intermediate*)	Contacts mucosa	Hand instruments Mouth props Plastic prophy angles Rubber dam frames	Heat sterilization Single-use disposables Chemical sterilization[a]
Non-critical (**intraoral contact**) (*Low*)	May contact skin and/or mucous membranes of dental personnel Contacts patient after fabrication, handling or repair	Impressions Prostheses Splints Other appliances	Thorough rinsing followed by disinfection[b] Also rinse and disinfect when item is returned to the patient
Non-critical (**no intraoral contact**) (*Low*)	Contacts unbroken skin	Blood pressure cuffs Face mask (e.g. NO_2)	Sanitize with detergent (no blood or saliva) Disinfect[b] (when blood or saliva present) Removable surface covers
Environmental surfaces (**patient care**) (*Very low*)	Usually contacts dental personnel, but not patients	Dental unit surfaces Laboratory equipment X-ray equipment	Sanitize with detergent (no blood or saliva) Disinfect[b] (when blood or saliva present) Removable surface covers
Environmental surfaces (**housekeeping**) (*Minimal*)	Rarely contacts dental personnel or patients	Floors Walls Work tops	Sanitize with detergent (no blood or saliva) Disinfect[b] (when blood or saliva present) Surface covers for worktops

Fig. 10.12 Classification and management of contaminated dental instruments and surfaces. [a]Only for items destroyed by heat. [b]For example, iodophors, synthetic phenolics, or sodium hypochlorite. (Designed from materials in Spaulding 1971; Cottone, *et al.* 1991; Miller and Palenik 1994, pp. 172–95.)

Key facts

- Any items used in a patient's mouth must be cleaned and sterilized before reuse on another patient.

- Cleaning contaminated items prior to disinfection or sterilization is essential.

- Packaging instruments prior to sterilization keeps them in functional groups and maintains asepsis after sterilization, but UK authorities do not recommend prepacking if a downward displacement sterilizer is used.

- Sterilization is a process which kills all microbes; sterility is an absolute state.

- Disinfection is a process which greatly reduces the number of disease-producing microbes but does not kill all microorganisms present, for example bacterial spores.

- Heat sterilization may be achieved with steam, dry heat, or unsaturated chemical vapour.

- Cold chemical sterilization is inherently less reliable than heat sterilization and should only be used for heat-sensitive items, of which there are very few in dental practice.

- Sterilization monitoring can be undertaken with biological monitors (spores), chemical monitors (process indicators and integrators), or by physical monitoring.

- Other methods of sterilization include ethylene oxide and gamma irradiation, although neither are used in dental practice.

- The two approaches to surface asepsis are the use of disposable coverings which are changed between patients, and cleaning and disinfecting surfaces between patients.

- Disinfectants chosen for use should have appropriate official approvals for safety and effectiveness, be tuberculocidal in addition to killing other bacteria, and kill hydrophilic viruses.

- Contaminated impressions and appliances should be cleaned and disinfected before they are sent to a laboratory.

References and further reading

Block, SS (1991). *Disinfection, sterilization and preservation* (4th edn). Lea and Febiger, Philadelphia.

Cottone, JA, Terezhalmy, GT, and Molinari, JA (1991). *Practical infection control in dentistry*, pp. 118–30. Lea Febiger, Philadelphia.

Lowbury, EJL, Ayliffe, GAJ, Geddes, AM, and Williams, JD (ed.). (1992). *Control of hospital infection* (3rd edn). Chapman and Hall, London.

Miller, CH (1992). Sterilization and disinfection: what every dentist needs to know. *Journal of the American Dental Association*, 123, 46–54.

Miller, CH (1993a). Update on heat sterilization and sterilization monitoring. *Compendium of Continuing Education in Dentistry*, 14, 304–16.

Miller, CH (1993b). Cleaning, sterilization, and disinfection: basics of microbial kill for infection control. *Journal of the American Dental Association*, 124, 48–56.

Miller, CH (1996). Infection control. *Dental Clinics of North America*, 40, 437–56.

Miller, CH, and Palenik, CJ (1994). *Infection control and management of hazardous materials for the dental team*. Mosby Year Book, St Louis.

Mims, C, Playfair, J, Roitt, I, Wakelin, D, and Williams, R (1998). Hospital infection, sterilization and disinfection. In *Medical microbiology* (2nd edn), Chapter 34. Mosby, London.

Russell, AD, Hugo, WB, and Ayliffe, GAJ (1992). *Principles and practice of disinfection, preservation and sterilization* (2nd edn). Blackwell, Oxford.

Spaulding, EH (1971). Chemical disinfection and antisepsis in the hospital. *Journal of Hospital Research*, 9, 5–31.

Section 2

11

Epidemiology

Epidemiology

Introduction

Epidemiology is the study of the occurrence, spread, and control of disease. It relies upon the collection of detailed statistical information recording the diseases affecting a population and, in the case of infectious diseases, may help to identify their causes and modes of transmission. It may also predict the future likelihood of infection, identify risk factors, and help in the planning of control measures involving chemotherapy and vaccination.

This chapter discusses the determinants of infectious diseases from an epidemiological viewpoint. An understanding of how and why infectious diseases occur requires consideration of not only the specific determinants themselves, but also how they interact. The three basic determinants are:

- the number of microbes entering the body (*dose*);
- the ability of the microbe to cause disease (*virulence*);
- the ability of the body to defend itself against the specific microbe (*resistance*).

The occurrence of disease or maintenance of health is determined by the interaction of these three factors. High dose, high virulence, and low resistance result in the greatest chance for developing disease. Thus, prevention of disease focuses on lowering the dose of the microbes that contaminate our bodies (for example by wearing gloves, masks, eyewear, and gowns at the dental chairside) and increasing body resistance by vaccination.

It should be stressed that many factors other than mere exposure to a pathogenic microbe must be satisfied for clinically evident infection to result. Thus, there are several stages in the development of an infectious disease, starting with the source of a microbe and ending with a harmful infection in a new host. These stages will be described in the next section.

DEVELOPMENT OF INFECTIOUS DISEASE	
Stage	**Example: occupationally acquired hepatitis B infection**
Source of the microbe	Dental patient infected with hepatitis B virus
⇓	
Escape from the source	Blood is liberated during extraction of a tooth
⇓	
Spread to a new host	Blood contaminates the surgical instruments and gloves of the dentist
⇓	
Entry into the host	Patient moves during the final stages of the extraction and a blood contaminated surgical instrument pierces the skin of the dentist's thumb
⇓	
Infection of the host	Virus survives, reaches the liver, and begins to replicate
⇓	
Damage to the host	Sufficient liver cells are killed to result in symptoms

Fig. 11.1 Stages in the development of an infectious disease, illustrated by the development of hepatitis B following occupational exposure in the dental surgery.

Stages in the development of infectious diseases

There are six stages in the development of infectious diseases (Fig. 11.1). To help explain these steps, Fig. 11.1 shows how hepatitis B might develop as an occupationally acquired infection in a dentist who had not been successfully vaccinated. Each of the various stages will now be described in detail.

Source of the microbe

Microbes are ubiquitous in nature, existing almost everywhere. Most pathogenic microbes that infect humans actually come from other humans, but some, for example rabies, come from animals (zoonoses). Other human pathogens originate from the environment, for example *Clostridium tetani* spores in soil. Contaminated objects or surfaces (fomites) are another environmental source.

Identifying the source of an infectious agent causing disease in a single individual is usually difficult, because the infected person has typically had contact with many other humans as well as the environment. By contrast, establishing the source of an infectious agent involved in an outbreak (a sudden occurrence of a disease in a defined group of people) is usually easier, though only if a common exposure incident can be identified. In a dental surgery the main source of pathogenic agents is the patient's respiratory tract and mouth, together with their associated secretions which may contain blood. In the example quoted (Fig. 11.1), a patient with hepatitis B infection served as the source.

Escape from the source

Microbes must escape from the source in order to contaminate a new host. The mechanisms of escape vary depending upon the source. In the case of the human body, microbes are shed in many ways (Fig. 11.2). The actual mode of escape may be natural (for example coughing or sneezing) or artificial (for example by donating blood or through the creation of salivary aerosols with a high-speed dental handpiece). These various modes of escape can result in contaminated fluids, tissues, or excreta leaving the body prior to entering a new host, but infection can also result from microbes being removed from contaminated body surfaces by direct contact with a new host. In the example illustrated (Fig. 11.1), the mode of escape of the hepatitis B virus is in blood liberated into a patient's mouth during the extraction of a tooth.

Spread to a new host

This step involves contamination, which is the mere presence of a microbe on a body surface or on the surface of an inanimate object. When a microbe spreads to a new host, the new host is said to be contaminated. Such contamination may occur in four different ways, as follows:

1. *Direct spread*. If there is direct spread from the microbial source, such as touching a patient's tongue without wearing gloves or drinking contaminated water, then the mode of escape and mode of spread are usually the same.

HOW MICROBES ESCAPE FROM THE BODY
• Tears
• Nasal secretions
• Saliva
• Blood in saliva
• Respiratory fluids and sputum
• Blood and tissue fluids exiting through small breaks in the skin or through injuries
• Contact with the skin
• Breast milk
• Faeces
• Intestinal fluids
• Semen
• Vaginal secretions
• Urine

Fig. 11.2 Table summarizing the methods by which microbes may escape from the human body.

2. *Indirect spread*. Indirect spread occurs if a secondary inanimate microbial source (fomite) is involved in the transmission of microbes to a new host. This may occur when dental instruments (secondary source) used in the patient's mouth (primary source) are not properly sterilized before being used on another patient. A key issue with this mode of spread is whether the microbes can survive in a viable form on a fomite for long enough to cause disease when they are transferred to a new host.

3. *Air-borne spread*. The third mode is air-borne spread, also called droplet infection (see Fig. 28.8). If a person with influenza sneezes, causing microbes to escape from the source, another person may inhale some of those contaminated droplets or aerosols, which may then establish infection.

4. *Vector-borne spread*. This mode of spread involves insects. This may be external, when the microbes simply contaminate the outside of the insect, for example flies crawling on faeces. Internal vector-borne spread occurs when the microbe is ingested by the insect, for example rat fleas ingesting *Yersinia pestis* and then depositing the organism on the skin of a new host. As the flea bites the new host it frequently defecates or regurgitates and the host scratches the irritation, thus rubbing the contaminated material into the skin.

Entry into the new host

Transmission from mother to developing fetus is termed vertical transmission and other modes of spread from person to person are

ROUTES OF MICROBIAL ENTRY	
Route	**Example**
Ingestion	*Salmonella* spp.
Inhalation	*Mycobacterium tuberculosis*
Injection	Hepatitis B virus
Across mucous membranes	*Treponema pallidum*
Into the ear	*Pseudomonas aeruginosa*
Transplacental	Cytomegalovirus

Fig. 11.3 Table summarizing the various routes of entry of microbes into the human host.

called horizontal transmission. There are six routes through which microbes may enter the body (Fig. 11.3). The route of entry into the body can determine if disease will subsequently occur. Some microbes must reach certain body sites before they are able to colonize the host tissues and subsequently cause disease. For example, swallowing the hepatitis B virus is not known to cause disease, but injection through the skin (for example, a contaminated sharps injury) providing 'blood-to-blood' contact provides a high risk for disease.

Skin is constantly being contaminated with microbes from the environment and from other people. However, these microbes usually fail to penetrate the skin, either because they do not produce factors to facilitate invasion of skin or due to the absence or low level of trauma that occurs (see Chapter 7). The hepatitis B example (see Fig. 11.1) illustrates entry through the skin.

Infection

Infection is the survival and multiplication of a microbe in a defined environment. We are seldom contaminated with a high-enough microbial load that effectively would result in immediate sickness. Disease, which is the clinical expression of an infection that causes damage to the body, usually results only after the contaminating microbes have multiplied to a level that causes harm. A key aspect in this step is the number of contaminating microbes involved – the dose or load. If the dose is high, a harmful level of microbes in the body may be reached more quickly. Conversely, if the dose is low, the body defences will have a better chance of destroying the invader before it can reach a harmful level.

In some instances of food poisoning the microbe may not even need to multiply in the body before harm occurs. For example, if *Staphylococcus aureus* has multiplied in food stored at room temperature and produced a large amount of enterotoxin, ingestion of such food may result in the toxin being absorbed from the gastro-intestinal tract and exerting its effects within a very few hours, with minimal multiplication of the organism within the body. This type of disease is more properly referred to as an intoxication, where true infection by living micro-organisms is not necessarily required.

Disease (damage to tissues)

The last step in the development of an infectious disease is the occurrence of actual damage to the new host, with clinically detectable signs and symptoms. This occurs when host defences fail to control the microbe and its multiplication results in tissue damage (Chapter 4).

Incubation period

The time between contamination and the development of symptoms is called the incubation period, and varies widely for different infections (Fig. 11.4). In some instances a contaminating microbe (for example most viruses) multiplies at the site of entry and then invades a specific target organ or body site to cause actual disease. Thus, a combination of the site of entry and the suitability of that site to support microbial growth, as well as assisting the agent to evade the host defences, determines the length of the incubation period and whether disease occurs or not.

Longer incubation periods (for example 1–6 months with hepatitis B) may result if the microbe is slow to reach the organ where damage occurs (target organ), or if multiplication or damage to tissues is slow in the body. Shorter incubation periods occur for the opposite reasons. Thus, influenza has an incubation period of only 1–3 days because the respiratory epithelial cells are infected very early in the course of virus spread through the body. These cells serve as both the site of initial virus replication and as a target 'organ' for this virus. From an epidemiological point of view, long incubation periods create longer time periods when the infecting microbe may be spread to others, resulting in a greater spread of the disease because of more human contacts.

During an incubation period the microbe is multiplying, even if at a slow rate. This is in contrast to the latent phase of a disease, in which the microbe stops multiplying after an initial acute infection and becomes latent or dormant in the host tissues for months or years. The agent may later be reactivated with subsequent replication and host damage. Examples of latency are shingles, cold sores, and reactivation tuberculosis.

INCUBATION PERIOD FOR VARIOUS DISEASES	
Disease	**Incubation period**
Hepatitis A	15 – 40 days
Hepatitis B	30 – 180 days
Hepatitis C	30 – 150 days
Hepatitis D	21 – 90 days
Influenza	1 – 3 days
Mumps	12 – 26 days
Gonorrhoea	2 – 9 days
Measles	About 11 days
Chickenpox	10 – 21 days

Fig. 11.4 The range of incubation periods for selected diseases.

Endogenous and exogenous infections

In many instances infection does not lead to disease. This has resulted in the establishment of our normal body flora, that survives and multiplies on various body surfaces usually without causing damage. However, some members of the normal flora can cause disease, referred to as an endogenous disease, if they are allowed to accumulate to 'harmful levels' (for example, periodontal disease and dental caries), or if they become displaced to another body site or are allowed to invade deeper tissues (for example, cervicofacial actinomycosis and postsurgical infections).

In contrast, diseases caused by microbes from external sources, for example influenza and gonorrhoea, are called exogenous infections.

Subclinical infections and the carrier state

Subclinical or asymptomatic infections are those that produce no clinically detectable symptoms but may result in an immune response that allows serological detection of the infection. For example, many infections with the Epstein–Barr virus are subclinical.

A carrier (commonly called an asymptomatic carrier) is an infected person with no clinical evidence of disease, though the signs and symptoms of the disease may have been evident earlier. Carriers are very important in the spread of diseases because they (as well as their contacts) are usually unaware of their infectious nature. Carriage of blood-borne viruses, such as hepatitis B and HIV, is a prime example of the importance of chronic carriage in the spread of infection.

Occurrence of diseases

Infections may occur as occasional cases at irregular intervals (sporadic occurrence), as a low number of cases at regular intervals (endemic occurrence), or as a high number of cases appearing suddenly (epidemic occurrence). A pandemic is an epidemic that has spread between continents.

The prevalence of a disease refers to the proportion of the population affected, or to the numbers of cases that are active at a particular time. This differs from the incidence of a disease which is a rate, indicating the number of cases within a specific population in a defined time period.

Epidemiological studies

There are two main analytical epidemiological methods available. In a case-controlled study, the investigation starts with a clinical effect and attempts to identify the cause of that effect. This is also referred to as a retrospective study – going back in time to determine what caused a specific effect. In a cohort study, also referred to as a prospective study, a population exposed to a presumed cause is followed to identify if and when disease supervenes and the outcome.

CONDITIONS THAT CONTRIBUTE TO THE EMERGENCE OF DISEASES	
Ecological changes	Lyme disease (increase in deer populations)
	Hantavirus pulmonary syndrome in Southwest USA (mild and wet weather increased rodent population and increased exploration of the wild by humans)
Changes in human demographics or behaviours	Tuberculosis (overcrowded housing and homelessness)
	AIDS (injection drug abuse)
Technology	Outbreaks of bacterial food poisoning (mass production of food)
	Legionnaires' disease (contamination of air-conditioning cooling towers leading to aerosolization of the causative bacterium present in water)
	Transfusion-related hepatitis (transfusion of contaminated blood or blood products)
Microbial changes	Influenza (genetic changes in virus making previous years' vaccine obsolete)
	Infections with antibiotic-resistant bacteria
Breakdown in public health measures	Diphtheria (relaxation of vaccination programme in the new independent states of former Russia)

Fig. 11.5 Conditions that contribute to the emergence of infectious diseases. (Based on Morse 1995.)

An additional method is a cross-sectional study which looks at the population at a specific timepoint to describe the prevalence relationships outlined above.

Emerging diseases

Emerging diseases are either previously unrecognized diseases or are known diseases with changing patterns. These occur when microbes and man come together in new or different ways. Conditions that contribute to disease emergence are listed in Fig. 11.5.

Changes in ecological conditions may enhance contacts between humans and animal or insect microbes, resulting in insect-borne or zoonotic diseases. For example, ecological conditions that cause an increase in deer populations increase the numbers of the deer tick, which in turn is the vector of Lyme disease in humans. This presents as a skin rash followed later by inflammatory changes in the nervous system, joints, and heart, and is caused by the spirochaete *Borrelia burgdorferi*.

Changes in human demographics and behaviours have contributed to the existence of the AIDS epidemic world-wide, involving spread by injection drug abuse and sexual contact. International travel and commerce allow a rapid spread of microbes associated with the human body or with products shipped around the world.

Sometimes technological advances bring humans and microbes together in ways not previously imagined. For example, the technology of blood transfusion has saved many lives but has also created a very efficient route of spread for blood-borne pathogens such as hepatitis B, hepatitis C, and HIV if donated blood is not screened.

Another obvious contributor to emerging diseases is genetic change in the microbe. This periodically creates infective agents with new immunological properties, new patterns of resistance to antimicrobial agents, and sometimes new virulence properties.

Finally, breakdown in public health measures may allow previously controlled microbes to contact and cause disease in humans. For example, failure of certain components at a water treatment plant in Milwaukee, Wisconsin, USA, in 1993 caused about 400 000 cases of diarrhoea because *Cryptosporidium parvum*, in ground water contaminated with animal faeces, was not removed from the drinking water. Another notable breakdown in public health measures was a relaxation of the vaccination programme during the formation of the 'independent states' of Russia in 1994 and 1995, resulting in about 100 000 cases of diphtheria.

References and further reading

Coggan, D, Rose, G, and Barker, DJP (1997). *Epidemiology for the uninitiated* (4th edn). BMJ Publishing Group, London.

Mausner, JS and Kramer, S (1985). *Epidemiology – an introductory text*. W.B. Saunders, Philadelphia.

Key facts

- Epidemiology is the study of the occurrence, spread, and control of diseases.

- The three factors determining whether an infectious disease is established are the dose and virulence of the organism and the host resistance.

- Most human pathogens are contracted from other humans, but some are from animals (zoonoses) and some from the environment.

- Microbes may contaminate a new host by direct spread, indirect spread, air-borne spread, or vector-borne spread.

- Transmission from mother to fetus is termed vertical transmission. Other modes of spread from person to person are called horizontal transmission.

- Microbes may enter the body by ingestion, inhalation, percutaneously, across mucous membranes, through the ear, and across the placenta.

- Infection is the survival and multiplication of a microbe in a given environment.

- Asymptomatic carriers are infected but have no clinical evidence of disease. They are usually unaware of their infectious nature and are very important in the spread of infection.

- Diseases may be sporadic (occasional cases at irregular intervals), endemic (low number of cases at regular intervals), or epidemic (large number of cases appearing suddenly).

- Prevalence refers to the proportion of the population affected, or the number of active cases at a particular time.

- Incidence is a rate, indicating the number of cases in a specific population over a defined time.

- Epidemiological studies may be retrospective or prospective.

- Emerging diseases may result from ecological changes, changes in human demographics or behaviour, new technology, microbial changes, or breakdown in public health measures.

Mims, C, Playfair, J, Roitt, I, Wakelin, D, and Williams, R (1998). Entry, exit and transmission. In *Medical microbiology* (2nd edn), Chapter 8. Mosby, London.

Morse, SS (1995). Factors in the emergence of infectious diseases. *Emerg. Infect. Dis.*, 1, 7–15.

12

Diagnostic microbiology

- General principles
- Diagnosis of oral infections

Diagnostic microbiology

The accurate diagnosis of infections is essential if they are to be treated appropriately. The main aims of a diagnostic microbiology laboratory are to identify any causative organisms and, if possible, to provide guidance on appropriate antimicrobial therapy. Antimicrobial sensitivity testing has already been discussed in Chapter 9. In the present chapter, the wide range of laboratory methods employed to diagnose infection will be summarized. Laboratory diagnosis of infections in the head and neck region poses particular problems, which will be described in the last section of this chapter.

General principles

Microbiological specimens

Types

It is important for clinicians to recognize that the accuracy of a microbiological report can only be as good as the quality of the specimen on which it is based. Whilst laboratories are able to provide advice and appropriate specimen containers, it is the responsibility of the clinician to obtain the correct sample. If possible, the specimen should be collected before antimicrobial therapy is prescribed.

There are three main categories of specimen (Fig. 12.1). In specimens collected for culture, maintenance of viability of the organisms is essential. For this reason, swabs are not ideal and collection of actual fluid or tissue provides a far greater chance of successful culture. Swabs also become readily contaminated with organisms of the normal flora, making interpretation of the plates difficult.

There is increasing interest in methods which detect microbial products or genome, but although rapid they do not permit determination of antimicrobial sensitivity patterns.

Antibody detection (serology) is used mainly for the diagnosis of infections with non-cultivable organisms such as hepatitis B virus or with organisms for which culture poses a major hazard to laboratory staff.

SPECIMEN TYPES	
For culture	Essential to maintain viability of organism Fluid (e.g. pus or urine) or tissue Ideally collect actual fluid, not swabs Collect specimen into sterile container Transport specimen rapidly to laboratory
For detection of microbial products	Do not require maintenance of viability of organism Rapid results Examples: detection of cell-wall antigens and toxins Gene sequence detection by DNA probes now possible
For detection of antibodies	Samples of serum, cerebrospinal fluid or saliva For non-cultivable or very hazardous organisms Detect four-fold rise in IgG antibody titre between acute-phase and convalescent serum (10–14 days apart) Detection of specific IgM response allows diagnosis from single serum specimen

Fig. 12.1 Categories of specimens submitted to diagnostic microbiology laboratories.

Specimen labelling and request forms

Careful and accurate labelling of specimens by the responsible clinician is essential, to ensure that all samples are attributed to the correct patient. Laboratories must also maintain a strict protocol for identifying specimens during their passage through the diagnostic process.

The request form submitted by the clinician must also provide the necessary clinical details to allow laboratory staff to process the specimen in the appropriate manner and to permit the reporting microbiologist to compile a meaningful report. The latter should then be entered in the patient's records.

Transportation

All specimens should be transported to the laboratory as quickly as possible. In some specimens, for example urine, bacteria and fungi may multiply rapidly, resulting in falsely high counts if there is a delay before culture. Such overgrowth may also result in more fastidious organisms remaining undetected.

Conversely, in other specimens, such as throat swabs, delicate organisms, for example *Neisseria* species, survive poorly and a delay in specimen transportation may result in a false-negative result.

Fluids and tissue specimens can be transported to the laboratory in a sterile container without the addition of a preservative solution. Never place such a specimen into the histological fixative formol saline, since this will kill any organisms present.

It is best to transport swabs in a medium which will preserve the viability of the organisms but not allow them to multiply. Various transport media are available for swabs taken for bacterial culture. Most, such as Stuart or Amies transport media, contain a sloppy agar with other additives such as charcoal to adsorb toxic agents.

In the case of swabs collected for viral culture, a viral transport medium should be employed. These contain antibiotics which help to reduce bacterial contamination of the specimen.

Sampling and the normal flora

Some specimens are collected from sites which are normally sterile in health, for example blood or cerebrospinal fluid. In these cases, any organisms isolated are significant. Other specimens are collected from sites which have a normal flora, for example the mouth, skin, or gastrointestinal tract. A further complication is that some specimens from sites which are normally sterile, for example bladder urine, are collected through sites that have a normal flora and may contaminate the specimen. Clinicians must, therefore, take as many precautions as possible to collect uncontaminated specimens, whilst the microbiologist must interpret each specimen in the light of its source and type.

Laboratory processing of specimens

As indicated earlier, a wide range of specimen types is submitted to a diagnostic microbiology laboratory. Similarly, there are many different ways of processing these specimens (Fig. 12.2). A flow chart, which illustrates the interrelationships between these tech-

SPECIMEN PROCESSING	
Non-cultural methods	**Microscopy:** Light microscopy Electron microscopy Detection of microbial antigens Detection of microbial genes
Cultural methods	**Bacteria and fungi:** Range of solid or liquid culture media **Viruses:** Tissue culture cells
Antibody detection methods	Several techniques e.g. ELISA

Fig. 12.2 Summary of methods available for processing microbiological specimens.

niques of specimen processing and gives some indication of timescale, is provided in Fig. 12.3. Historically, culture of microorganisms has been the mainstay of microbiological diagnosis, but the methods are labour-intensive and slow. In addition, some micro-organisms cannot be grown in artificial media. Some of the newer non-culture methods, such as antigen detection or the detection of microbial genome, are very rapid and in the long term are likely to supplant many of the currently employed culture techniques.

Microscopy

Microscopy is an important element of diagnostic microbiology. Light microscopy is employed for visualizing bacteria, fungi, and parasites whilst electron microscopy is necessary for the detection of viruses.

LIGHT MICROSCOPY

The commonest form of light microscopy is called bright-field microscopy and may be used to examine either wet preparations or stained preparations. Wet preparations allow the demonstration of micro-organisms in fluid specimens such as urine or faeces and are also used to detect fungi in skin. The motility of microbes, for example *Proteus* species, can also be detected.

In dark-ground microscopy, the micro-organisms appear brightly lit against a dark background. The method is useful for visualizing very thin cells such as spirochaetes, since the reflection of the light makes them appear larger. Motility can also be seen. Dark-ground microscopy is used in the rapid diagnosis of syphilis (*Treponema pallidum*) and has also been employed by dental researchers to examine for spirochaetes in specimens collected from periodontal pockets.

More frequently, the microbiologist produces stained preparations of dried material that has been fixed to the microscope

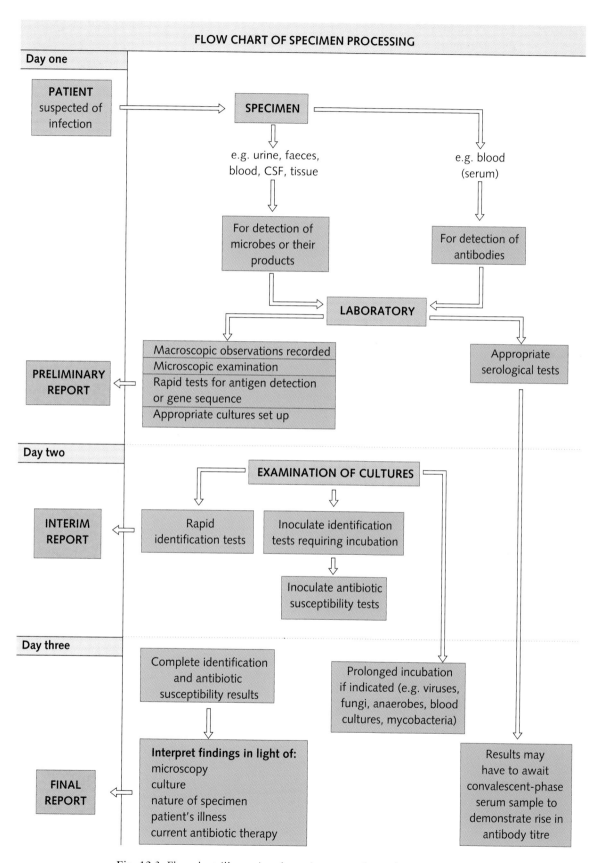

Fig. 12.3 Flow chart illustrating the various stages in specimen processing.

slide and which is examined at a magnification of 1000 × through an oil-immersion lens. The most important staining technique in bacteriology is the Gram stain (see Fig. 2.2), which allows the division of bacteria into two broad groups. Gram-positive bacteria stain purple (Fig. 12.4 (a)) and Gram-negative bacteria stain pink (Fig. 12.4 (b)). Some bacteria do not take up the Gram stain and require special staining techniques. For example, mycobacteria have a waxy cell wall and are stained with the Ziehl–Neelsen stain, in which the red dye fuchsin is forced into the cells by heating and the cells subsequently withstand decolorization with acid and alcohol (Fig. 12.5). Other staining techniques may be employed to demonstrate particular features of cells such as spores.

Finally, fluorescence microscopy is a valuable tool. Specific antibodies tagged with fluorescent dyes are now used widely in microbiology, for example in antigen detection tests. Specimens are examined through a microscope fitted with an ultraviolet light source.

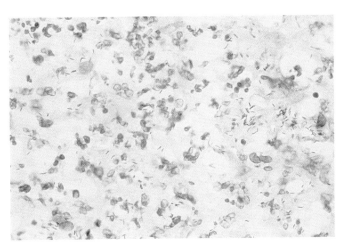

Fig. 12.5 A Ziehl–Neelsen stained smear of sputum from a patient with pulmonary tuberculosis, showing acid- and alcohol-fast bacilli which appear red.

ELECTRON MICROSCOPY

Electron microscopy allows the rapid detection of virus particles by direct examination of specimens. It is especially useful for viruses that are non-cultivable. Electron-dense stains such as osmium tetroxide are applied to the specimen to improve contrast (Fig. 12.6). Electron microscopy alone is often insufficient to allow accurate identification of a virus, but both the sensitivity and specificity can be increased by reacting the specimen with specific antiviral antibody which results in clumping of the virus particles.

Detection of microbial antigens

These tests are more rapid than culture tests although they often lack sensitivity. There are two main types of assay. First, some antigens (for example *Streptococcus pneumoniae* capsule) can be detected by their interaction with specific commercially available

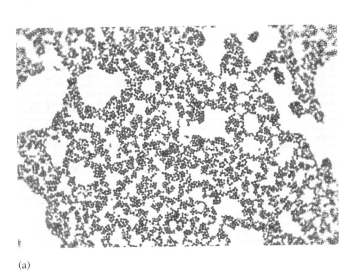

(a)

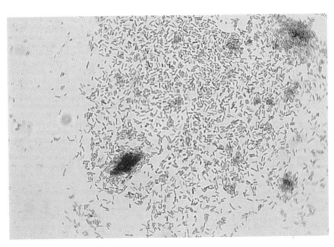

(b)

Fig. 12.4 Gram-stained films of (a) *Staphylococcus aureus* (Gram-positive cocci) and (b) *Escherichia coli* (Gram-negative bacilli).

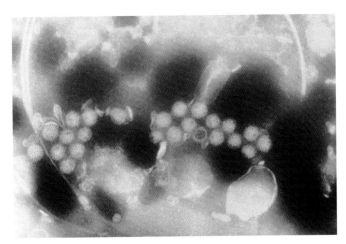

Fig. 12.6 An electron micrograph of rotavirus in a stool specimen from a child with diarrhoeal disease. (Courtesy of Ian Miller.)

antibodies. The specificity of this form of test has been increased greatly with the availability of monoclonal antibodies (see Fig. 7.13). The antibodies are often coated onto latex particles or red blood cells and used in agglutination assays (see Fig. 7.21). Alternatively, the antibodies may be labelled with a radioisotope, an enzyme, or a fluorescent marker to permit detection of the antigens to which they have bound.

The second type of assay detects microbial toxins. These include both exotoxins (for example *Clostridium difficile* cytotoxin) and endotoxin (detected by the limulus lysate assay). Toxins may be detected either by their antigenic properties or by demonstrating their action in appropriate bioassays.

Detection of microbial genes

A gene probe is a nucleic acid molecule which, when in a single-stranded state and appropriately labelled, can be used to detect a complementary sequence of DNA by hybridization (Fig. 6.11). The label may be either a radioactive isotope, or an enzyme which produces a colour change in a substrate when it is included in the reaction mixture.

If probes are produced for virulence factors such as toxins, organisms carrying these genes can be detected in specimens without the need for culture. Such technology is especially useful for organisms that are slow or difficult to grow in the laboratory, and increasing numbers of gene probes are likely to be developed. However, detection of small numbers of organisms can be a limiting factor. This problem can be overcome through gene amplification using the polymerase chain reaction (PCR) in which a specific DNA sequence can be amplified to produce millions of copies within a few hours (see Chapter 6). Confirmation of the identity of the product is by subsequent gene probing or sequencing. Whilst PCR is still largely a research tool, it is already employed as the 'gold standard' method in virology laboratories for confirmation of infection with hepatitis C virus.

Diagnosis of oral infections

The accurate diagnosis of oral infections poses several difficulties for clinical microbiologists. Many oral infections are endogenous (caused by members of the normal oral flora). The size and complexity of the oral flora (Chapter 20) means that this can complicate the interpretation of results, especially if specimens have been collected incorrectly and are contaminated with organisms from the normal flora. In addition, many of the bacteria involved in purulent oral infections are strict anaerobes with fastidious growth requirements, often requiring prolonged incubation times for colonies to develop. It is essential that there is good understanding and communication between the dentist treating the patient and the microbiologist handling the specimen, if the outcome is to be successful.

Specimens submitted to an oral microbiology laboratory can be broadly divided into three categories. First, there are those collected from purulent infections, for example a dental abscess. Second, specimens relating to oral mucosal infections such as can-

didosis or herpetic stomatitis are often examined. Finally, specimens may be collected to help in the management of periodontal disease and dental caries. These will be dealt with in turn.

Diagnosis of purulent infections

The microbiology of purulent infections in the head and neck region is described in Chapter 24. If possible, clinicians should submit an aspirate of pus (Fig. 12.7), rather than a swab. This prevents contamination of the specimen and maintains viability of anaerobic organisms. The needle should be removed with appropriate precautions and the hub of the syringe protected with a small plastic cover. Alternatively, the needle can be re-sheathed using a re-sheathing device and the sheath taped to the barrel of the syringe during transportation.

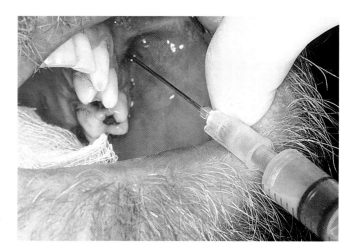

Fig. 12.7 The direct aspiration of pus from a dental abscess into a sterile syringe. This is the ideal method for sampling purulent infections. (Courtesy of Dr M.A.O. Lewis.)

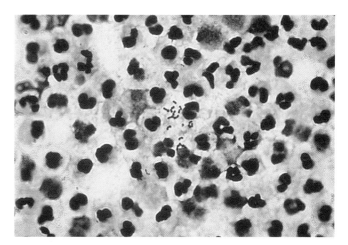

Fig. 12.8 A Gram-stained film prepared from an aspirate of pus collected from a dental abscess. Polymorphonuclear leucocytes and Gram-positive cocci are both seen.

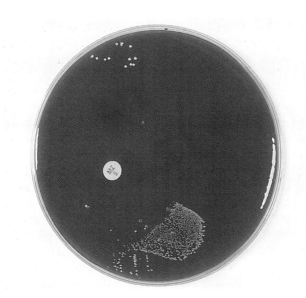

Fig. 12.9 The zone of inhibition around the metronidazole disc on this primary plate indicates the presence of anaerobes in the specimen.

Once the specimen has been received by the laboratory and booked in, an immediate Gram film is prepared (Fig. 12.8). If large numbers of leucocytes are seen, this confirms that an infection is present. The morphology of any bacteria visualized may also give early information on the types of organism present.

The specimen is next inoculated onto blood agar plates for aerobic and anaerobic incubation and into a bottle of sterile broth. Additional nutrients, such as vitamin K and haemin, are required in media for the growth of anaerobes. A metronidazole disc is usually placed on the anaerobic plate (Fig. 12.9) to help in the detection of anaerobic bacteria. Primary antibiotic sensitivity plates are also set up with the neat specimen, to allow an early indication of which antimicrobial agents the clinician should choose for treatment.

All cultures are examined after 48 hours' incubation. Purity plates are prepared of representative colony types for identification and antibiotic sensitivity testing.

Diagnosis of oral mucosal infections

Fungal infections

These are described in detail in Chapter 26. Yeasts can be cultured readily from the oral cavity. Specimens may be cultured from specific sites on the oral mucosa by swabbing. Alternatively, the presence of yeasts can be determined by collecting an oral rinse, in which patients swill their mouths with sterile saline and expectorate it. The rinse can then be inoculated onto media selective for yeasts. An advantage of the oral rinse is that that it can also be inoculated onto media for the isolation of other potential pathogens, for example *Staphylococcus aureus* and coliforms. It also provides a semi-quantitative result.

Sabouraud's agar is the most widely used isolation medium for yeasts, but most species have the same colonial morphology when grown on this medium (Fig. 12.10 (a)). This is unfortunate, because although *Candida albicans* is the commonest yeast isolated from the mouth, other species are also frequently present and patients often carry more than one species simultaneously. It is important, therefore, to use an additional agar on which different species produce different types of colony, for example CHROMagar® (Fig. 12.10 (b)).

Following incubation, yeast colonies are picked off the primary plates. All are subjected to a germ-tube test (Fig. 12.11) which identifies isolates of *Candida albicans*. Germ-tube negative yeasts are identified on the basis of further tests, for example sugar assimilation or sugar fermentation tests. Commercial kits are also available for yeast identification.

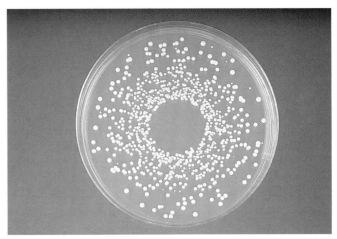

(a)

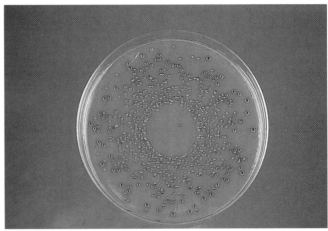

(b)

Fig. 12.10 Photograph illustrating *Candida albicans* and *Candida glabrata* growing on (a) a Sabouraud's agar plate and (b) a CHROMagar® plate. The value of CHROMagar® in allowing detection of different species is self-evident (*C. albicans* colonies: green; *C. glabrata* colonies: purple).

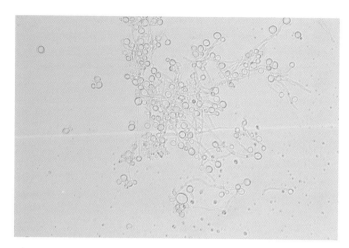

Fig. 12.11 Microscopy of a wet film illustrating the production of germ tubes by *Candida albicans* following 2 hours' incubation in serum.

Antifungal sensitivity tests can be undertaken. The reproducibility of these tests is questionable and the laboratory methods used are technically demanding, but surveillance of antifungal resistance, particularly to the azoles, is becoming increasingly important.

Viral infections

Herpes simplex virus is the commonest cause of viral infection of the oral mucosa. This virus can be cultured readily in tissue culture cells from a viral swab of lesional tissue and a result may be available within 48 hours. However, with the advent of specific antiviral drugs, a more rapid result is desirable and this may be achievable through the use of rapid antigen detection tests such as those based on immunofluorescence. Serological techniques are of little use in the clinical setting, because they are too slow for diagnosing primary infections and there are no serological markers of reactivation disease.

The diagnosis of shingles is usually made clinically, but may be confirmed by laboratory tests. Antigen detection and serology are the most valuable methods.

Diagnoses of herpangina and of hand, foot, and mouth disease are also usually made clinically, but isolation of the relevant coxsackieviruses can be attempted in tissue culture, ideally from stool specimens.

Diagnosis of caries and periodontal disease

Bacteria are very important factors in the aetiology of both caries and periodontal disease, but the role of a microbiology laboratory in the management of these infections is limited.

In the case of dental caries, salivary counts of lactobacilli (on Rogosa agar) and *Streptococcus mutans* group organisms (on MSB agar) can be undertaken (Chapter 22). Such counts, however, are poor predictors of future caries activity if taken in isolation. More recently, there has been renewed interest in caries activity tests based not only on bacterial counts, but also taking into account factors such as dietary analysis and salivary buffering capacity. Lactobacillus counts are a useful marker of patient compliance to a low carbohydrate diet.

The microbiology of periodontal disease is extremely complex (Chapter 23). The examination of a deep gingival smear to demonstrate the fusospirochaetal complex (Fig. 23.4) is a useful aid to the diagnosis of acute necrotizing ulcerative gingivitis. However, for other forms of periodontal disease there is still no consensus on which organisms are the key pathogens. Plaque can be screened for putative periodontal pathogens, including *Porphyromonas gingivalis*, *Prevotella intermedia*, and *Actinobacillus actinomycetemcomitans*, using methods such as anaerobic culture, antigen detection tests, and gene probes. However, for the present, the treatment of periodontal diseases is based largely on non-specific plaque-control measures, with the use of antimicrobial agents in certain circumstances.

Key facts

- Diagnostic microbiology laboratories identify organisms causing infections and undertake antimicrobial sensitivity testing to guide clinical treatment.

- The accuracy of a microbiological report can only be as good as the quality of the specimen submitted.

- Specimens can be collected for analysis by culture, antigen or genome detection, or serological techniques.

- Specimens must be transported to the laboratory as quickly as possible, making use of appropriate transport media.

- Care must be taken to avoid contamination of specimens with organisms from the normal flora.

- An aspirate of pus is the most appropriate specimen for microbiological analysis of purulent infections in the head and neck region.

- Swabs or oral rinses can be collected for diagnosing candidal infections of the oral mucosa.

- Viral infections of the oral mucosa can be diagnosed by tissue culture or antigen detection tests.

- Salivary counts of lactobacilli and mutans streptococci can be undertaken as a component of caries activity tests.

- A deep gingival smear with demonstration of the fusospirochaetal complex is useful for the confirmation of acute necrotizing ulcerative gingivitis.

Further reading

De la Maza, LM, Pezzlo, MT, and Baron, EJ (1997). *Color atlas of diagnostic microbiology*. Mosby Year Book, St Louis.

Mims, C, Playfair, J, Roitt, I, Wakelin, D, and Williams, R (1998). Diagnostic principles of clinical manifestations. In *Medical microbiology* (2nd edn), Section 13. Mosby, London.

Murray, PR, Rosenthal, KS, Kobayashi, GS, and Pfaller, MA (1998). General principles of laboratory diagnosis. In *Medical microbiology* (3rd edn), Section III. Mosby Year Book, St Louis.

Samaranayake, LP (1987). The wastage of microbial samples in clinical practice. *Dental Update*, 14, 53–61.

13

Infections of the skin and soft tissues

- The normal skin flora
- Bacterial infections of the skin and soft tissues
- Fungal infections of the skin
- Viral infections of the skin

Infections of the skin and soft tissues

The normal skin flora

The skin provides an excellent defence for the underlying tissues against invading, pathogenic micro-organisms (Chapter 7). Important factors in this protection are the normal skin's acid pH, the limited amount of moisture present, and excreted chemicals such as sebum, fatty acids, and urea. In addition, the skin is colonized by a large number of bacterial species which comprise the resident normal flora. This resident flora includes coagulase-negative staphylococci, micrococci, propionibacteria, and diphtheroids and plays an important defence role through the prevention of colonization by exogenous pathogens.

In addition to the resident flora, the skin may become colonized for short periods of time by a wider range of organisms known as the transient flora. Good examples include *Staphylococcus aureus* and enterobacteria. These organisms may survive for several hours if the skin is not washed and dried effectively, a fact of considerable importance in relation to hospital infection control and wound infection.

Staphylococcus aureus may be carried asymptomatically in the anterior nares or on other moist areas of the skin such as the axilla or groin. The prevalence of such carriage is much higher (up to 60%) in hospital staff than in the general population (10–30%), and is again relevant to hospital-acquired infections.

Bacterial infections of the skin and soft tissues

Figure 13.1 summarizes several ways in which the skin may become infected and damaged. *Staphylococcus aureus* and *Streptococcus pyogenes* (a group A beta-haemolytic streptococcus) are by far the most frequent causes of skin infections (Fig. 13.2) and will be discussed individually. In some instances, bacterial infections which become established in skin subsequently spread to involve deeper tissues and may also have significant systemic effects by virtue of toxin production. These features will become evident in the following sections.

Staphylococcal skin infections

Minor skin infections, such as boils, are commonly caused by *Staphylococcus aureus*, but this organism is also important in more

---

MODES OF INFECTION OF SKIN
Breach of intact skin
Permits infection from outside the skin
Skin manifestations of systemic infections
Blood-borne spread, for example typhoid
Direct extension, for example actinomycosis
Toxin-mediated skin damage
Microbial toxin produced at a distant site

Fig. 13.1 Mechanisms of skin infection.

serious wound infections. Infection may be either endogenous, for example transfer of organisms from the anterior nares to another body site, or exogenous whereby infection is acquired from an outside source, usually another person.

Staphylococci are catalase-positive Gram-positive cocci, the cells of which are typically arranged in clusters. The species *Staphylococcus aureus*, an important medical pathogen, produces the enzyme coagulase together with a range of exotoxins. Beta-lactamase stable penicillins are the treatment of choice, though resistance to methicillin is an increasing problem.

Boils and carbuncles

Boils (furuncles) result from a superficial infection with *Staphylococcus aureus* in and around a hair follicle (Fig. 13.3). There is an intense acute inflammatory response, with neutrophil infiltration and pus formation. However, fibrin is deposited, the site walled off, and the infection normally remains localized. Carbuncles are larger and deeper than boils and result from infection of multiple hair follicles. Typically they continue to expand until they erode the overlying skin, 'point', and then drain.

Diagnosis is usually clinical and treatment is by drainage, though antibiotics, for example flucloxacillin, may be needed if the infection is severe and/or the patient is febrile. Patients experiencing recurrent boils should be examined for chronic staphylococcal carriage and receive treatment of any carriage sites with topical antimicrobial agents such as neomycin or mupirocin. In addition, diabetes mellitus should be excluded as an underlying predisposing factor.

STAPHYLOCOCCAL AND STREPTOCOCCAL SKIN INFECTIONS

Breach of skin surface

Structure	Infection	Cause
Epidermis	Impetigo	*S. aureus* and/or *S. pyogenes*
Dermis	Erysipelas	*S. pyogenes*
Hair follicle	Folliculitis Boils Carbuncles	*S. aureus*
Subcutaneous tissues	Cellulitis	*S. pyogenes*
Fascia	Necrotizing fasciitis	*S. pyogenes* ± *S. aureus*

Toxin-mediated skin manifestations

Organism	Disease	Skin manifestation
S. pyogenes	Scarlet fever	Erythematous rash
S. aureus	Toxic shock syndrome	Rash and desquamation

Fig. 13.2 Table summarizing the range of skin infections caused by *Staphylococcus aureus* and *Streptococcus pyogenes*.

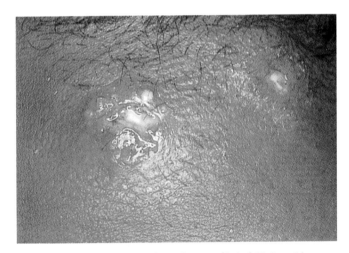

Fig. 13.3 Carbuncles caused by infection of hair follicles with *Staphylococcus aureus*. (Courtesy of Dr C. Gemmell.)

Toxic-shock syndrome

This serious systemic illness is caused by strains of *Staphylococcus aureus* which produce an exotoxin called toxic-shock syndrome toxin. The major clinical features are fever, skin rash (diffuse macular erythema), hypotension, and desquamation, the latter occurring 1–2 weeks after onset and affecting particularly the palms and soles. Many other body systems may be involved. Most physicians became aware of the disease in the early 1980s, when it was described primarily in healthy, young, menstruating women using tampons which became infected with *S. aureus*. Although this classic form of staphylococcal toxic-shock syndrome still occurs, it is now recognized in many other patients and clinical settings. Any clinical condition possibly involving staphylococcal infection or colonization may result in toxic-shock syndrome and it has been reported as a complication of virtually all types of surgical procedure.

Streptococcal skin infections

Streptococci are catalase-negative Gram-positive cocci, the cells of which are typically arranged in chains. They can be divided into three groups on the basis of the pattern of haemolysis seen on blood agar, namely beta (complete haemolysis), alpha (partial haemolysis), and gamma (no haemolysis). They can also be divided, on the basis of group-specific carbohydrate antigens, into the Lancefield groups (A to S).

Streptococcus pyogenes (Group A beta-haemolytic streptococcus) is responsible for most streptococcal skin infections. These infections are typically spreading in nature, because the organism produces a number of toxic products and enzymes, such as hyaluronidase. In many cases there is co-infection with *Staphylococcus aureus* (Fig. 13.2).

Impetigo

This is a superficial infection of the epidermis, usually due to *Streptococcus pyogenes* and seen most commonly in children. The infection is highly communicable. It is characterized by vesicles which later form golden crusts, occurring typically on the limb extremities or face (Fig. 13.4). Vesicle fluid, which contains the organism, infects adjacent skin areas. Secondary infection often

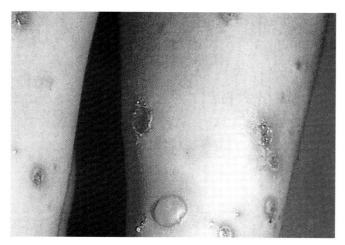

Fig. 13.4 Bullous impetigo affecting the skin of the legs. (Courtesy of Dr C. Gemmell.)

occurs with *Staphylococcus aureus*. Penicillin is the treatment of choice, or erythromycin for penicillin-allergic patients.

Certain strains of *Streptococcus pyogenes* (nephritogenic strains) are associated with the development of acute glomerulonephritis, as an autoimmune phenomenon. This complication occurs more frequently after skin infections than after throat infections. By contrast, rheumatic fever rarely follows streptococcal skin infections.

Cellulitis and erysipelas

Cellulitis presents as a spreading and marked erythema which is often painful. There is a brawny thickening of the skin and swelling of the subcutaneous tissues. Previous trauma or an underlying skin lesion predispose to cellulitis. It is a serious disease because of the propensity of the infection to spread via the lymphatics and bloodstream with development of marked constitutional upset and septicaemia. *Streptococcus pyogenes* is the commonest cause, though *Staphylococcus aureus* may also be implicated, often as a co-infecting organism. Penicillin is the treatment of choice, but if a staphylococcal element is suspected then flucloxacillin should be prescribed.

Erysipelas is a distinctive type of superficial cellulitis of the skin due to infection with *Streptococcus pyogenes*. There is prominent involvement of the lymphatics. Clinically it is a painful lesion with a bright red, oedematous, indurated appearance and an advancing raised border that is sharply demarcated from the surrounding normal skin. The face is frequently affected (Fig. 13.5), when there is often a typical butterfly distribution involving the cheeks and the nose. Lesions are also common on the lower extremities. Penicillin or erythromycin are the treatments of choice.

Necrotizing fasciitis

The last decade has seen an increase in serious *Streptococcus pyogenes* infections and the media have reported many cases of rapidly pro-

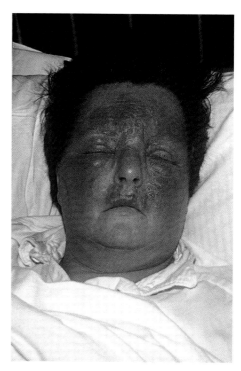

Fig. 13.5 Erysipelas involving the skin of the face.

gressing cutaneous infections involving skin, fascia, and muscle, often associated with this organism.

The term necrotizing fasciitis includes two different entities, dependent on the bacteriology (Fig. 13.6). Type I are mixed infections, including at least one strict anaerobe, whilst Type II infections are those from which *Streptococcus pyogenes* is isolated, either alone or in combination with other species, typically *Staphylococcus aureus*. These infections occur primarily in the limbs, although occasionally they are found in the head and neck region, with primary sites in the orbit or mouth.

Type II necrotizing fasciitis may follow minor trauma, stab wounds, or surgery, particularly in patients with diabetes and peripheral vascular disease. Major presenting features include

---

NECROTIZING FASCIITIS

Type I

Mixture of organisms

One strict anaerobe (commonly *Bacteroides* or *Peptostreptococcus* spp.) plus at least one facultative anaerobe (often Enterobacteriaceae)

Type II

Streptococcus pyogenes ± *Staphylococcus aureus*

Fig. 13.6 The two forms of necrotizing fasciitis.

fever, confusion, tachycardia, hypotension, and multiorgan failure. These infections can develop rapidly, run a fulminant course, and prove fatal within 24 hours. They are often associated with particular strains of *Streptococcus pyogenes*, notably those producing pyrogenic exotoxins, and it is believed to be exotoxin release rather than bacteraemia that is responsible for the severe complications. Development of tissue necrosis in a streptococcal soft-tissue infection is a late feature and results from local thrombosis of the arterioles supplying the skin. Management entails both surgery and antibiotic administration.

Infection of burns

Bacterial infection of burns is very common and causes significant mortality. Organisms implicated include *Staphylococcus aureus* and Gram-negative bacilli. Whilst these infections are often superficial and mild, they may also infect deeper tissues and cause septicaemia. *Pseudomonas aeruginosa* frequently infects burns. Not only can this organism prevent grafts from taking successfully but it may also cause pseudomonas septicaemia, which has an extremely high mortality.

All patients with burns should be nursed in isolation, with strict attention paid to good aseptic technique. Without such measures, cross-infection is very likely to occur.

Gas gangrene

Wounds, whether resulting from accidental trauma or surgery, may become infected with organisms of the genus *Clostridium*, particularly in the presence of muscle injury. Clostridia are Gram-positive anaerobic spore-forming rods. They are widely distributed in soil and in the gut of man and animals. Their pathogenicity is dominated by the production of enzymes and potent exotoxins.

Though gas gangrene may be caused by several species of clostridia, the most common is *Clostridium perfringens*, which may enter wounds from the patient's own faecal flora or from the environment. Infection tends to develop in areas of the body with a

poor blood supply because of the associated anaerobic conditions. The organisms multiply initially within the subcutaneous tissues, producing gas in the tissues and an anaerobic cellulitis. Subsequently they invade deeper into the muscle, which undergoes rapid disintegration (Fig. 13.7).

Clinically, the onset of the disease is acute, progressing rapidly in a matter of hours. Pain, often excruciating, is an early symptom and because of the severe toxaemia patients rapidly become extremely unwell. Ensuing complications include shock, jaundice, and acute renal failure. The mortality rate is high.

Much of the tissue damage results from the production by *Clostridium perfringens* of a lecithinase enzyme (alpha toxin) which hydrolyses lipids in cell membranes to cause cell lysis and death. This enzyme can be detected in the laboratory by the Nagler reaction (Fig. 13.8).

Microbiological diagnosis requires the collection of pus, wound swabs, and blood cultures for the preparation of anaerobic cultures on blood agar and, where appropriate, Gram films. Identification relies on biochemical tests and the Nagler reaction.

Treatment entails prompt and extensive surgery to excise infected and dead tissue. Antibiotic administration, typically penicillin, is an important adjunct to surgery. Treatment in a hyperbaric oxygen chamber, to increase oxygenation of the tissues, has been recommended but its efficacy is still under debate.

In view of the severity of this infection, prevention is important. Wounds should be cleaned and debrided as soon as possible to remove dead and poorly perfused tissue which favours the growth of anaerobes. Prophylactic antibiotics should be administered preoperatively to patients undergoing elective surgery of body sites liable to contamination with faecal flora, particularly in diabetic patients with ischaemic arterial disease.

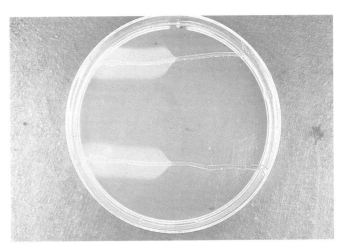

Fig. 13.8 The Nagler reaction. The alphatoxin produced by *Clostridium perfringens* is a lecithinase. Here the organism is growing on a medium containing lecithin. The alphatoxin has produced opacity around the line of growth on the left side of the plate. This has been inhibited by application of anti-alpha toxin to the right side.

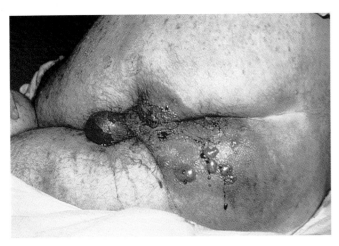

Fig. 13.7 Gas gangrene, caused by *Clostridium perfringens*, involving the buttock. (Courtesy of Dr C. Gemmell.)

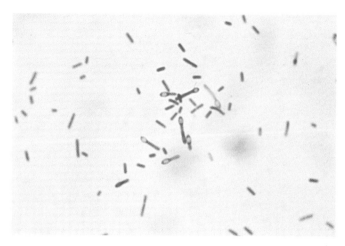

Fig. 13.9 A Gram-stained film of *C. tetani*. Note the terminal spores.

Tetanus

Clostridium tetani also establishes infection through broken skin. Spores of the organism (Fig 13.9), originating from animal faecal material, are found in soil and may then enter a wound. Under appropriate anaerobic conditions the organism multiplies locally and releases an exotoxin called tetanospasmin. Deep or penetrating wounds in avascular sites are most likely to become complicated by tetanus, particularly in the presence of a foreign body. However, the disease may occur following a trivial injury and in some cases there is no history of a previous wound.

The powerful exotoxin is responsible for all the features of this disease. The toxin is carried in peripheral nerve axons to the central nervous system, where it binds to the presynaptic terminals of inhibitory spinal neurones, blocks the release of inhibitory mediators, and causes excessive activity of motor neurones. This results in the muscular spasms typical of tetanus.

Patients develop exaggerated reflexes, muscle rigidity, and uncontrolled muscle spasms. Lockjaw (trismus) is a characteristic early feature of the disease. Muscular spasm also causes dysphagia (difficulty swallowing), 'risus sardonicus' of the face, and opisthotonus (arching of the back) (Fig. 13.10). Death, which occurs in up to 50% of cases, results from exhaustion and respiratory failure.

Treatment involves the prompt administration of antitetanus immunoglobulin, excision of the wound, and provision of penicillin to inhibit bacterial replication. Skilled intensive care management in a specialist centre gives patients the best hope of survival.

Prevention of such a serious infection is critical. Although more common in developing countries, the disease is now rare in developed countries (less than 100 new cases per year in Britain). Universal immunization with tetanus toxoid (Chapter 8) could eliminate the disease altogether.

FACTORS INFLUENCING WOUND SEPSIS
Type of wound
'Clean' wound
No incisions through gastrointestinal, respiratory, or genitourinary tracts
Sepsis rate: 2–5%
Usually *Staphylococcus aureus*
'Contaminated' wound
Surgery involving site with known normal flora for example colon
Sepsis rate: 10–40%
Gram-negative bacilli and anaerobes predominate
'Infected' wound
For example drainage of an abscess
Sepsis rate: 100%
Presence of foreign body or prosthesis
Increases risk of infection
Infection with low-grade pathogens
Surgical team
Lower sepsis rate for skilled surgeons
Carriers of *Staphylococcus aureus* in operating team increase likelihood of wound infection
The patient
Elderly and debilitated have higher wound infection rates
Short preoperative stay reduces risk
Appropriate peroperative antibiotic prophylaxis may reduce wound infection rates

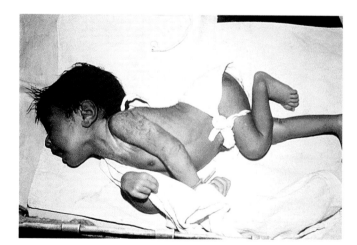

Fig. 13.10 Tetanus in a child. Note the arching of the back (opisthotonus). (Courtesy of Dr C. Gemmell.)

Fig. 13.11 The range of factors influencing the risk of wound infection.

Surgical wound infection

Surgical wound infections account for about a quarter of all hospital-acquired infections. Whilst some wound infections are caused by cross-infection in the operating theatre or ward, many are endogenous and derived from the patient's own flora. The factors influencing wound sepsis are summarized in Fig. 13.11, of which the most important is the type of surgical wound.

The most obvious clinical feature of an infected wound is the discharge of pus. Major wound sepsis may result in delayed wound healing, in dehiscence of the wound, or the spread of infection to deeper structures such as bones, joints, or the peritoneal cavity. It may also result in the failure of skin grafts.

Prevention of wound infections depends on skilled surgical technique, careful nursing with due attention to the risks of cross-infection, and the judicious use of antibiotic prophylaxis for appropriate cases.

Fungal infections of the skin

Fungal infections of the skin may be confined to the outer layer (superficial mycoses) or may penetrate into the epidermis or dermis (subcutaneous mycoses).

Superficial mycoses

Dermatophyte infections

Dermatophytes are keratin-loving organisms which invade the keratinized layers of the skin, nails, or hair to cause tinea infec-

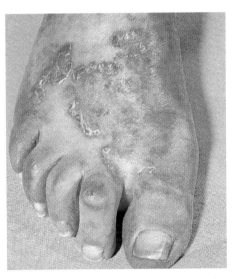

Fig. 13.12 Dermatophyte infection of the skin of the foot, caused by *Trichophyton rubrum*. (Courtesy of Dr M. Richardson.)

COMMON DERMATOPHYTE INFECTIONS	
Infection	**Common causes**
Tinea capitis (Scalp ringworm) Disease of childhood Scaling of scalp skin, erythema, and inflammation Hair loss is characteristic but not permanent	*Microsporum audouinii*
Tinea pedis (Athlete's foot) Peeling, maceration, and cracking of skin between toes May spread to involve sole of foot	*Trichophyton rubrum* *Trichophyton mentagrophytes (interdigitale)*
Tinea corporis (Body ringworm) Often misdiagnosed Most lesions have prominent scaling margin with pustules or papules and a less inflamed centre Commonly affects trunk and legs	Mainly *Trichophyton* spp.
Tinea cruris Scaling and irritation in the groin, extending onto anterior thigh Mainly young adult males	*Trichophyton rubrum* *Epidermophyton floccosum*
Onchomycosis (Ringworm of the nails) Yellow discoloration at side of affected nails Nails become brittle and thickened	*Trichophyton rubrum*

Fig. 13.13 Summary of the common dermatophyte infections.

tions (ringworm) (Fig. 13.12). These infections are among the most common in humans and frequently affect the hands and feet. There are three important genera of dermatophytes, namely *Trichophyton*, *Microsporum*, and *Epidermophyton*. They are categorized as zoophilic, anthropophilic, or geophilic depending on whether the original source is animal, human, or soil, respectively. Infections are spread by contact with arthrospores, the thick-walled spores formed by dermatophyte hyphae. These are shed from the primary host in skin scales and hair. Details of the commonest dermatophyte infections are given in Fig. 13.13.

DIAGNOSIS

Some dermatophytes fluoresce under ultraviolet light. This can be a useful clinical diagnostic aid, particularly for tinea capitis.

Scrapings or clippings from the lesions are collected. Initially, these are examined by direct microscopy after 'clearing' the tissue in warm potassium hydroxide so that fungal hyphae and spores can be seen. Specimens are also cultured on Sabouraud's agar, often requiring prolonged incubation. Confirmation of identity depends on the colonial (Fig. 13.14 (a)) and microscopic (Fig. 13.14 (b)) characteristics of the cultured organism.

TREATMENT

Topical treatment, including both antifungal and keratolytic agents, is used as far as possible, but nail and hair infections are better treated by the oral administration of antifungal drugs. The oral agent used most commonly is griseofulvin. Azole antifungals (Chapter 9) are also active against the common dermatophyte fungi.

Superficial candidosis

Candida albicans is the most important cause of superficial forms of candidosis (Chapter 26). Whilst organisms of the genus *Candida* can be isolated from the mouth and intestinal tract of up to 50% of the general population, they are found in only low numbers on healthy, intact skin. However, they can rapidly colonize damaged skin and apposed skin sites which are moist and chafed.

Lesions of superficial cutaneous candidosis (intertrigo) usually begin as vesicles and pustules in the groin and other skin folds. The pustules rupture and develop into erythematous areas with an irregular margin. Interdigital lesions arise as small fissures in the interdigital folds and are usually seen in those whose occupation entails prolonged immersion of the hands in water. Such individuals often also complain of nail and nail-fold infections with *Candida* species.

The term chronic mucocutaneous candidosis describes a group of uncommon conditions in which individuals with congenital immunological or endocrine disorders develop mucosal, cutaneous, or nail infections with *Candida albicans*. A more detailed description is given in Chapter 26. The mouth is involved first, but lesions subsequently appear on the scalp, trunk, hands, and feet, often involving the nails.

Subcutaneous mycoses

Subcutaneous mycoses are rare and will not be described in detail. They usually develop following traumatic implantation of the causative fungus into the skin.

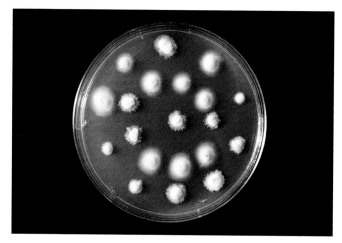

(a)

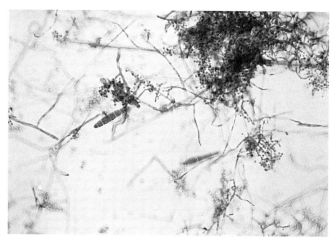

(b)

Fig. 13.14 Culture (a) and microscopy (b) of the dermatophyte *Trichophyton rubrum*. (Courtesy of Dr M. Richardson.)

The most common type is sporotrichosis, a subacute or chronic infection caused by the fungus *Sporothrix schenckii*. Because the organism is found in soil, on plants, and on sphagnum moss, it is an occupational hazard for those such as gardeners and florists. It typically affects exposed sites, especially the hands and fingers, most commonly presenting as a localized cutaneous or subcutaneous nodule with a series of secondary nodules along draining lymphatics. Diagnosis is confirmed by culture, and treatment is with oral potassium iodide or itraconazole.

Viral infections of the skin

There are two types of mucocutaneous lesions caused by viruses. In the first type, the virus remains localized to the site of initial infection, for example the papillomaviruses which cause warts. The second category includes those in which the virus causes

COMMON VIRAL SKIN LESIONS		
Virus	**Lesion**	**Virus shedding from lesion**
Localized infections		
Papillomaviruses	Common, plantar and genital warts	✔
Molluscum contagiosum	Fleshy papule	✔
Systemic spread		
Herpes simplex	Vesicular (neural spread and latency)	✔
Varicella zoster		
Coxsackievirus A16	Vesicular (hand, foot, and mouth disease)	✔
Human parvovirus B19	Facial rash: 'slapped cheek syndrome'	
Human herpesvirus 6	Exanthem subitum	
Measles	Maculopapular rash	
Rubella	Maculopapular rash	

Fig. 13.15 The common skin lesions caused by viruses.

mucocutaneous lesions after spreading systemically through the body, for example chickenpox, caused by varicella zoster virus. Furthermore, some viral infections result in a skin rash (exanthem), the lesions of which are non-infectious and immunologically mediated, such as measles and rubella.

The common cutaneous lesions caused by viruses are summarized in Fig. 13.15. Viral infections of the oral mucosa are discussed in detail in Chapter 27.

Papillomavirus infections

There are more than 70 types of human papillomaviruses and are the cause of skin papillomas (warts) as well as some intraoral lesions. At least five types are responsible for sexually transmitted genital warts (Chapter 14), with other types related to plantar warts and those on the knees and fingers. They may be transmitted by direct contact or indirectly. Warts eventually regress under the influence of the immune response, but treatment with dry ice or liquid nitrogen is regularly employed.

Molluscum contagiosum

A pox virus is responsible for molluscum contagiosum. The virus, which spreads by direct contact, infects epidermal cells resulting in a fleshy lesion with an umbilicated centre. These lesions disappear spontaneously within a few months.

Herpes simplex virus infection

Orofacial infections with herpes simplex virus are described in Chapter 27. On the skin, herpes simplex virus is responsible for recurrent cold sores and genital lesions. The skin of the finger may also become infected to cause an herpetic whitlow (Fig 13.16). This was an important occupational disease of dentists prior to the universal wearing of protective latex gloves.

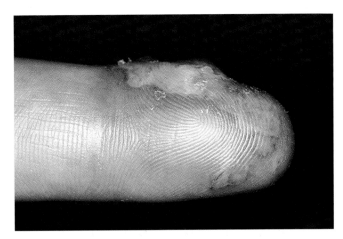

Fig. 13.16 An herpetic whitlow caused by herpes simplex virus type I on the finger of a recently qualified dental surgeon.

Herpetic infection of areas of eczematous skin can lead to severe disease in young children, requiring prompt and vigorous treatment. Similarly, primary or reactivated herpes simplex virus infections in immunocompromised hosts can be very serious.

The antiviral drug aciclovir (Chapter 9) has revolutionized the treatment of herpes simplex virus infections, especially in those at risk of serious disease.

Varicella zoster virus infection

Primary infection with varicella zoster virus causes chickenpox. Following initial infection of the respiratory tract, the virus infects mononuclear cells and is transported to the lymphoreticular tissues where it multiplies. The virus then enters the blood and is distributed to epithelial sites, with subsequent development of vesicles in the skin, particularly of the trunk, face, and scalp, and in some mucosal sites, including the mouth. The vesicles typically appear in 'crops', develop into pustules, and then break down before they scab over.

During the primary infection, varicella zoster virus enters sensory nerve endings and establishes a latent infection within nerve ganglia. Reactivation later in life causes shingles. Since this painful disease affects only the dermatome at the site of reactivation, the vesicular eruption is strictly unilateral (Fig 13.17). Increasing age and immunosuppression both predispose to shingles. Whilst the disease is commonest in the thoracic region, it also occurs in the head and neck; a detailed description of the clinical features of the condition is given in Chapter 27. Treatment is with high-dose aciclovir.

Other viral infections of the skin

Figure 13.15 lists several other viral infections involving the skin. Coxsackievirus infections are most common in children and cause a variety of skin rashes and lesions on mucosal surfaces. Two such infections, herpangina and hand, foot, and mouth disease, are considered in Chapter 27.

Human parvovirus B19 causes a febrile disease in children. Because of the characteristic maculopapular rash on the skin of the face, it has been termed 'slapped cheek syndrome' or 'erythema infectiosum'. However, symptomless infection is common and half the population have serological evidence of previous infection.

Human herpesvirus 6 infects nearly all infants in the first few months of life. It is commonly present in the saliva of adults, which is the probable source of infection. In a small proportion of infected infants it causes a mild febrile disease with a maculopapular rash, known as exanthem subitum.

Key facts

- *Staphylococcus aureus* and *Streptococcus pyogenes* are the commonest bacterial causes of skin infections.

- *Staphylococcus aureus* typically causes localized, purulent skin infections, for example boils.

- Skin infections caused by *Streptococcus pyogenes* are often spreading in nature, for example impetigo, erysipelas, and cellulitis.

- Bacterial superinfection of burns, for example with *Pseudomonas aeruginosa*, is a common clinical problem.

- Gas gangrene, caused by the spore-forming organism *Clostridium perfringens*, develops in damaged, poorly perfused tissue.

- Much of the tissue destruction in gas gangrene is a result of lecithinase production by *Clostridium perfringens*.

- The clinical features of tetanus, caused by infection with *Clostridium tetani*, are a result of the release of the exotoxin tetanospasmin.

- Development of wound sepsis relates to the type of wound, the presence of foreign bodies, the skill of the surgical team, and the medical status of the patient.

- The important fungal infections of skin are those caused by dermatophytes and those caused by *Candida albicans*.

- Skin manifestations of viral infection may represent either localized infections, for example warts, or systemic infections such as chickenpox.

- Herpes simplex and varicella zoster viruses cause both primary and reactivation skin lesions and are an important cause of disease in the head and neck region.

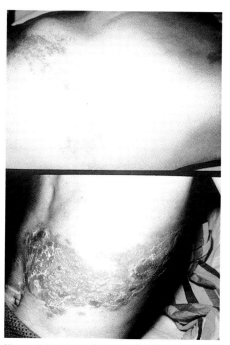

Fig. 13.17 Zoster (shingles) of the trunk, illustrating the unilateral, 'belt-like' distribution of the vesicular eruption. It follows reactivation of the virus in a dorsal root ganglion.

Further reading

Mims, C, Playfair, J, Roitt, I, Wakelin, D, and Williams, R (1998). Infections of the skin, muscle, joints, bone and hemopoietic system. In *Medical microbiology* (2nd edn), Chapter 23. Mosby, London.

Murray, PR, Rosenthal, KS, Kobayashi, GS, and Pfaller, MA (1998). Superficial, cutaneous and subcutaneous mycoses. In *Medical microbiology* (3rd edn), Chapter 69. Mosby Year Book, St Louis.

Shanson, DC (1989) Skin infections and infestations. In *Microbiology in clinical practice* (2nd edn), Chapter 16. Butterworth–Heinemann, Oxford.

Genitourinary tract infections

- Sexually transmitted diseases
- Urinary tract infections

Genitourinary tract infections

Sexually transmitted diseases

Introduction

Several infectious diseases are transmitted mainly or entirely by sexual intercourse. Often the causal organisms are delicate and do not remain viable outside the body for long. Transmission of the infective agents by direct contact between mucosal surfaces is essential. The primary lesion tends to be on the genitalia but several infections give rise to systemic manifestations. The prevalence of sexually transmitted diseases (STD) increased during the 1970s and early 1980s, but by the late 1980s and early 1990s a decline occurred, particularly in relation to gonorrhoea. Fear of AIDS and the promotion through the media of 'safe sex', particularly using condoms, may have played a part in this. Variations in sexual behaviour and practices can result in sexually transmitted diseases producing primary lesions in the rectum or oropharynx (Chapter 27). The spread of STDs is inextricably linked with sexual behaviour, and as such there are far greater opportunities for the control of such infections than in the case of respiratory infections. Infected but asymptomatic individuals play an important role, as does promiscuity. Transmission between heterosexuals or male homosexuals can take place following oral or anal intercourse, and it is not surprising that genital lesions or ulcers increase the risk of acquiring infections such as HIV. STDs do not necessarily come singly and the possibility of multiple infection, for example syphilis and gonorrhoea, should always be considered.

The top nine sexually transmitted diseases are listed (Fig. 14.1) together with brief details of treatment. The organisms respons-

COMMON SEXUALLY TRANSMITTED DISEASES			
Organism	Diseases	Comment	Possible treatments
Papillomaviruses	Genital warts, dysplasias	Commonest of all STDs. Associated with cancer of the cervix and penis	Podophyllin, surgical removal. No chemotherapy available
Chlamydia trachomatis (D–K serotypes)	Non-specific urethritis (NSU)	Increasing incidence	Tetracycline
Candida albicans	Vaginal thrush, balanitis	Very common. Several predisposing factors	Nystatin, clotrimazole, fluconazole
Trichomonas vaginalis	Vaginitis, urethritis	Very common	Metronidazole
Herpes simplex viruses types 1 and 2	Genital herpes	Increasing incidence. Problem of latency and reactivation	Aciclovir
Neisseria gonorrhoeae	Gonorrhoea	Decreasing incidence in developed countries	Penicillin, cefotaxime, spectinomycin
Human immunodeficiency virus	AIDS	Lethal. Incidence increasing world-wide	Azidothymidine (AZT) and other antiretroviral drugs
Treponema pallidum	Syphilis	Decreasing incidence in developed countries	Penicillin
Hepatitis B virus	Hepatitis	Particularly male homosexuals, but incidence decreasing	None but prevention by effective vaccine

Fig. 14.1 Table summarizing the 'top nine' sexually transmitted diseases.

ible for a number of these infections are described in other chapters, for example HIV (Chapter 19), hepatitis B (Chapter 18), *Candida albicans* (Chapter 26), and herpes simplex virus (Chapter 27). Some produce oral manifestations, for example *Treponema pallidum* and *Neisseria gonorrhoeae* (Chapter 27). A brief mention of all these infections will be included in this chapter, but more detailed coverage will be limited to those which have relevance to dentistry.

Syphilis

Syphilis is now a relatively rare disease, but it is still important because of its severity and long-term effects if inadequately treated. The causative agent is *Treponema pallidum* which is a motile helicobacterium. Spirochaetes have a unique helico structure: a central protoplasmic cylinder which is bounded by the cytoplasmic membrane and a cell wall of similar structure to that of Gram-negative bacteria (Fig. 14.2). Between a thin peptidoglycan layer and the outer membrane run the axial filaments, now regarded as internal flagella. These filaments are fixed at the extremities of the organism and meet to overlap in the middle of the cell. They constrict and distort the bacterial cell body to give rise to the typical structure and motility.

The pathogenesis of syphilis is complex and is summarized in Fig. 14.3. The treponemes enter the body through minute abrasions on the skin or mucous membranes and after multiplication at the site of infection spread to the regional lymph nodes. Typically the course of infection is divided into three stages – primary, secondary, and tertiary syphilis. However, a substantial proportion of individuals remain permanently free of the disease after suffering the primary or secondary stages of infection. The secondary stage may be followed by a latent period of 3–30 years, after which the disease may recur. The organism can survive in the body for many years despite a substantial immune response. A

typical primary chancre on the penis is shown in Fig. 14.4. The oral manifestations of syphilis are summarized in Fig. 14.3 and discussed in detail in Chapter 27.

Treponema pallidum is one of the few bacteria capable of crossing the placental border to infect the fetus and so cause congenital syphilis. Transmission usually occurs after the first three months of pregnancy. Manifestations of the disease range from serious infection resulting in intrauterine death to congenital abnormalities which may be obvious at birth, or to silent infections which may not be apparent until about two years of age. Amongst the latter are the dental abnormalities associated with infection of the developing tooth germs by *T. pallidum*. Since the deciduous teeth are usually well developed by the time the spirochaetes invade the developing dental tissues, these teeth are minimally affected. The first permanent molar teeth are usually involved and have roughened hypoplastic occlusal surfaces with poorly developed cusps and are smaller in size than normal. The upper central incisors may also be affected (Hutchinson's incisors), with crescentic notches in the middle of their incisal edge and a greater width gingivally than at the incisal edge, giving a 'screwdriver' appearance (Fig. 14.5).

The laboratory diagnosis of syphilis is illustrated in Fig. 14.6. Dark-ground microscopy is not commonly performed and the diagnosis is generally based on the results of serological tests. The Venereal Disease Reference Laboratory (VDRL) test contains a non-specific antigen which can produce biological false-positive reactions. Antibodies to this antigen disappear with treatment. The other tests employ specific treponemal antigens and while they give fewer false-positive reactions they remain positive after treatment.

Penicillin is the drug of choice and in primary infections large doses are continued for 2 or 3 weeks. In late or latent syphilis large doses for 3 weeks usually followed by 10 injections at weekly

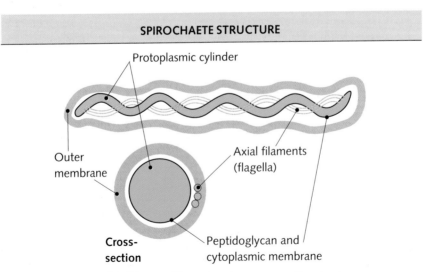

SPIROCHAETE STRUCTURE

Fig. 14.2 Diagram illustrating the structure of a spirochaete.

THE PATHOGENESIS OF SYPHILIS			
Stage of disease	**Signs and symptoms**	**Pathogenesis**	**Oral manifestations**
Initial contact ⇩ 2–10 weeks (depends on inoculum size) ⇩	Primary chancre at site of infection. Usually penis and vulva	Multiplication of treponemes at site of infection Associated host response	Chancre of lip, tongue, angles of mouth Infectious lesions
Primary syphilis ⇩ 1–3 months ⇩	Enlarged inguinal nodes Spontaneous healing	Proliferation of treponemes in regional lymph nodes	Cervicofacial lymph node enlargement Spontaneous healing
Secondary syphilis ⇩ 2–6 weeks ⇩	Flu-like illness Myalgia, headache, fever Mucocutaneous rash: dull red, macular or papular spots Spontaneous resolution	Multiplication with production of lesions in lymph nodes, liver, joints, muscles, skin, and mucous membranes	Greyish white glistening patches on gum, tonsil, soft palate, tongue, cheek
Latent syphilis ⇩ 3–30 years ⇩		Treponemes dormant in ?liver and spleen Re-awakening and multiplication of treponemes	
Tertiary syphilis	Neurosyphilis: general paralysis of the insane, tabes dorsalis Progressive destructive disease Cardiovascular syphilis: aortic lesions, heart failure	Further dissemination, invasion and host response (cell-mediated hypersensitivity) Gummas in skin, bone, testis	'Gumma' of palate, rarely osteomyelitis. Syphilitic leukoplakia with risk of oral carcinoma

Fig. 14.3 The clinical features, pathogenesis, and oral manifestations of syphilis.

intervals are recommended. Erythromycin or tetracycline can be used if the patient is hypersensitive to penicillin.

Gonorrhoea

Gonorrhoea is a bacterial infection caused by the Gram-negative coccus *Neisseria gonorrhoeae*. This organism causes natural infection only in humans and thus its only reservoir is in humans. Transmission is through sexual contact from person to person, and since it is sensitive to drying and survives poorly outside the human host, intimate contact is necessary for spread. The main reservoir is asymptomatic infected individuals, usually women.

The usual site of entry of *N. gonorrhoeae* into the body is via the vagina or the urethral mucosa of the penis, but other sexual practices may deposit the pathogen in the mouth or rectum. The structure and virulence factors of *N. gonorrhoeae* are diagrammatically represented in Fig. 14.7. The organism possesses adhesive properties (pili) which allow it to attach to mucosal cells and thereby evade removal by washing, by micturition, or vaginal discharge. Following attachment, the organism proliferates and

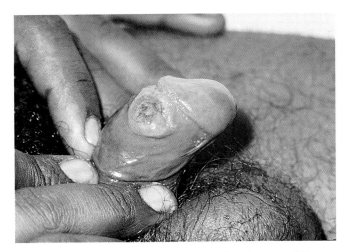

Fig. 14.4 A penile chancre of primary syphilis. (Courtesy of Gower Medical Publishing.)

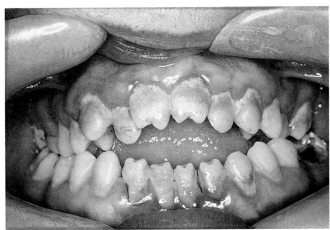

Fig. 14.5 Hutchinson's incisors: an oral manifestation of congenital syphilis. (Courtesy of Prof. D.G. MacDonald.)

DIAGNOSIS OF SYPHILIS

Microscopy

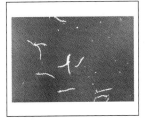

Dark-ground microscopy
of *Treponema pallidum* in fluid
from a chancre x 1000

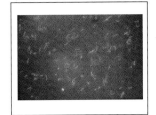

Fluorescent Treponema
Antibody Absorbed
(FTA Abs)

Culture

Treponema pallidum cannot be cultured *in vitro*. It can be propagated in animals, for example rabbit testes. This allows organisms to be prepared for serological tests

Serological tests

Stage of disease	VD Reference Laboratory (VDRL)	Treponema Pallidum Haemagglutination (TPHA)	Fluorescent Treponema Antibody Absorbed (FTA(Abs))
Primary	+ or -	-	+
Late primary	+	+ or -	+
Secondary and tertiary	+	+	+
Late (quaternary)	+	+	+
Latent	+ or -	+	+
Treated syphilis	-	+	+
Congenital syphilis	+	+	+

Fig. 14.6 Summary of the laboratory methods for diagnosing syphilis.

STRUCTURE OF *NEISSERIA GONORRHOEAE*

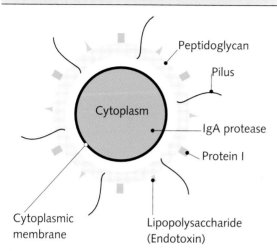

Fig. 14.7 Structure and virulence factors of *Neisseria gonorrhoeae*.

spreads through the cervix in women and up the urethra in men. Spread is facilitated by various virulence factors and the organism protects itself from the host's secretory antibodies by means of an IgA protease. An acute inflammatory reaction with pus formation ensues, and while the infection usually remains localized, bacteria can invade the bloodstream and cause disseminated infections.

In the male, symptoms are characterized by a urethral discharge and pain on passing urine, whereas in female patients a vaginal discharge occurs. While symptoms develop within 2–7 days, at least half of all women infected have mild symptoms or are completely asymptomatic. Complications in men are unusual; but infertility, resulting from damage to the fallopian tubes and other chronic pelvic inflammatory conditions, is not

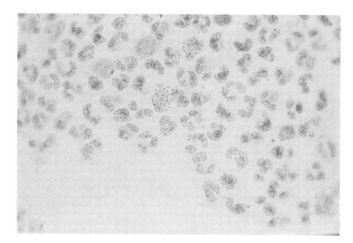

Fig. 14.8 Gram-stained film of urethral discharge from a male patient with gonorrhoea, illustrating the intracellular Gram-negative diplococci.

uncommon in women who receive no treatment. Both primary and secondary infection of the oral mucosa by *Neisseria gonorrhoeae* can occur (Chapter 27) and may be asymptomatic.

The laboratory diagnosis of gonorrhoea rests on microscopy and culture of urethral and vaginal discharges. The typical appearance of a Gram-stained film of a urethral discharge from a symptomatic male is shown in Fig. 14.8. It is essential that the diagnosis of gonorrhoea is confirmed by culture and identification. Additional antibiotic susceptibility tests should be performed. The standard treatment of gonorrhoea consists of a large single dose of amoxycillin, along with probenecid to delay its renal excretion. Ciprofloxacin (for infections complicated by chlamydia) may also be used. For extragenital infections, for example oropharyngeal gonorrhoea, 5–7 days' therapy may be necessary. *Neisseria gonorrhoeae* is extremely sensitive to penicillin but resistant strains of the pathogen are present in the population. Penicillin-resistant gonorrhoea can be treated with a number of drugs, for example ciprofloxacin or erythromycin.

Non-specific urethritis or cervicitis

The chlamydiae are very small bacteria which are obligate intracellular parasites. They have a complicated life cycle because they exist in different forms. The elementary body (EB) is adapted for extracellular survival and for initiating infection, while the reticulate body (RB) occurs in intracellular multiplication (Fig. 14.9). Certain serotypes of *Chlamydia trachomatis* cause genital infection and are acquired during sexual intercourse. Asymptomatic infection is common, especially in women, and non-specific urethritis is now the commonest sexually transmitted disease in Britain.

The clinical features in the male consist of an acute purulent urethral discharge which is indistinguishable clinically from that of gonorrhoea. Sometimes cervicitis is present in females but the disease is usually symptomless. Since infection with chlamydia is indistinguishable from other causes, a definitive diagnosis requires laboratory tests. The diagnosis is dependent on the demonstration of chlamydia elementary bodies or of antigen by indirect immunofluorescence with a monoclonal antibody. The drug of choice is tetracycline for 7–10 days but relapses are common. Alternatively, ciprofloxacin can be used.

Genital herpes

There are two types of herpes simplex virus: type 1 (HSV 1) which usually causes primary oropharyngeal infection; and HSV 2 which is transmitted by the venereal route and produces genital lesions. Although HSV 2 causes the majority of genital infections, HSV 1 is implicated in about a quarter of cases.

The primary lesion of infection with HSV 2 is vesicular. The vesicles soon break down to form painful, shallow ulcers on the penis and vulva about 5 days after infection. Local lymph nodes are enlarged and other symptoms include headache, fever, and malaise. Healing may take 2 weeks, and during this time the virus travels up sensory nerve endings to establish latent infection in dorsal route ganglion neurones. The latent virus can be reacti-

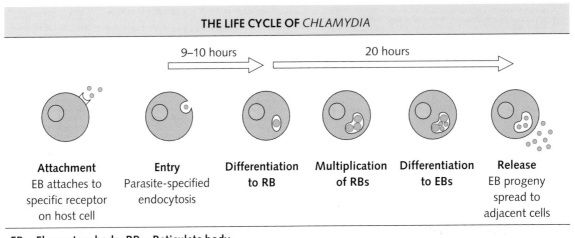

THE LIFE CYCLE OF *CHLAMYDIA*

9–10 hours   20 hours

Attachment	Entry	Differentiation to RB	Multiplication of RBs	Differentiation to EBs	Release
EB attaches to specific receptor on host cell	Parasite-specified endocytosis				EB progeny spread to adjacent cells

EB = Elementary body. RB = Reticulate body

Fig. 14.9 Diagram illustrating the life cycle of *Chlamydia*.

vated from this site, travel down nerves to the same area, and cause recurrent lesions (genital 'cold sores'). In addition, aseptic meningitis can occur in adults as a rare complication. Diagnosis is generally made by clinical examination but, if necessary, a sample of the vesicle fluid or a swab from the ulcer can be collected and HSV 1 or HSV 2 detected by tissue-culture or by immunological techniques.

Topical aciclovir can be beneficial for severe or early lesions and the drug can be given intravenously when systemic complications occur. Some patients experience troublesome recurrent attacks and in a percentage of individuals long-term low-dose treatment with oral aciclovir may reduce the frequency of symptoms.

Papillomavirus infection

There are about 70 distinct types of human papillomavirus that infect the skin or mucosal surfaces of humans. Many are adapted to specific regions of the body, for example Types 6, 12, 18, and 31 are transmitted by the venereal route. Infection by these viruses results in the appearance of warts on the penis, vulva, and perianal regions after an incubation period of 1–6 months. The lesions may be present for many months and can be treated with podophyllin. Flat areas of dysplasia form on the cervix and because of the association with cervical cancer (especially types 16 and 18) these lesions are best removed by laser.

Trichomoniasis

The causative agent of this infection inhabits the vagina in women and the urethra in men and is transmitted during sexual intercourse. *Trichomonas vaginalis* is a pear-shaped protozoan, which is motile by four flagella (Fig. 14.10). In women, infection is usually symptomatic, but varies from an acute severe vaginitis with typically a copious, offensive, greenish-yellow discharge; while in men, infection is usually asymptomatic, but sometimes causes a mild urethritis. The clinical diagnosis can be confirmed

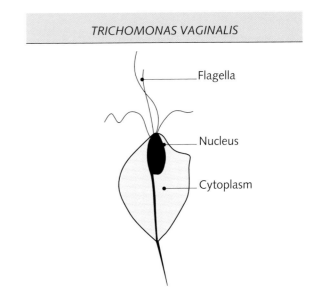

TRICHOMONAS VAGINALIS

Flagella

Nucleus

Cytoplasm

Fig. 14.10 *Trichomonas vaginalis*: this protozoan is motile by means of its four flagella.

by examining a direct wet film of the discharge which shows typical motile protozoa. The organism can also be cultured. Treatment is with oral metronidazole for 7 days, although a large, single dose is recommended for symptomatic infections. In addition, regular male partners of symptomatic women should also be treated with metronidazole to prevent reinfection.

Vaginal thrush (candidosis)

Yeasts, especially *Candida albicans*, normally inhabit the female vagina but in certain circumstances, which are not always clearly understood, the numbers of *Candida* increase and produce itching and irritation of the vulva or vagina (vaginal thrush). The infection is therefore endogenous, since it is caused by microbial agents from the individual's own microflora. White, membranous patches are usually present with a thick, white – or sometimes watery – discharge. Urethritis and dysuria may also be present. About 10% of male partners of females with vulvovaginal candidosis develop balanitis. The mycology, laboratory diagnosis, and treatment of candidosis is described in detail in Chapter 26, which deals with the oral form of the disease. Vaginal candidosis can usually be diagnosed on clinical grounds, but laboratory confirmation involves the examination of a Gram film and culture of a sample of the discharge. Treatment is with an oral antifungal, such as fluconazole, or a topical preparation such as nystatin.

Urinary tract infections

As indicated above, a number of sexually transmitted diseases have important oral manifestations. This is not the case for urinary tract infections, and the following section gives only a brief overview of this type of infection.

The urinary tract is a common site for bacterial infection, particularly in women, of whom a significant number have recurrent episodes. Most are acute and short-lived, but severe infections may result in loss of renal function and serious long-term complications.

Aetiology

In most cases, bacterial infection occurs via the ascending route from the urethra to the bladder and potentially to the kidney. Most are caused by *Escherichia coli*, but other Gram-negative rods, for example *Proteus*, *Klebsiella*, and *Serratia* spp. as well as *Pseudomonas aeruginosa*, are also associated with urinary tract infections (UTI), particularly in hospitalized patients. In relation to Gram-positive organisms, *Staphylococcus saprophyticus* may cause UTI in young, sexually active women, whilst *Staphylococcus epidermidis* and *Enterococcus* spp. are more often the cause in hospitalized patients. Non-bacterial causes of UTI are extremely rare and will not be discussed further.

Pathogenesis

Mechanical factors are important in the aetiology of UTI. Any factors that disrupt normal urine flow, prevent the bladder from emptying, or facilitate access of organisms to the bladder will predispose to infection. Thus, because of the shortness of the female urethra, women are more susceptible than men to UTI. Catheterization is also a major predisposing factor for UTI, as are pregnancy, prostatic hypertrophy, calculi, tumours, and strictures, all of which obstruct bladder emptying.

The virulence factors of urinary tract pathogens are incompletely understood. Most of the organisms originate from the faecal flora and certain serogroups of *E. coli* seem to be associated with UTI. Some urinary tract pathogens have specific adhesins which allow them to bind to uroepithelial cells. The production of haemolysin by certain species of *E. coli* and of urease by *Proteus* spp. are further suggested pathogenic determinants.

Clinical features

Lower urinary tract infections

The key clinical features are rapid onset of dysuria (burning pain when passing urine), urgency, and frequency of micturition. The urine is cloudy because of the presence of pus cells and bacteria. It may also contain blood. Laboratory examination of a urine specimen (see below) is essential to confirm the diagnosis.

Upper urinary tract infections

These can only be distinguished from lower urinary tract infections by examining urine obtained directly from the ureter by catheterization. Patients with a kidney infection (pyelonephritis) usually have a fever in addition to lower tract symptoms. Staphylococci are a frequent cause and there may be renal abscess formation.

Laboratory diagnosis

The urinary tract is normally sterile. However, the distal portion of the urethra is colonized with commensal organisms, which often include periurethral and faecal organisms. Specimen contamination is, therefore, common. To overcome this problem, quantitative culture methods are used and bacteriuria is only considered to be 'significant' if a properly collected midstream specimen of urine contains $>10^5$ organisms per ml. In a true infection there is usually only one bacterial species present, whereas contaminated urine often contains multiple species.

Urine is a good growth medium for some organisms. Rapid transportation of specimens to the laboratory is, therefore, essential to avoid multiplication of bacteria within the urine and false-positive results. All specimens should be examined microscopically for leucocytes, red cells, renal casts, and bacteria. Culture using quantitative or semi-quantitative methods is routine and antibiotic sensitivity tests are set up for all significant isolates.

Treatment

Uncomplicated UTI should be treated with oral antibacterial agents, which include amoxicillin, augmentin, cephalexin, trimethoprim, nitrofurantoin, nalidixic acid, and ciprofloxacin. Ideally, the choice of agent should be based on the results of susceptibility tests, though in the community such prescribing is often on a 'best guess' basis. Follow-up cultures should be undertaken to ensure eradication of the organism. Patients should also be encouraged to drink large volumes of fluid.

Initially, pyelonephritis must be treated with a systemic antibacterial agent to which the organism is known to be sensitive. After the symptoms subside, treatment can continue with an oral agent.

Key facts

- A variety of infectious diseases caused by viruses, bacteria, yeasts, and protozoa are transmitted by sexual intercourse (sexually transmitted diseases; STDs).

- Variations in sexual practices can produce STDs in the oropharynx and rectum.

- Promiscuity and asymptomatic carriers play an important role in the spread of STDs.

- Vaccines are not available for STDs, except hepatitis B.

- Syphilis is caused by *T. pallidum*.

- The primary, secondary, and tertiary stages of syphilis are characterized by the specific clinical features of (1) chancre, (2) skin rash and mucosal patches, and (3) gumma and neurosyphilis, respectively.

- *T. pallidum* cannot be cultured routinely; the diagnosis is made by serological tests. Treatment is with penicillin.

- Gonorrhoea is caused by *N. gonorrhoeae*, which enters the urethral mucosa of the penis or the vagina and produces a purulent discharge. Asymptomatic infection is common in females.

- Clinical diagnosis of gonorrhoea is confirmed by culture, identification, and antibiotic sensitivity testing. Amoxycillin is commonly prescribed.

- Both syphilis and gonorrhoea may affect the mouth.

- Non-specific urethritis (NSU) has a similar clinical presentation to that of gonorrhoea, but is caused by an intracellular parasite called *C. trachomatis*.

- Laboratory diagnosis is essential in NSU and treatment is with tetracycline.

- Primary and recurrent herpes of the genitalia can occur, mainly due to herpes simplex type 2 virus, though type 1 is also implicated.

- Some types of human papillomavirus are transmitted by the venereal route and produce warts on the penis, vulva, and perianal area.

Key facts – (*cont.*)

- Dysplasia can occur on the cervix of the uterus following infection with papillomaviruses, and is associated with the development of cervical cancer.

- Symptomatic trichomoniasis is seen mainly in women, and is characterized by an offensive discharge caused by *T. vaginalis*. Treatment is with metronidazole.

- The reservoir of *T. vaginalis* may be an asymptomatic male partner.

- Acute vaginal candidosis is usually an endogenous infection and is characterized by a white discharge.

- *Escherichia coli* is the commonest cause of urinary tract infections (UTI).

- Factors that disrupt normal urine flow or complete bladder-emptying, or that facilitate the access of organisms to the bladder, predispose to UTI.

- Bacteriuria is considered to be 'significant' if a properly collected midstream specimen of urine contains $>10^5$ organisms per ml.

Further reading

Greenwood, D, Slack, R, and Peutherer, J (ed.) (1992). *Medical microbiology* (14th edn). Churchill Livingstone, Edinburgh.

Mims, C, Playfair, J, Roitt, I, Wakelin, D, and Williams, R (1998). Urinary tract infections; Sexually transmitted diseases. In *Medical microbiology* (2nd edn), Chapters 18 and 19. Mosby, London.

Mindell, A (ed.) (1990). Sexually transmitted diseases. *Current Opinion in Infectious Diseases*, 3, 1–38.

Shanson, DC (1989). Infections of the urinary tract; Sexually transmitted diseases. In *Microbiology in clinical practice* (2nd edn), Chapters 19 and 20. Butterworth–Heinemann, Oxford.

Siegel, MA (1996) Syphilis and gonorrhea. *Dental Clinics of North America*, 40, 369–83.

Gastrointestinal infections

15

- Food-borne infections and food poisoning
- Pathogenesis of bacterial gastrointestinal infections
- Prevention of gastrointestinal infections
- *Helicobacter pylori*

Gastrointestinal infections

In this chapter gastrointestinal infections are defined as diseases caused by micro-organisms which affect the stomach, small intestine, or large intestine and are usually characterized by the symptoms of vomiting and/or diarrhoea. The acquisition of the infecting agent is usually either via the faecal–oral route or through consuming contaminated food or drink. However, more rarely, contaminated medical devices have been implicated in transmitting gastrointestinal infections, most notably *Clostridium difficile* colitis (see later) which has been transmitted through inadequately sterilized endoscopes.

The faecal–oral transmission route occurs largely because of inadequate personal hygiene, contaminated hands being the normal vehicles. Prevention is by proper handwashing and through disinfection of faecally contaminated surfaces.

Food-borne infections and food poisoning

The ingestion of food or drink containing pathogenic micro-organisms is probably the most significant cause of gastrointestinal disease. It is, of course, totally preventable if normal hygiene procedures are observed during food production, preparation, cooking, and storing, and if a clean water supply is used. In the developing world the latter does not always exist, and diarrhoeal diseases cause many millions of deaths, especially among the young, in poor countries in the tropics.

A distinction should be made between food-borne infections – where the food or drink is simply a vehicle for transmitting the pathogens – typified by cholera; and food poisoning, where the micro-organisms grow in the food or drink, thereby boosting the numbers of pathogens to an infectious dose and/or a toxin to a toxic dose, for example *Salmonella enteritidis* or *Clostridium perfringens*.

Other infections are also typically transmitted through food and drink, but their effects are systemic. If one follows the definition given at the beginning of this chapter then these are not true infections of the gastrointestinal tract, for example enteric fever (caused by *Salmonella typhi* and *S. paratyphi*), poliomyelitis, and hepatitis A.

Botulism, caused by the ingestion of *Clostridium botulinum* toxin and listeriosis, caused by *Listeria monocytogenes*, are not infec-

tions of the gastrointestinal tract, but are included in this chapter as they are both associated with ingesting bacterially contaminated food. In the case of botulism, the potent neurotoxin is produced by the organism growing in the food. *Listeria monocytogenes* is usually thought of as a food-borne infection, but the organism usually multiplies in the food before ingestion, which can occur in food stored in a refrigerator. Listeriosis is a mild, almost symptomless disease in a healthy individual, but can cause severe neurological disease in immunosuppressed patients, and can cause abortion if acquired during pregnancy.

Typical food/water-borne micro-organisms and the types of gastrointestinal infections they cause are summarized in Fig. 15.1. Classical forms of food-poisoning and the causative micro-organisms, together with botulism and listeriosis, are summarized in Fig. 15.2.

Pathogenesis of bacterial gastrointestinal infections

Although each micro-organism which causes an infection of the gastrointestinal tract has its own set of pathogenic mechanisms, there are several concepts or themes that are common to more than one pathogen. These mechanisms are primarily involved with evading the immune defences of the host, and causing harm.

The initial consideration must be the infective dose of micro-organisms required to cause disease. This is dependent on the ability of the organism to survive the gastric acid barrier of the stomach and other innate defences, which in turn are often dependent on the nutritional status of the host and the vehicle in which the pathogen is being carried, namely liquid or solid food. Some micro-organisms such as *Shigella* spp. and *E. coli* O157 typically require very few organisms to cause disease (< 100), while others such as *Salmonella* and *Campylobacter* spp. require more than 10^4–10^5.

Adhesion and toxin production

The periodic flushing action of the gastrointestinal tract is dependent on peristalsis and the flow rate of food, drink, saliva, and gastric, hepatic, pancreatic, and succus entericus secretions passing through the gut. The mucous lining of the epithelium also tends to prevent organisms inhabiting the upper small intestine. In normal health the flow rate in the small intestine is faster

FOOD/WATER-BORNE MICRO-ORGANISMS	
Micro-organism	**Disease : symptoms; pathogenesis**
Vibrio cholerae	**Cholera:** vomiting and diarrhoea – rice water stools; motility through mucus, adhesion in the small intestine with enterotoxin production
Shigella dysenteriae *S. flexneri, S. boydii, S. sonnei*	**Dysentery:** scant diarrhoea with blood and mucus – the bloody flux; invasion and killing of colonic epithelium. Shiga (vero) toxin
Escherichia coli **(enterotoxigenic) (ETEC)**	**Travellers' diarrhoea:** cholera-like; adhesion through fimbriae (colonisation factor antigens: CFAs); two enterotoxins—heat-labile and heat-stable toxins (LT and ST)
Escherichia coli **(O157) (verotoxin-producing) (VTEC)**	**Haemorrhagic colitis and haemolytic uraemic syndrome:** bloody diarrhoea, renal failure; invasion and killing of colonic epithelium. Production of vero toxin
Campylobacter jejuni	**Diarrhoea, abdominal cramps:** probably the most common cause of diarrhoea in the developed world; multifactorial and poorly understood
Rotavirus	**Infantile diarrhoea, low-grade diarrhoea and vomiting:** in young children; faecal–oral transmission
Small, round-structured viruses (Norwalk agent)	**Vomiting and diarrhoea:** associated with eating shell fish. Filter-feeders concentrate virus from sewage-polluted waters
Giardia lamblia	**Diarrhoea:** protozoan parasite associated with water contaminated by faeces of wild animals. Cysts are resistant to chlorine and must be removed from drinking water by filtration
Cryptosporidium	**Diarrhoea:** cause of diarrhoea in calves but has recently become recognized as a cause of very serious diarrhoea in AIDS patients. A protozoan found in water contaminated with cattle faeces. Can cause large-scale outbreaks of diarrhoea of short duration in previously healthy individuals

Fig. 15.1 Food- and water-borne micro-organisms commonly responsible for gastrointestinal infections.

than the division rate of micro-organisms, so any bacteria entering this section of the gut tend to be washed through. To cause disease at this site the organism must be able to penetrate the mucus – this is accomplished by being motile – and to adhere to the mucosal border by means of fimbriae (pili). Organisms typically able to do this are *Vibrio cholerae*, enterotoxigenic *E. coli* (ETEC), and *Campylobacter jejuni*. Once attached, many of the organisms produce an exotoxin – enterotoxin – which is responsible for the symptoms of the disease.

Diarrhoea and vomiting are the result of different biochemical mechanisms, and more than one enterotoxin may be involved. However, three main types of response occur in the small intestine:

1. Some enterotoxins are cytotonic toxins and cause the normal absorptive processes to be reversed, resulting in a watery, secretory diarrhoea. This is typified by the 'rice-water stools' of cholera and ETEC diarrhoea. Cholera toxin and the closely related heat-labile toxin (LT) and the heat-stable toxin (ST) of *E. coli* are responsible for the symptoms.

2. A painful, cramping diarrhoea results because the cells at the tips of the villi are destroyed by cytotoxic enterotoxins, for example *Clostridium perfringens* diarrhoea. Absorption is prevented due to loss of the surface integrity.

3. Enterotoxins, for example some of those produced by *Staphylococcus aureus*, cause vomiting by acting on the vagus nerve in the mesentery. This stimulates the vomiting centre in the brain, resulting in an acutely intense response.

TYPICAL FOOD POISONING BACTERIA	
Micro-organism	**Implicated foods: symptoms; pathogenesis**
Salmonella enteritidis, *S. typhimurium*	**Eggs, poultry, meat, and meat products:** responsible for 80% of reported cases in UK and 57% in USA. 6–48 hours after ingestion — nausea, vomiting and diarrhoea, fever, abdominal pain. Lasts 1–7 days; multifactorial, poorly understood
Clostridium perfringens	**Bulk, cooked meat, stews:** responsible for 15% of reported cases in UK and 5% in USA. 8–22 hours after ingestion — abdominal pain and diarrhoea. Lasts 1–2 days; enterotoxin produced following sporulation in ileum — destruction of villus tips
Staphylococcus aureus	**Dairy products, salted meats:** responsible for 4% of reported cases in UK and 8% in USA. 1–6 hours after ingestion — acute vomiting and/or diarrhoea; several different enterotoxins produced in the food. Stimulation of vomiting centre via vagus
Bacillus cereus	**Cooked rice allowed to stay warm, typically lightly fried rice:** 1+ hours after ingestion — acute vomiting followed several hours later by diarrhoea; production of two enterotoxins (heat stable) in the food following spore germination
Yersinia enterocolitica, *Y. pseudotuberculosis*	**Meat and milk:** diarrhoea, fever, headache, severe abdominal pain; organism can grow at 4°C
Vibrio parahaemolyticus	**Associated with shellfish and other seafood:** found in contaminated estuarine waters. Most common cause of gastroenteritis in Japan; 24 hours after ingestion — abdominal pain, vomiting, watery stools similar to cholera
Clostridium botulinum	**Home-preserved (or improperly preserved) meat, fish, and vegetables:** generalized flaccid paralysis usually fatal unless intensive care with artificial ventilation; potent neurotoxin
Listeria monocytogenes	**Soft cheese, coleslaw:** organism can grow in food in the refrigerator. Neurological disease in immunosuppressed. Abortion. Can proliferate in macrophages

Fig. 15.2 Bacteria commonly responsible for food poisoning.

In the colon, bloody diarrhoea with mucus, or dysentery, is caused by *Shigella* spp. The symptoms are caused by bacterial invasion followed by destruction of the cells lining the epithelial mucosa. After a cell has been invaded, the bacteria multiply in that cell and then move laterally into neighbouring cells, thus killing them. The haemorrhagic colitis caused by certain strains of *E. coli* (e.g. O157) has a very similar aetiology to shigellosis. Shiga toxin, also known as vero toxin because of its ability to kill vero cells, is involved in the damage to the kidney seen in the haemolytic uraemic syndrome typical of *E. coli* O157 — the largest cause of acute renal failure in children in many developed countries.

Adhesion mechanisms are not important for organisms which produce toxin in the food prior to ingestion, for example in food poisoning (or intoxications) caused by *Clostridium botulinum*, *Staphylococcus aureus*, and *Bacillus cereus*.

Toxin genes and genetic control

It is well recognized that many toxin genes can be located on a prophage or a plasmid (Chapters 4 and 6). The best-known examples are *Clostridium botulinum* and *Corynebacterium diphtheriae* (both prophage encoded) and ETEC labile toxin (plasmid encoded). Other genes on such virulence plasmids or prophages can also code for other virulence factors such as adhesins, and their expression is co-ordinately regulated.

Recently, the genes encoding cholera toxin have also been shown to be carried on a bacteriophage which has lysogenized the bacterium. The production of cholera toxin is co-regulated with the pilus (the toxin co-regulated pilus) which is involved in adherence of the bacterium to the ileal mucosa.

Colonization resistance

In sites with an extensive normal bacterial flora, in this chapter the colon, there is protection from pathogens by a phenomenon known as colonization resistance: the normal indigenous bacteria occupy all available niches and prevent colonization by pathogens.

An important infection, recognized fairly recently, is thought to result from a disturbance of the normal flora of the colon by antibiotics. The result is the development of antibiotic-associated colitis (pseudomembranous colitis) or antibiotic-associated diarrhoea. *Clostridium difficile* is the aetiological agent of this condition. The symptoms of diarrhoea with or without blood or mucus, and sometimes destructive enough to result in perforation of the bowel, are thought to be caused by the action of two toxins: Toxin A an enterotoxin and Toxin B a cytotoxin. The disease is becoming increasingly common especially in the elderly, and is now endemic in certain hospitals and nursing homes. Although a strict anaerobe and a difficult organism to work with in the laboratory, *Clostridium difficile* produces resistant spores and this is one of the reasons for its apparent persistence in the environment. This infection was originally thought to be due to overgrowth of *Clostridium difficile* following antibiotic treatment, directly from the patient's own normal bowel flora, where it was assumed to be present normally at low levels. It is likely, however, that most cases arise in a patient with lowered colonization resistance due to antibiotic treatment, by acquisition from either an infected patient, or from spores contaminating the environment.

Prevention of gastrointestinal infections

Virtually all infections of the gastrointestinal tract are preventable, yet in most parts of the world their incidence is increasing. In the developed world this is due to a general relaxation in standards of food production, with more reliance being placed on the mass preparation of food and the trend towards lightly preserved and chilled fresh foods.

Steps to prevent food-borne infections and food poisoning include drinking clean water, cooking food thoroughly, and educating food handlers. Avoiding the contamination of cooked foods by keeping them separate from uncooked food – especially meat and other animal products – and storing food safely in a refrigerator are also important food safety measures.

Helicobacter pylori

Although not a cause of typical gastrointestinal disease, this spiral-shaped Gram-negative bacterium was first recognized in 1982 and proposed to be a cause of peptic ulcers. Despite much disbelief, it is now recognized as the causative agent of the majority of gastric and duodenal ulcers. *Helicobacter pylori* has the ability to live in the harsh acid environment of the stomach. It survives there by living beneath the layer of mucus which protects the stomach mucosa from acid. It also produces a highly active urease which decomposes urea to ammonia, creating a local alkaline environment. The ulceration is likely to be triggered by the creation of a local inflammatory reaction. Antibiotic therapies have now been developed to eradicate the organism from the stomach. If eradication of the *Helicobacter pylori* is successful then the ulcer is also cured.

Key facts

- Diarrhoea and vomiting are the classic symptoms of gastrointestinal infections.

- Gastrointestinal infections are transmitted via the faecal–oral route, or through the ingestion of contaminated food and drink.

- Food-poisoning results from the ingestion of food or drink contaminated with micro-organisms and/or their toxins, following growth of the micro-organism in the food – the food acts as a booster stage.

- Adhesion – to prevent the pathogen being flushed from the small intestine – and enterotoxin production are common attributes of micro-organisms affecting the gastrointestinal tract.

- In the colon, colonization resistance prevents access by some pathogenic micro-organisms.

- *Clostridium difficile* is the aetiological agent of antibiotic-associated diarrhoea and colitis (pseudomembranous colitis).

- Most infections of the gastrointestinal tract are preventable with good hygienic procedures, especially when producing and preparing food.

- *Helicobacter pylori* is the cause of gastric and duodenal ulcers.

Further reading

Blaser, MJ and Parsonnet, J (1994). Parasitism by the "slow" bacterium *Helicobacter pylori* leads to altered gastric homeostasis and neoplasia. *Journal of Clinical Investigation*, 94, 4–8.

Mims, C, Playfair, J, Roitt, I, Wakelin, D, and Williams, R (1998). Gastrointestinal tract infections. In *Medical microbiology* (2nd edn), Chapter 20. Mosby, London.

Shanson, DC (1989). Infections of the gastro-intestinal tract. In *Microbiology in clinical practice* (2nd edn), Chapter 14. Butterworth–Heinemann, Oxford.

16

Respiratory tract infections

- Introduction
- Upper respiratory tract infections
- Lower respiratory tract infections

Respiratory tract infections

Introduction

Although inhaled air contains many particles, including micro-organisms, the host defence mechanisms in the respiratory tract frequently prevent infection. In the upper respiratory tract these non-specific defence mechanisms include a mechanical washing mechanism, the cough response, and the mucociliary tree. There are additional barriers in the lower respiratory tract (see below). However, infection may ensue if there are large numbers of pathogenic organisms within the inspired air or if the host defences are compromised. There are 'professional invaders' which can infect healthy respiratory mucosa, for example *Streptococcus pyogenes*. In addition, there are 'secondary invaders' which only infect if the host defences are weakened, for example *Pneumocystis carinii* in AIDS patients.

Respiratory tract infections may be caused by bacteria, viruses, protozoa, or fungi and are important in dentistry because the causative agents may be spread through respiratory and oral fluids. Thus, both patients and the dental team are exposed to these microbes during treatment, particularly when splatter and aerosols are generated.

In this chapter, upper and lower respiratory tract infections will be described separately. However, it is important to remember that the respiratory tract is a continuum as far as micro-organisms are concerned and many can cause infection in both parts.

Upper respiratory tract infections

Common cold, pharyngitis, and tonsillitis

Both viruses and bacteria cause pharyngitis and tonsillitis, although approximately 70% of acute sore throats are caused by the former (Fig. 16.1). Pharyngitis often occurs as part of the common cold or influenzal syndromes. The other specific viral causes are covered elsewhere in this book (Chapter 27) and include Epstein–Barr virus, herpes simplex virus, and certain coxsackie A viruses (herpangina and hand, foot, and mouth disease).

The common cold is caused by several families of viruses, especially rhinoviruses which have 100 different antigenic types. Symptoms are usually mild and self-limiting, but nevertheless the disease is a significant cause of industrial and school absenteeism. Patients experience sneezing, sore throat, and cough,

CAUSES OF UPPER RESPIRATORY TRACT INFECTIONS		
Organisms	**Examples**	**Comments**
Viruses	Rhinoviruses (100 antigenic types), coronaviruses	Mild symptoms in the common cold
	Adenoviruses	Pharyngoconjunctival fever
	Parainfluenza viruses	Common cold and lower respiratory tract infection
	Influenza viruses	Pharyngitis and lower respiratory tract infection
	Coxsackie A and other enteroviruses	Small vesicles, for example herpangina
	Epstein–Barr virus	In 70–90% of glandular fever patients
	Herpes simplex types 1 and 2	May be severe, with palatal vesicles or ulcers
Bacteria	*Streptococcus pyogenes*	Causes 10–20% of cases of acute pharyngitis
		Sudden onset, mostly in 5–10-year-old children
	Corynebacterium diphtheriae	Pharyngitis often mild, but toxic illness can be severe
	Haemophilus influenzae	Epiglottitis
	Oral *Spirochaetes* plus fusobacteria	Vincent's angina. Commonest in adolescents and adults

Fig. 16.1 Summary of the viral and bacterial causes of upper respiratory tract infections. Some of these organisms may also cause lower respiratory tract infections.

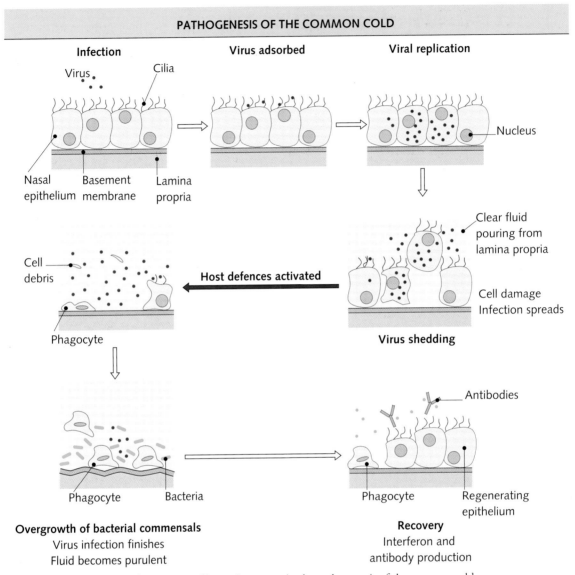

Fig. 16.2 Diagram illustrating stages in the pathogenesis of the common cold.

together with nasal discharge and obstruction. Other symptoms include hoarseness and headache.

The pathogenesis of the common cold is summarized in Fig. 16.2. The incubation period is between 2 and 4 days. A flow of virus-rich fluid from the nasopharynx is induced by the infection and, when sneezing is triggered, large numbers of viral particles are expelled into the air. Transmission by aerosol is, therefore, important but these viruses are also spread via contaminated hands. Diagnosis is based on clinical features and treatment is symptomatic.

Streptococcus pyogenes is the commonest bacterial cause of sore throat. Mild redness of the tonsillar tissue and pharynx may occur, but the classical picture is of an infection involving the fauces and soft palate with acute follicular tonsillitis (Fig. 16.3). Infection is common in children (5–8-year-olds especially) but less so in adults. In severe cases, complications include peritonsillar abscess, and extension of the infection to involve the sinuses and middle ear (Fig. 16.4). The complications of untreated infections are now relatively uncommon in industrialized countries, but the involvement of *Streptococcus pyogenes* in rheumatic heart disease (see below) is an important issue for dentists.

Ulcerative tonsillitis (Vincent's angina) is associated with an overgrowth of endogenous spirochaetes and fusobacteria within the tonsillar crypts; a smear from the lesions has a characteristic appearance that is diagnostic. The infection is uncommon and is sometimes present in medically compromised patients.

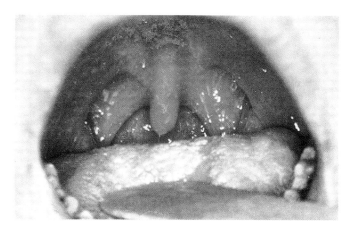

Fig. 16.3 Streptococcal tonsillitis caused by a group A β-haemolytic streptococcus. (Courtesy of Dr C. Gemmell.)

Rheumatic fever

The disease is caused by certain strains of Group A streptococci (*Streptococcus pyogenes*). These contain cell-membrane antigens that trigger the production of antibodies which cross-react with human heart-tissue antigens. The cross-reaction causes immunological damage to the tissues, and is not a direct infection of the heart. Acute rheumatic fever generally affects younger age groups, typically between the ages of 5–15 years. In developed countries the disease is now quite rare, probably due to the wide availability of penicillin.

Typically, the disease is associated with a bout of severe streptococcal tonsillitis 1–4 weeks earlier. Confirmatory evidence of streptococcal infection includes scarlet fever, isolation of *Streptococcus pyogenes* from a throat swab, or an increase in the antistreptolysin O titre (ASOT) from a blood sample.

Clinical features include fever, a migratory polyarthritis, subcutaneous nodules, Sydenham's chorea (jerky involuntary movements involving the head, face, or limbs), and inflammation of all parts of the heart (endocardium, myocardium, and pericardium). Characteristically, this pancarditis leads to the formation of small granulomas called Aschoff nodes, which consist of a central area of necrotic collagen surrounded by inflammatory cells and fibroblasts. When the lesions heal they are replaced by scar tissue. The heart valves become inflamed and swollen, with the development of small fibrin thrombi on their surfaces. When healing occurs the valves become thickened and fibrosed with concomitant contraction. Depending on the severity of the disease, valvular damage can be minor or severe, with narrowing (stenosis) and incompetence. Individuals with valves compromised in this way have detectable heart murmurs and run a life-long risk of developing infective endocarditis (Chapter 17).

COMPLICATIONS OF STREPTOCOCCAL SORE THROAT	
Complication	**Comments**
Peritonsillar abscess (quinsy)	May follow untreated infection Uncommon
Otitis media or sinusitis	Local spread
Scarlet fever	Generalized punctate erythematous rash, beginning on face and spreading to most of body Tongue initially furred, but later red Mediated by erythrogenic toxin
Rheumatic fever	Indirect complication Antibodies to antigens in streptococcal cell wall cross-react with the sarcolemma of human heart
Rheumatic heart disease	Repeated attacks of *Streptococcus pyogenes* infection can result in damage to heart valves Future attacks prevented by penicillin prophylaxis in childhood
Acute glomerulonephritis	Specific antibodies bind to streptococcal components to form circulating immune complexes. These are deposited in the glomeruli with resultant local inflammation Caused by 4 to 5 specific 'nephritogenic' strains Second attacks are rare

Fig. 16.4 The potential complications of a sore throat caused by *Streptococcus pyogenes*.

Acute rheumatic fever is generally treated with penicillin and bed rest. However, the disease tends to recur leading to increased cardiac damage with mitral stenosis. Recurrences can be prevented with long-term penicillin prophylaxis. Additional antibiotic cover is also required during certain clinical procedures to prevent infective endocarditis (Chapter 17).

Diphtheria

Diphtheria is caused by toxin-producing strains of the Gram-positive bacillus *Corynebacterium diphtheriae*. The genes encoding toxin production are carried by a bacteriophage. Widespread immunization with toxoid has made this infection rare in developed countries, but it is still common in many other parts of the world. Toxigenic strains colonize the pharynx, larynx, and nose. The toxin destroys epithelial cells and polymorphs and an ulcer forms, covered with a necrotic exudate – the 'false membrane'. There is local inflammation and swelling and the cervical lymph nodes may be enlarged. When the larynx is involved it can result in life-threatening respiratory obstruction.

In addition to local effects, diphtheria toxin is absorbed into the lymphatics and blood, resulting in the following systemic effects:

* constitutional upset, including fever and exhaustion;

* myocarditis, possibly resulting in cardiac failure;

* polyneuritis, often several weeks after the onset of illness; involvement of the glossopharyngeal nerve may cause paralysis of the soft palate.

Diphtheria is a potentially fatal disease and rapid diagnosis is, therefore, essential. Once suspected clinically, the patient is isolated and treatment with antitoxin begun. Penicillin or erythromycin are given as an adjunct. Tracheotomy may be required to maintain the airway.

Otitis and sinusitis

The air spaces associated with the upper respiratory tract include the sinuses, the middle ear, and mastoid. Acute infection of the middle ear or sinuses is often due to secondary bacterial infection following a viral infection of the respiratory tract, e.g. measles. Primary infection with mumps virus or respiratory syncytial virus can occasionally cause vestibulitis or temporary deafness.

Acute otitis media is a common cause of earache in infants and small children. The tympanic membrane may rupture with the discharge of pus. There may also be generalized symptoms and otitis media should be considered in any child with unexplained fever, diarrhoea, or vomiting. At least 50% of attacks are viral. The bacterial invaders are most commonly *Streptococcus pneumoniae*, *Haemophilus influenzae*, or *Streptococcus pyogenes*. Treatment is usually with amoxycillin.

The infection may become chronic and other bacterial species may superinfect – some perhaps through the external ear, such as *Staphylococcus aureus* or enteric Gram-negative bacilli, or from the mouth, for example strictly anaerobic Gram-negative rods.

Treatment of chronic infections with antimicrobial agents is often disappointing.

Acute sinusitis

The aetiology and pathogenesis are similar to otitis media, but clinical features include facial pain and localized tenderness. Treatment is usually empirical with supportive treatment and antibiotics such as amoxycillin.

Laboratory diagnosis of throat and pharyngeal infections

The laboratory diagnosis of this wide range of bacteria and viruses is complex and outside the scope of this book. Good clinical samples are necessary and consist of one or more of the following: throat swabs, oral washings, nasal secretions for culture, and blood samples for serology. Generally, samples are cultured in tissue culture for viruses and on solid nutrient media for bacteria. *Streptococcus pyogenes* is isolated on blood agar and identified by Lancefield grouping, while *Corynebacterium diphtheriae* is cultured on a selective medium (blood tellurite) and its identity confirmed by demonstrating toxin production in a gel-diffusion precipitin reaction known as the Elek test. However Vincent's angina is diagnosed from a stained smear since the spirochaetes cannot be easily cultured.

Lower respiratory tract infections

The range of micro-organisms involved in lower respiratory tract infections is very wide, and only a selected few will be discussed in this chapter. Infections may be acute or chronic, limited to the bronchial tree (bronchitis), involve the lung alveoli (pneumonia), or be a mixture of these (bronchopneumonia). Some forms of disease, such as tuberculosis, are always caused by the same species, while others can be caused by a range of different organisms.

Harmful infections of the lungs occur only after the micro-organisms have negotiated a formidable host defence system. The non-specific mechanisms in the upper respiratory tract include a mechanical washing mechanism, the cough response, anatomical barriers, and the mucociliary tree. In the lower respiratory tract additional barriers include the frequent branching of the pulmonary tree (to effect aerodynamic filtration) and the restrictive size (0.3 to 5.0 μm) of the alveolus opening. If micro-organisms do reach the alveolus, they must resist the activity of phagocytes, immune-response cells, and other antimicrobial defence factors.

Whooping cough

Whooping cough (or pertussis) is a severe disease of childhood caused by *Bordetella pertussis* (Fig. 16.5), which is spread by airborne droplets. The organism infects the ciliated epithelial layer of the respiratory tract without invading deeper, resulting in an acute tracheobronchitis. Tissue damage is caused by a range of toxic factors, and the clinical features are listed in Fig. 16.5.

PERTUSSIS — WHOOPING COUGH	
Causative agent	*Bordetella pertussis:* Specific adhesins that attach to ciliated epithelium Toxic factors released, e.g. adenylate cyclase and pertussis toxin
Clinical features	Insidious onset Catarrhal stage with common cold symptoms (2 weeks) Paroxysmal coughing (2 weeks) Residual cough (4–6 weeks)

Fig. 16.5 The major features of whooping cough.

EXACERBATIONS OF CHRONIC BRONCHITIS	
Bacterial	*Haemophilus influenzae* (unencapsulated) *Streptococcus pneumoniae* *Moraxella (Branhamella) catarrhalis*
Viral	Influenza A Parainfluenza Coronavirus Rhinovirus Herpes simplex virus

Fig. 16.6 Causes of infective exacerbations of chronic bronchitis.

However, the diagnostic feature is the paroxysmal cough which is characterized by a series of short coughs followed by a severe inspiratory gasp of air, thus producing a 'whooping' sound. Vomiting is common, and, although morbidity is high, fatality is low; the disease is confined mainly to infants. There is a significant risk of developing subsequent chronic chest disease, for example bronchiectasis.

Diagnosis is usually based on the clinical signs and symptoms. Samples from the respiratory tract are cultured on a selective medium (charcoal blood agar) and colonies identified with specific antisera. Antimicrobial therapy is of most value if given within the first 10 days of infection, during the catarrhal stage, when the diagnosis may not be suspected. Erythromycin is the drug of choice for treatment and prevention is by active immunization (Chapter 8).

Bronchitis

Acute bronchitis

Acute bronchitis is an inflammatory condition of the tracheo-bronchial tree, usually associated with infection. In a patient with a healthy respiratory tract the disease is often a mild complication of upper respiratory tract infections due to common viruses such as rhinovirus and coronavirus, as well as less common agents, for example influenza and adenoviruses. The degree of damage to the respiratory epithelium varies with the infectious agent, and secondary bacterial infection with *Streptococcus pneumoniae* and *Haemophilus influenzae* may also play a role in pathogenesis. A cough, initially dry and painful but later productive with the expectoration of greenish sputum, is a prominent presenting symptom. Treatment is largely symptomatic if the disease is mild, and although antibiotics are usually prescribed their value is uncertain, unless the identity and sensitivity of the causative agent(s) are known.

Chronic bronchitis

Chronic bronchitis is a disease in which cough and excessive secretion of mucus are present in the tracheobronchial tree but are not attributable to specific diseases such as tuberculosis and asthma. Aetiological factors include infection, cigarette smoking, and the inhalation of toxic dust or fumes. Infection does not appear to initiate the disease, but is significant in prolonging it and producing the acute exacerbations which increasingly damage lung tissue and which may lead to death. Both viruses and bacteria are commonly associated with acute bouts of infection (Fig. 16.6). However, interpretation of the results of the microbiological analysis of sputum from patients with acute exacerbations is difficult, because many of these agents are present in the flora of the upper respiratory tract and can contaminate sputum during collection. Therapy is complex, and depends on the severity of the exacerbation and the causative agents.

Pneumonia

In pneumonia, the lung alveolar spaces become filled with components of oedema fluid, accompanied by an inflammatory reaction in the lung parenchyma. Bacteria may gain access to the lung tissue by inhalation or through aspiration of oropharyngeal fluid. The latter is thought to be the route of most bacterial pulmonary infections. Pneumonia remains a significant cause of death in infancy (usually viral in origin), in the elderly, and in immunocompromised patients (more commonly bacterial), although antibiotic therapy has transformed the prognosis in many cases. Pneumonia may be classified as lobar (consolidation of lung tissue limited to one lobe or segment), bronchopneumonia (consolidation scattered throughout the lung but concentrated mainly at the bases), and atypical (patchy consolidation).

The main clinical features of pneumonia are listed in Fig. 16.7. Pneumonia can be acquired either in the community (about 90% of cases) or uncommonly in hospitals – a selection of the wide range of microbial causes are presented in Fig. 16.8. Pneumonias caused by *Streptococcus pneumoniae*, viruses, or *Mycoplasma pneumoniae* are most common in healthy individuals, with low numbers of cases attributed to other bacteria. Patients with underlying disease may also develop community-acquired pneumonia caused by these and other agents, including *Staphylococcus aureus*, *Haemophilus influenzae*, *Klebsiella pneumoniae*, or *Pneumocystis carinii*.

CLINICAL FEATURES OF PNEUMONIA

- Sudden or insidious onset
- Fever, rigors, malaise
- Shortness of breath, rapid shallow breathing, cyanosis
- Cough producing purulent sputum
- Consolidation of lungs, on clinical and radiographic examination

Fig. 16.7 The clinical features of pneumonia.

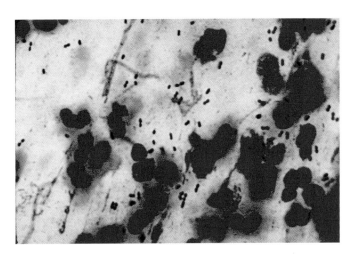

Fig. 16.9 A Gram-stained smear of sputum, demonstrating pus cells and Gram-positive diplococci, in a patient with pneumococcal pneumonia.

Hospital-acquired pneumonias are commonly associated with aerobic or facultative Gram-negative bacilli. *Staphylococcus aureus* is the most common Gram-positive bacterium involved (Fig. 16.8). Modes of transmission of hospital-acquired pneumonia include the contaminated hands of health-care workers, together with instruments and equipment.

Pneumococcal pneumonia

Streptococcus pneumoniae (the pneumococcus) causes at least one-third of all community-acquired pneumonias and about one-half of the pneumonias that develop in the elderly as sequelae to influenza. Although pneumococcal pneumonia can occur in persons of all ages, those aged over 65 years are 3–5 times more susceptible than younger adults. The most important pathogenic property of *Streptococcus pneumoniae* is its interference with phagocytosis, mediated by its large and well-defined polysaccharide

capsule, of which there are 81 different antigenic types. *Streptococcus pneumoniae* is carried asymptomatically in the pharynx of some children and some adults, who serve as the sources of infection for others. Most pneumococcal and other Gram-positive bacterial pneumonias result from the aspiration of oropharyngeal fluids containing colonized bacteria.

The first symptom is commonly a sudden dramatic rigor followed by high fever lasting for about 3 days and accompanied by chest pain. Chills may occur, and most patients produce purulent sputum. The presence of large numbers of Gram-positive, lancet-shaped cocci/diplococci in sputum is very helpful in diagnosing pneumococcal pneumonia (Fig. 16.9), especially if these cells show a positive capsular swelling reaction. This occurs when pneumococci are exposed to polyvalent capsular antiserum and methylene

CAUSES OF PNEUMONIA

Community-acquired pneumonias	*Streptococcus pneumoniae* Viruses *Mycoplasma pneumoniae* *Haemophilus influenzae* *Legionella pneumophila* *Chlamydia pneumoniae* *Moraxella (Branhamella) catarrhalis* *Pneumocystis carinii*
Hospital-acquired pneumonias	*Staphylococcus aureus* Gram-negative bacilli e.g. *Pseudomonas* spp. *Klebsiella pneumoniae* *Escherichia coli* *Legionella pneumophila*

Fig. 16.8 Summary of the major causes of community-acquired and hospital-acquired pneumonia.

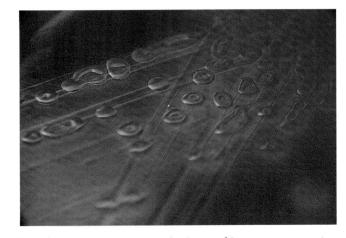

Fig. 16.10 Draughtsman-shaped colonies of *Streptococcus pneumoniae* on blood agar, illustrating α-haemolysis. (Courtesy of Dr C. Gemmell.)

blue stain on a slide and examined microscopically. Colonies of *Streptococcus pneumoniae* on blood agar are alpha-haemolytic and have a characteristic 'draughtsman shape' morphology (Fig. 16.10), though this is less obvious for very mucoid strains. Pneumococci are differentiated from many species of oral streptococci by being sensitive to optochin and soluble in bile. Bacteraemia occurs in about 25% of cases and blood culture may help in the diagnosis.

Antibiotic sensitivity testing should be performed so that penicillin-resistant strains can be identified and appropriate drugs prescribed. A vaccine is available and is composed of polysaccharides from the 23 most common disease-producing capsular types of *Streptococcus pneumoniae*. Generally, it is recommended for medically compromised individuals with an increased risk of infection, for example those with splenic dysfunction, diabetes mellitus, or chronic cardiopulmonary disease.

Legionella pneumonia

Legionella pneumophila is a Gram-negative bacillus that causes an atypical pneumonia called Legionnaires' disease. This potentially life-threatening disease was first recognized in 1976 following an outbreak of pneumonia among guests attending an American Legion convention at a hotel in Philadelphia, Pennsylvania, USA.

Legionella pneumophila and 33 other species of *Legionella* are water bacteria that are widely distributed in nature and sometimes exist inside free-living amoebae. However, most cases of Legionnaires' disease (about 70% of which are caused by *Legionella pneumophila*) are associated with pieces of apparatus that aerosolize *Legionella*-contaminated water and so disseminate the disease. These include cooling towers, humidifiers, and respiratory therapy equipment. Inhalation of the bacterium, and perhaps aspiration, may initiate disease in the lung. No person-to-person transmission of Legionnaires' disease has been documented. The main features of this disease are presented in Fig. 16.11.

From a dental point of view it is interesting to note that *Legionella pneumophila*, together with other *Legionella* spp., have been detected in dental unit water in several studies involving clinics in the USA, Austria, England, and Germany. For example, in one American study, *Legionella pneumophila* was detected in 8% of water samples taken from the dental units in 28 offices distributed over a 4-state area. There is a theoretical risk of infection during dental treatment, and the indirect evidence from published serological studies tends to support this conclusion. However, to date, there is no scientific evidence that water from a dental unit has ever caused Legionnaires' disease.

Atypical pneumonia

There are a number of other causes of atypical pneumonia, especially *Mycoplasma pneumoniae* and, to a lesser extent, *Chlamydia* spp. Generally, atypical pneumonia in adults presents with marked headache, nasopharyngeal symptoms, and a non-productive or minimally productive cough. *Mycoplasma pneumoniae* is a bacterium without a cell wall that causes respiratory tract infections in all age groups, but is most common in schoolchildren and young adults. The majority of individuals who become infected with *Mycoplasma pneumoniae* only develop pharyngitis or bronchitis, but about 10% succumb to pneumonia which is usually self-limiting. The bacterium causes about 15% of all pneumonias in persons over the age of 40 years and is seen in 'enclosed populations' such as college students, prisoners, or military personnel. This type of pneumonia is usually acquired by inhaling respiratory droplets from an infected person. Treatment of mycoplasmal pneumonia is with tetracyclines or erythromycin.

LEGIONNAIRES' DISEASE	
Transmission	Inhalation of aerosols from contaminated water Aspiration of oropharyngeal colonized bacteria
Symptoms	Initially influenza-like which progress to a severe pneumonia Other features include mental confusion, renal failure, and gastrointestinal symptoms
Diagnosis	Culture and identification or demonstration in tissue or body fluids by immunofluorescence or DNA probes Measurement of antibody levels Chest radiograph
Therapy	Erythromycin is drug of choice Unresponsive to penicillin
Case mortality	5% in treated patients 20–30% in untreated otherwise healthy patients 24% in treated immunocompromised patients 80% in untreated immunocompromised patients

Fig. 16.11 The important features of Legionnaires' disease.

Tuberculosis

Disease characteristics

In 1995, *Mycobacterium tuberculosis* killed about 3.1 million people world-wide (World Health Organization) and tuberculosis (TB) remains the largest single cause of death from any infectious disease. It is estimated that one-third of the world's population is infected with *Mycobacterium tuberculosis*, and it is fortunate that only about 10% of those infected actually develop TB during their lifetime. However, this percentage increases if high-risk factors are involved, for example the risk for a person infected with HIV of developing TB goes from 10% in a lifetime to 8% per year of life. The clinical features of TB are presented in Fig. 16.12.

Pathogenesis

Tuberculosis is spread by aerosols from human to human and the course of the disease is modified by the host response (Fig. 16.13). Infection leads most commonly to asymptomatic cases that are radiograph-negative and skin-test positive, but in whom small numbers of *Mycobacterium tuberculosis* may remain viable and may be involved in the reactivation of TB. Some infections lead to the development of symptomatic primary TB that starts as exudative lesions in the lower respiratory tract, which progress to a productive lesion once cell-mediated immunity (type IV hypersensitivity) develops and tubercles form. Healing may occur at this point or the lesions may expand with caseation necrosis. This could heal or result in the massive destruction of lung tissue causing cavity formation.

Haematogenous spread of *Mycobacterium tuberculosis* from the lungs to other body sites occurs in about 15% of otherwise normal patients, but this increases to 50–70% in HIV-infected patients. Such spread is facilitated by the ability of *Mycobacterium tuberculosis* to establish intracellular infection. Early in the course of the disease, cells of *Mycobacterium tuberculosis* are engulfed by phagocytes, but they survive intracellular digestion and can even multiply within and destroy the phagocytes. However, the development of cell-mediated immunity produces 'activated' macrophages that can destroy the bacterium. Tuberculosis can

TUBERCULOSIS (TB)	
Transmission	Inhalation of aerosolized respiratory droplet nuclei from infected person with active pulmonary TB Low infectivity among casual contacts Higher infectivity among long-term contacts especially in crowded conditions or closed air systems
High-risk factors	Close contact with known active TB case Residency in prison, nursing home, mental institution, some health-care facilities HIV infection Injection drug abuse Alcoholism Contact with persons from high prevalence TB countries (Africa, Asia, Latin America)
Symptoms	Malaise Productive cough for more than 3 weeks Headache, fever Weight loss, night sweats Blood in sputum
Diagnosis	AFB (acid-fast bacilli) in sputum (Ziehl–Neelsen) Isolation of *Mycobacterium tuberculosis* from sputum (Lowenstein–Jensen medium) Skin testing (tuberculin testing) with purified protein derivative (PPD) to determine infection Chest radiograph
Preventive therapy	BCG vaccine (not provided routinely in USA) In PPD-positive, X-ray-negative cases: isoniazid (INH) daily for 6 to 12 months

Fig. 16.12 Summary of the main epidemiological and clinical features of tuberculosis.

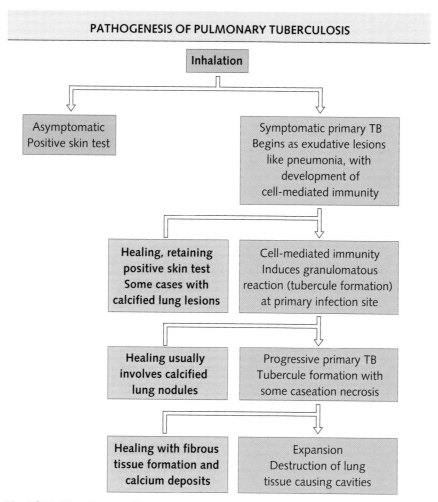

PATHOGENESIS OF PULMONARY TUBERCULOSIS

Inhalation

Asymptomatic
Positive skin test

Symptomatic primary TB
Begins as exudative lesions
like pneumonia, with
development of
cell-mediated immunity

**Healing, retaining
positive skin test
Some cases with
calcified lung lesions**

Cell-mediated immunity
Induces granulomatous
reaction (tubercle formation)
at primary infection site

**Healing usually
involves calcified
lung nodules**

Progressive primary TB
Tubercle formation with
some caseation necrosis

**Healing with fibrous
tissue formation and
calcium deposits**

Expansion
Destruction of lung
tissue causing cavities

Fig. 16.13 Flow diagram illustrating stages in the pathogenesis of pulmonary tuberculosis.

recur later in life due to tubercle bacilli that remained viable but inactive in the body as a result of a previous primary infection. The WHO estimates that about two-thirds of all new active cases of TB actually result from the reactivation of a healed primary infection.

Diagnosis, treatment, and drug resistance

The diagnosis of TB is based on the microscopic detection of acid and alcohol-fast bacilli and the culture of *Mycobacterium tuberculosis* from sputum (see Fig. 12.5), together with skin testing. Culture is undertaken on a special agar called Lowenstein–Jensen medium and is extremely slow (4–8 weeks). For this reason, the value of new molecular techniques in diagnosing the disease is being actively investigated.

The Mantoux test consists of an intradermal injection in the arm of purified protein derivative (PPD) from cultures of *Mycobacterium tuberculosis*. A positive test (a 'hard' lesion 10 mm or more in diameter at the site of the injection after 48 to 72 hours) indicates either active disease or past infection. A negative test does not definitively rule out TB, as some false-negatives may occur.

Patients with TB are usually treated with three drugs to prevent the emergence of resistant strains during the prolonged treatment period. Isoniazid (INH), rifampicin, and pyrazinamide are usually prescribed for 6 to 9 months. However, within the last decade, multiple drug-resistant strains of *Mycobacterium tuberculosis* (MDRTB) have emerged, about 20% of which are resistant to both INH and rifampicin. Secondary drugs (less effective and generally more toxic) include ethambutol, para-aminosalicylic acid, and streptomycin.

Immunization

A live, avirulent, bovine *Mycobacterium* strain named bacillus Calmette–Guérin (BCG) has been used almost world-wide (although not in the USA) for vaccination against TB in PPD-negative persons. Unfortunately, protection has been shown to be variable; it appears to be strongest in children and less effective in adults. A drawback to vaccination is that while it may or may not give protection, it will cause a positive skin test which eliminates the skin test as a means of detecting early infection.

Cases of occupational TB can occur in health-care workers following exposure to patients with known active or unsuspected pulmonary infection with *Mycobacterium tuberculosis*. Although transmission of TB to members of the dental profession has not been a particular problem, some care is required. Emergency dental care of a patient with active disease should be performed in a hospital environment where isolation facilities exist.

Non-tuberculous mycobacteria

There are additional members of the *Mycobacterium* genus (non-tuberculous mycobacteria, NTM) that may be pathogenic in children and compromised hosts e.g. AIDS patients. Since they have been recovered from a variety of environmental sites (soil, waters, house dust, birds, animals, foods), it is likely that they enter the lung from environmental sources, although the exact modes of transmission are not known; two of the NTM most commonly involved in pulmonary disease are the *M. avium* complex and *M. kansasii*.

Viral pneumonias

A range of viruses cause pneumonia. As a group, viruses cause most of the pneumonias in infants and children but probably no more than 10% of the pneumonias in adults (Fig. 16.14). It is often difficult to differentiate clinically between viral and bacterial pneumonias in the absence of laboratory culture data and in presumed cases of viral pneumonia – a specific viral agent is identified in only about one-half of the cases. Even when viruses do not themselves cause pneumonia, for example measles virus, they prepare the way for secondary bacterial pneumonia by damaging the respiratory defences.

Influenza

The influenza viruses cause endemic, epidemic, and pandemic infections. There are two different types of RNA myxoviruses that infect man (A and B), both of which undergo genetic change as they spread through the host species. Virus A is the principal cause of epidemic influenza, while virus B causes milder outbreaks in the winter months. Transmission of influenza is by droplet inhalation. The viral particles attach to sialic acid receptors on superficial epithelial cells of the upper and lower respiratory tract and, as a result of proliferation, kill the cells. Cytokine release from host cells causes chills, malaise, fever, and muscular aches. Influenza A rarely causes primary pneumonia, and damage to the lung is due usually to secondary bacterial infection by *Streptococcus pneumoniae*, *Staphylococcus aureus*, or *Haemophilus influenzae*.

Vaccines are available, but they do need to be reviewed annually in relation to the genetic changes that have occurred in viruses circulating the previous year. They provide protection in up to 70% of vaccinees and are valuable for protecting high-risk individuals, especially the elderly and those with chronic cardiopulmonary disease. Genetic changes are of two types – antigenic shift and drift. The former involves a major genetic re-assortment of the RNA segment that codes for the viral surface haemagglutinin, thus creating a new virus to which human populations have little or no protection; world-wide epidemics may well result. Antigenic drift is due to spontaneous mutation with minor changes in the haemagglutinin, which allows the virus to infect partially immune hosts. Amantidine hydrochloride inhibits the replication of influenza A virus. If given within 1 to 2 days of disease onset it may reduce the severity of the infection, but is more valuable as a prophylactic agent.

VIRAL PNEUMONIAS	
Influenza virus	**Children:** more commonly involved in febrile upper respiratory tract infections **Adults:** most common cause of viral pneumonia
Respiratory syncytial virus (RSV)	**Children:** causes 40–60% of pneumonias in those aged 6 months to 3 years **Adults:** more commonly involved in benign upper respiratory tract infections
Parainfluenza virus	**Children:** most often associated with common cold symptoms, tracheobronchitis, and croup. May cause pneumonia **Adults:** lower respiratory tract infections are rare
Pneumonia as part of systemic viral diseases	**Measles:** commonly causes respiratory symptoms. Some cases progress to pneumonia **Varicella zoster:** commonly causes respiratory symptoms. 10–20% of adolescents and adults with chickenpox may have pneumonia, but this is rare in children **Cytomegalovirus (CMV):** most cases of CMV pneumonia occur in immunocompromised patients who have systemic CMV infection

Fig. 16.14 Summary of the viral causes of pneumonia. These are more common in children than in adults.

FUNGAL INFECTIONS OF THE LOWER RESPIRATORY TRACT	
Histoplasmosis	**Cause:** *Histoplasma capsulatum* (dimorphic fungus) Most infections are asymptomatic, undiagnosed, and primary lesions usually heal spontaneously Occurs world-wide About 200, 000 new infections a year in the USA Lung lesions usually heal with fibrosis and calcification as in tuberculosis **Diagnosis:** microscopic and cultural identification of the microbe from sputum, complement-fixing antibody detection and, in some instances, skin-testing with histoplasmin Some cases (most frequently the immunocompromised) have disseminated disease with haematogenous spread from the lung **Treatment:** IV amphotericin B and in some cases, ketoconazole
Blastomycosis	**Cause:** *Blastomyces dermatiditis* (dimorphic fungus) Endemic in southwest USA, Mexico, Africa. Sporadic in other parts of the world Lesions in lung are like tuberculosis and histoplasmosis **Diagnosis:** microscopic and cultural identification of the microbe from sputum May progress to acute pneumonia with haematogenous spread of microbes to internal organs, bone and skin **Treatment:** IV amphotericin B and in some cases, ketoconazole
Coccidiomycosis	**Cause:** *Coccidioides immitis* (dimorphic fungus) Endemic in southwest USA, northern Mexico, Central and South America About 60% of primary infections are asymptomatic, 40% result in mild to severe pulmonary disease, 0.3% progress to disseminated disease **Diagnosis:** microscopic and cultural identification of the microbe from sputum, complement-fixing antibody detection, and in some cases skin-testing with coccidiodin **Treatment:** IV amphotericin B and in some cases ketoconazole
Cryptococcosis	**Cause:** *Cryptococcus neoformans* (grows primarily as a yeast) Soil containing pigeon droppings frequently contains high numbers of this microbe and serves as a primary source of infection world-wide Most infections are asymptomatic, undiagnosed, and primary lesions usually heal spontaneously Pneumonia can lead to disseminated disease most commonly involving the brain and meninges **Diagnosis:** microscopic observation of yeast cells with large capsules in sputum, cultural identification, detection of capsular antibody **Treatment:** IV amphotericin B and in some cases 5-fluorocytosine
Other fungal diseases of the lung	Aspergillosis Zygomycosis

Fig. 16.15 Summary of the important fungal infections of the lower respiratory tract.

Fungal infections

There are a number of fungi that infect the lower respiratory tract and these are acquired by inhaling pathogenic fungal spores or yeast cells. Most cases are asymptomatic or undiagnosed, but some involve serious manifestations (Fig. 16.15).

Pneumocystis carinii is now believed to be a fungus (although some consider it to be a protozoan) that commonly invades the respiratory tract, usually causing asymptomatic infections. Some data on the measurement of specific antibody levels to *Pneumocystis carinii* suggest that about 80% of children are colonized by the age of four years. A few cases of *Pneumocystis carinii* pneumonia (PCP) occur in otherwise healthy children, but by far the most important expression of the disease is in the immuno-compromised, especially AIDS patients. About 70% of these patients develop PCP that recurs not infrequently following successful treatment. PCP has been the leading cause of death in

HIV disease. Diagnostic methods include demonstration of the microbe in sputum or lung biopsy tissue using indirect immuno-fluorescent staining with monoclonal antibodies. Treatment involves sulphamethoxazole/trimethoprim or pentamidine.

References and further reading

Bagg, J (1996). Tuberculosis: a re-emerging problem for health care workers. *British Dental Journal*, **180**, 376–81.

Mims *et al.* (1993). Mosby Year Book, Europe.

Mims, C, Playfair, J, Roitt, I, Wakelin, D, and Williams, R (1998). Upper respiratory tract infections; Lower respiratory tract infections. In *Medical microbiology* (2nd edn), Chapters 15 and 17. Mosby, London.

Phelan, JA, Jimenez, V, and Tompkins, DC (1996). Tuberculosis. *Dental Clinics of North America*, **40**, 327–41.

Shanson, DC (1989). Infections of the lower respiratory tract. *Microbiology in clinical practice* (2nd edn), Chapter 12. Butterworth–Heinemann, Oxford.

Van-Arsdall, JA, *et al.* (1983). The protean manifestations of Legionnaires' disease. *Journal of Infection*, **7**, 51–62.

Key facts

- Most acute sore throats are caused by viruses.

- *Streptococcus pyogenes* is the commonest bacterial cause of pharyngitis.

- Potential complications of a streptococcal sore throat include rheumatic heart disease and acute glomeru-lonephritis.

- Diphtheria is a life-threatening infection caused by toxin-producing strains of *Corynebacterium diphtheriae*, which can be prevented by immunization with toxoid.

- 'Whooping cough' is an acute tracheobronchitis caused by *Bordetella pertussis*, which can be prevented by immunization with a killed vaccine.

- *Haemophilus influenzae*, *Streptococcus pneumoniae*, and *Moraxella* (*Branhamella*) *catarrhalis* are the commonest causes of acute exacerbations of chronic bronchitis.

- Most community-acquired pneumonias are caused by *Streptococcus pneumoniae*, viruses, or *Mycoplasma pneumoniae*.

- Gram-negative bacilli, particularly *Pseudomonas aeruginosa*, cause up to 60% of all hospital-acquired pneumonias.

- Legionnaires' disease is a form of pneumonia caused by the Gram-negative bacillus *Legionella pneumophila* and is usually associated with water-handling systems.

- Most cases of atypical pneumonia in adults are caused by *Mycoplasma pneumoniae*.

- One-third of the world's population is infected with *Mycobacterium tuberculosis*.

- Tuberculosis is spread by inhaling respiratory droplet nuclei, and infection is commonly asymptomatic.

- Diagnosis of tuberculosis can be made by the detection of acid-fast bacilli in a Ziehl–Neelsen stained smear of sputum, culture, and the Mantoux skin test.

- Tuberculosis is treated with triple therapy, for example isoniazid, rifampicin, and pyrazinamide, but drug resistance is a growing problem.

- The BCG vaccine can be used to immunize against *Mycobacterium tuberculosis*, but protection is variable.

- Influenza viruses are myxoviruses, transmitted by droplet inhalation, which undergo genetic change (antigenic drift and shift) as they spread.

- *Pneumocystis carinii* pneumonia is a common problem in patients with AIDS.

17

Infective endocarditis and sepsis syndrome

- Infective endocarditis
- Sepsis syndrome

Infective endocarditis and sepsis syndrome

Infective endocarditis

Introduction

Infective endocarditis was first recognized in 1885 by Sir William Osler, who described the clinical appearance as 'malignant endocarditis', because of the rapid progress of the disease and multi-system involvement. Osler also described the valvular defects of endocarditis as vegetations and noted that: 'micrococci are constant elements in the vegetations'.

Endocarditis is an infection of the endocardial surface of the heart, most commonly affecting the heart valves. It is usually due to microbial colonization of thrombi formed over surface irregularities or defects. The thrombi consist of a meshwork of platelets and fibrin, which provide a suitable environment for micro-organisms to colonize and evade the host defences. The clinical features of the disease are due to embolic phenomena produced when infected thrombi are released into the bloodstream. Almost any micro-organism (possibly excluding viruses) may be causative.

Endocarditis continues to cause high morbidity and mortality. The incidence in the United Kingdom is approximately 1400 cases per year, with some 200 deaths annually. The modes of clinical presentation of the disease have changed over the last 30 years in developed countries. Rheumatic heart disease, previously the commonest predisposing factor in all age groups, now has a declining incidence in industrial countries, although it is a continuing problem in many other parts of the world. Congenital heart disorders remain important predisposing factors, but degenerative heart disease and prosthetic heart valves have become increasingly important risk factors, with the result that over 50% of patients with endocarditis are now over 50 years old. There is also a higher proportion of cases involving intravenous drug users, with the added complication of HIV infection. In addition, a new form of the disease secondary to modern therapeutic methods is emerging, termed nosocomial endocarditis. This is seen most frequently in hospitalized patients with intravenous catheters, pacemakers, and dialysis shunts, all of which may become infected and a source of bacteria in the bloodstream.

Infective endocarditis has particular relevance to dentistry, since it has been estimated that approximately 1 in 8 cases probably arise from bacteraemias caused by dental treatment in patients at risk from developing the condition.

Pathogenesis of infective endocarditis

The disease is initiated by haemodynamic changes resulting from structural abnormalities on the surface of the heart. The valves are most commonly affected, though any surface of the endocardium may be involved. Areas of turbulence are created in the blood flow across these surfaces; this allows platelets and fibrin to be deposited in the area, forming a thrombus. The structural defect and thrombus form a vegetation (Fig. 17.1), to which micro-organisms carried in the bloodstream may then adhere. Following adherence, the microbes can colonize and multiply within the protection of the vegetation leading to further damage of the heart valve. The vegetation usually enlarges by further platelet and fibrin deposition, together with continued bacterial proliferation. Occasionally small pieces (emboli) may dislodge and are carried into the circulation where they become impacted and may cause clinical symptoms.

Structural abnormalities of the heart predisposing to endocarditis may be of several types (Fig. 17.2). Historically, valvular damage caused by rheumatic fever was the most common, though as described earlier, others have now assumed greater importance.

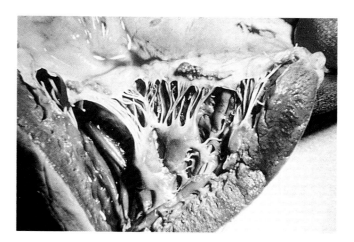

Fig. 17.1 This photograph illustrates vegetations on the mitral valve of a patient with infective endocarditis caused by *Streptococcus mitis*. (Courtesy of Mr L. Rawle.)

HEART DISEASES PREDISPOSING TO ENDOCARDITIS	
Require antibiotic cover	**Do not require antibiotic cover**
Rheumatic heart disease	Angina
Heart murmurs (take advice from consultant cardiologist)	Coronary artery by-pass
Prosthetic heart valve	Atherosclerosis
Congenital heart disease such as Downs, Marfans and Ehlers–Danlos Syndromes	Heart/kidney/liver transplant (providing no other indication)
Septal defects	Aortic aneurysm
Patent ductus arteriosus	
Previous history of endocarditis	

Fig. 17.2 Cardiac abnormalities that predispose to endocarditis and require antibiotic cover for medical and dental procedures which produce a bacteraemia.

Clinical features of infective endocarditis

Any procedure that causes a transient shower of bacteria into the bloodstream (bacteraemia), such as tooth extraction or genitouri-

INFECTIVE ENDOCARDITIS: CLINICAL FEATURES	
General points	
Many varied signs and symptoms	
Any organ system may be involved	
Four processes contribute to clinical picture: • The infection on the valve • Bland or septic embolization to many organs • Frequent bacteraemia, often with metabolic foci of infection • Circulating immune complexes and other immunopathological factors	
Physical findings	**%**
• Fever	90
• Heart murmur	85
• Embolic phenomena, e.g. splenic or renal infarction, cerebral emboli	>50
• Skin manifestations, e.g. Osler nodes, splinter haemorrhages, and petechiae	18–50
• Splenomegaly	20–57
• Septic complications, e.g. pneumonia, meningitis	20
• Mycotic (infective) aneurysm	20

Fig. 17.3 Diagram illustrating the important clinical features of infective endocarditis.

nary manipulation, may lead to endocarditis in susceptible patients. Nevertheless, in the majority of patients with endocarditis no precipitating cause can be found. The mitral valve followed by the aortic valve are most commonly affected in native valve endocarditis, with right-sided endocarditis more common in drug addicts.

There are four processes that contribute to the clinical picture (Fig. 17.3), of which bacteraemia and/or embolic septic thrombi are particularly important. The clinical features are hugely varied and may involve many organs. The common physical findings are summarized in Fig. 17.3.

The microbiology of endocarditis

Causative organisms

Most cases of endocarditis are bacterial and are frequently caused by streptococci which form part of the normal oral flora, or by enterococci. Staphylococci are the next most common cause. The important groups of organisms are summarized in Fig. 17.4. Several virulence factors have been suggested to account for the high prevalence of some bacterial species involved in endocarditis compared to others (Fig. 17.5).

Microbiological diagnosis

The diagnosis of endocarditis is made by a combination of observing clinical signs, echocardiography to visualize the heart lesions, and microbiological culture to identify the infecting organism and test its sensitivity to antimicrobial agents.

Blood culturing (Fig. 17.6) is an important investigation, because this will allow the most appropriate antibiotic to be chosen to eradicate the organism. In endocarditis there is usually a low-grade recurrent bacteraemia. Several sets of blood for culture, each at least 10 ml, should be collected before the start of antibiotic therapy and cultured under aerobic and anaerobic conditions. If no micro-organisms are detected, blood should

ORGANISMS INVOLVED IN ENDOCARDITIS		
Group	Species	Comments
Streptococci/ enterococci	Commonly referred to as viridans streptococci. These include the *Streptococcus oralis* group such as *S. oralis, S. sanguis, S. mitis, S. gordonii,* and *S. parasanguis*	Account for 40–50% of cases Primary habitat is the oral cavity and upper respiratory tract
	Enterococcus faecalis	May occur following genitourinary disease
	Streptococcus bovis	May occur following gastrointestinal disease
	Streptococcus pyogenes	Rare cause
Staphylococci	*Staphylococcus aureus*	Second most frequent cause of endocarditis. Rapid onset, high mortality, and common in intravenous drug addicts
	Coagulase-negative staphylococci	Common after heart surgery
Fungi	*Candida albicans*	Mostly affects prosthetic valves and drug addicts
Others	*Rickettsia burnetti* Anaerobes	Rare causes

Fig. 17.4 The major groups of organisms involved in endocarditis.

continue to be collected for culture during the course of the illness, preferably when the temperature of the patient rises, since this probably indicates fever due to bacteraemia.

Virtually any micro-organism is capable of causing endocarditis, therefore any agent isolated from at least two different blood culture sets should be considered as significant. Identification and antibiotic sensitivity tests are performed. Some patients will have negative blood cultures which may be due to previous antibiotic treatment, failure of the infecting organism to grow, or an incorrect clinical diagnosis.

Antimicrobial treatment

It is necessary to provide antibiotic treatment which is bactericidal, to ensure that all the organisms in the vegetations are killed as quickly as possible. Antibiotic therapy should be guided by the microbiological findings from blood cultures. However, these are frequently unavailable at the beginning of treatment and suitably high doses of relatively broad-spectrum antibiotics are initially combined, for example penicillin and gentamicin. It is important that combinations are not antagonistic and ideally should show synergistic activity. The antibiotic therapy can be altered, if necessary, when the results of laboratory sensitivity testing become available. Treatment usually lasts for 4 weeks but may be longer in cases of infected prosthetic heart valves.

During antibiotic treatment the levels of aminoglycoside antibiotics, for example gentamicin, must be measured regularly to avoid toxic effects to the patient, for example nephrotoxicity. In addition, cardiac monitoring is required, since emergency surgical valve replacement may be necessary if there is an inadequate response to antimicrobial treatment. Even in successfully treated cases, valve replacement may be required because of the extent of tissue damage caused by the infection.

Prevention of infective endocarditis

Since operative dentistry may cause a bacteraemia and subsequent endocarditis in patients with cardiac abnormalities, dental surgeons must be fully conversant with the appropriate preventive measures. The two main approaches are encouraging patients to have a very high standard of oral health and the use of appropriate antimicrobial drugs prior to specific dental procedures that cause significant bacteraemias (see Fig. 17.7).

The current British recommendations (from the Endocarditis Working Party of the British Society for Antimicrobial Chemotherapy) are summarized in Fig. 17.8. Special risk patients – who should be referred to hospital – are given more complex prophylactic antibiotic regimens, for example gentamicin in

VIRULENCE FEATURES OF ORGANISMS CAUSING ENDOCARDITIS

Virulence feature	Pathogenesis
Extracellular polysaccharide production	Many oral streptococci such as *Streptococcus sanguis* and *Streptococcus mutans* have the ability to produce dextrans. These may increase their adherence to thrombi, provide protection from host defences, and help bacteria resist the effects of antibiotics
Fibronectin binding	Fibronectin is a glycoprotein found in plasma and the extracellular matrix that binds to collagen, fibrin, and cell surfaces. Microbes with a high affinity for fibronectin, such as *Streptococcus mitis*, may colonize thrombi more easily
Stimulation of platelet aggregation	Some organisms such as *Staphylococcus aureus* and *Streptococcus mutans* promote platelet aggregation. This provides protection and increases the size of the thrombus

Fig. 17.5 Table summarizing the important virulence features of organisms involved in endocarditis.

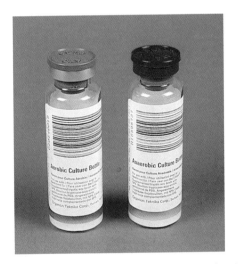

Fig. 17.6 A set of aerobic and anaerobic blood culture bottles. A positive blood culture permits identification and antibiotic sensitivity testing of the isolate causing the infection.

PREVENTION OF INFECTIVE ENDOCARDITIS

Maintenance of good oral health

Reduces bacteraemias during normal functions, e.g. chewing

Reduces the need for operative dental treatment

Prophylactic antimicrobial agents

- Chlorhexidine mouthwash
  Reduces microbial load prior to treatment

- Prophylactic antibiotic cover
  Required for dental procedures likely to cause bacteraemia:
  Dental extractions
  Subgingival scaling
  Periodontal surgery

Fig. 17.7 General principles for the prevention of infective endocarditis related to the oral flora.

combination with amoxycillin, teicoplanin, or vancomycin. Prophylactic cover should involve the use of bactericidal rather than bacteriostatic antibiotics at an adequate dose and at the right time. The most common organisms causing endocarditis from an oral source are streptococci, hence the common use of a penicillin to provide prophylaxis (Fig. 17.8).

The USA recommendations, made by the American Heart Association (AHA), were updated in 1997 and are only slightly different. They indicate 2.0 g rather than 3.0 g of amoxycillin for those not allergic to penicillin. For those allergic to penicillin,

the AHA recommendations add the alternatives of 500 mg of azithromycin or clarithromycin as alternatives to clindamycin. Other alternatives are 2.0 g of cephalexin or cefadroxil for those who do not have an immediate-type of hypersensitivity reaction to penicillin (urticaria, angioedema, or anaphylaxis).

It should also be borne in mind that transient bacteraemias will occur during chewing or toothbrushing, especially if the individual has poor periodontal support. An assessment of each individual's degree of risk, following consultation with the

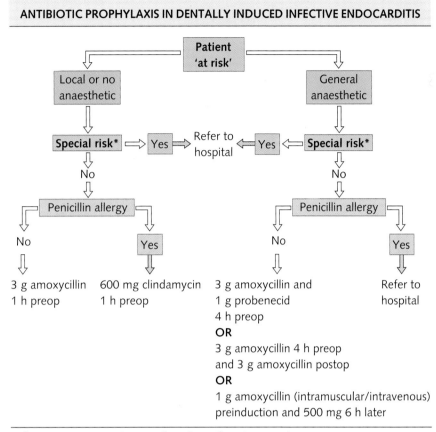

ANTIBIOTIC PROPHYLAXIS IN DENTALLY INDUCED INFECTIVE ENDOCARDITIS

All preparations are given orally unless otherwise stated
* Special-risk patients who should be referred to hospital are those:
  • who have had infective endocarditis before;
  • who require a general anaesthetic, and
  a) have a prosthetic heart valve or
  b) are allergic to penicillin or have had penicillin more than once in the previous month

Fig. 17.8 A flow chart summarizing the current recommendations made by the British Society for Antimicrobial Chemotherapy for prophylaxis against dentally induced infective endocarditis. The American regulations differ slightly (see text).

patient's medical practitioner or cardiologist, is recommended when considering prophylaxis for procedures with questionable degrees of exposure, such as endodontics and periodontal probing. It would seem prudent to use topical antimicrobial preparations such as chlorhexidine as a mouthwash or irrigant to reduce the bacterial load prior to any procedure.

Prophylactic antibiotic cover for certain dental procedures carried out on patients with artificial joints remains a controversial issue. Many orthopaedic surgeons consider that routine prophylaxis is essential. However, the advice of a Working Party of the British Society for Antimicrobial Chemotherapy is that patients with prosthetic joint implants, including total hip replacements, do not require antibiotic prophylaxis for dental treatment, since the risks of prophylaxis are believed to exceed

any benefits. Ideally, there should be liaison between orthopaedic surgeons and dentists before patients undergo joint replacement so that they can be rendered dentally fit before the operation. In any cases of doubt regarding prophylaxis, dentists should consult the patient's orthopaedic surgeon.

Sepsis syndrome

Introduction

When bacteria enter the bloodstream transiently and can be detected by laboratory blood culture techniques a bacteraemia is said to be present. There is a wide range of clinical responses to the presence of bacteria in the bloodstream, ranging from hypotension, fever, and rigors to shock, organ failure, and death. When the presence of bacteria in the bloodstream is persistent and correlates with clinical signs and symptoms then this is described as septicaemia.

Following invasion of the bloodstream by micro-organisms, the host can activate its defence mechanisms. In addition to localized defences, a systemic response to infection can be mediated by a cascade of inflammatory cytokines such as tumour necrosis factor α and interleukin-1 (Chapter 7). The release of these cytokines is stimulated by microbial products, usually lipopolysaccharide (endotoxin) from Gram-negative organisms, teichoic acid and peptidoglycan from Gram-positive bacteria, and exotoxins/superantigens from both Gram-positive and Gram-negative organisms. Generally, the cytokines act in concert to help eliminate the micro-organisms. However, excessive or prolonged activation of the cytokine system can lead to problems for the host, including the development of organ dysfunction and circulatory septic shock.

The resultant clinical responses to infection have been grouped together into a collection of signs and symptoms referred to as the systemic inflammatory response syndrome (SIRS) (Fig. 17.9). There may be organ dysfunction in severe cases, for example adult respiratory distress syndrome (ARDS). Oliguria, hypoperfusion, or acute renal failure may occur if the kidneys are involved. Occasionally the infection may trigger a pathological activation of the coagulation system (disseminated intravascular coagulation) due to the consumption of platelets and clotting factors, leading to severe bleeding disorders. The main groups of organisms responsible for the SIRS are indicated in Fig. 17.10, though it

should be stressed that the syndrome is not always due to a systemic bacterial infection but can be caused by other triggers such as ischaemia (especially of the gastrointestinal tract, which is a huge reservoir of Gram-negative bacteria), trauma, and tissue necrosis.

Predisposing factors for septicaemia

Examples of factors predisposing to septicaemia are shown in Fig. 17.11. Poor cross-infection control procedures and the overuse of broad-spectrum antibiotics in hospitals may encourage the spread of resistant bacteria, which compounds the problem.

Gram-negative septicaemia

The clinical features are precipitated by the release of endotoxin (Chapter 4) from the bacterial cell envelope. Gram-negative septicaemia is common in patients undergoing extensive surgery of the gastrointestinal tract, those receiving immunosuppressive chemotherapy, burn victims, and in the very young or very old. These infections are mostly hospital-acquired and are associated with the additional complication of infection by strains resistant to a wide range of antimicrobial drugs. The most common isolate is *Escherichia coli* which may arise from infections of the urinary, gastrointestinal, hepatobiliary, and respiratory tracts, and may cause serious disease in immunologically compromised patients with leukaemia or severe burns.

In normal individuals, especially younger age groups, the most common cause of septicaemia is *Neisseria meningitidis*. This infection can run a rapid course that progresses to meningitis, a

---

THE SYSTEMIC INFLAMMATORY RESPONSE SYNDROME (SIRS)

A clinical definition based upon 2 or more of the following findings

- Temperature > 38°C or < 36°C
- Heart rate > 90 beats per minute
- Respiratory rate > 20 breaths per minute or $PaCO_2$ < 4.3 kPa
- White blood cell count > 12 000 cells/mm³ or < 4000 cells/mm³

Fig. 17.9 Diagnostic features of the systemic inflammatory response syndrome (SIRS).

MAJOR CAUSES OF SEPSIS SYNDROME

Organisms	% Incidence	Example
Gram-negative bacteria	49	*Escherichia coli*
Gram-positive bacteria	40	*Staphylococcus aureus*
Anaerobic bacteria	7	*Bacteroides fragilis*
Non-bacterial causes	7	*Candida albicans*

Fig. 17.10 Table summarizing the important causes of sepsis syndrome.

PREDISPOSING FACTORS FOR SEPTICAEMIA	
Impaired host defences	**Examples:** leukaemia, diabetes mellitus, high-dose steroid treatment, trauma, burns, ischaemia
Instrumentation or surgery	**Examples:** manipulation of the urogenital tract or gastrointestinal system
Localized sepsis	**Example:** release of bacteria from collections of pus in the biliary tract

Fig. 17.11 Table summarizing the factors which predispose patients to septicaemia.

petechial rash, shock, and death in a few hours. Appropriate antibiotics should be given as quickly as possible to offset the sequelae. *Haemophilus influenzae* may also cause septicaemia and meningitis.

Gram–positive septicaemia

The clinical features are precipitated by teichoic acid and peptidoglycan from the cell wall or via the release of exotoxins such as staphylococcal toxic-shock syndrome toxin, a superantigen (Chapter 4). The most common organisms in this group are *Staphylococcus aureus* and *Streptococcus* spp. The bloodstream is usually infected via skin, respiratory tract, bone, or joint infections. In particular, *Streptococcus pneumoniae* can cause septicaemia from lung infections or meningitis, and coagulase-negative staphylococci may establish septicaemia following infection from in-dwelling venous catheters.

Fungal septicaemia

Fungal septicaemia is relatively rare and typically occurs in immunosuppressed individuals, for example those with haematological malignancies and individuals suffering from AIDS. The fungus most commonly isolated is *Candida albicans*.

Microbiological investigations for septicaemia

Blood cultures

One of the most important investigations is culture of blood samples to reveal the causative organism. Several separate blood samples should be collected by venepuncture to ensure that the micro-organism is detected and that positive cultures are not a result of contamination from the venepuncture site. Antimicrobial susceptibility testing of the invading organism can then be undertaken.

Culture of other infected sites

In order to determine the source of the infection it is also essential to take specimens from sites suspected to be causing the infection, for example urine from a suspected urinary tract infection or sputum from a chest infection.

Detection of microbial products in serum

Occasionally it may be difficult to culture the invading organism from blood cultures due to the presence of previously administered antibiotics. In this case it may be possible to detect bacterial antigens, such as pneumococcal antigen, in serum. Specific immunological reagents are available for this purpose. The detection of endotoxin and cytokines in the systemic circulation is an area of active research.

Treatment

Owing to the high mortality associated with septic shock (>50%) the condition must be treated aggressively in its early stages. Initially the haemodynamic status is stabilized using appropriate intravenous fluids, oxygen, and cardiogenic drugs. Ideally blood should be collected for culture before antibiotic treatment starts.

When the patient has been stabilized, high-dose antibiotics must be prescribed that cover the most likely invading organism. In the first instance, the choice of an appropriate antibiotic regimen is usually decided without appropriate microbiological data, and a 'best guess' must be made on clinical grounds as to the most likely bacteria involved. Following culture of the offending organism, the antibacterial therapy can be modified, if necessary, to provide more appropriate cover.

The source of the septicaemia should also be identified and removed. This may involve the removal of foreign bodies such as intravenous catheters or the addition of appropriate antibiotics.

Occasionally, septicaemia is slow to respond to treatment or recurs. This may be due to the presence of a collection of pus that requires surgical drainage, the presence of a foreign body such as a prosthetic hip joint, antibiotic resistance, or impaired host resistance such as in leukaemic patients.

Key facts

- Endocarditis is an infection of the endocardial surface of the heart, most commonly the heart valves, usually due to microbial colonization of microthrombi formed on the surface of defects.

- Surface defects may be due to damaged valves (rheumatic fever), congenital defects, and prosthetic heart valves.

- Endocarditis may follow any procedure that causes a bacteraemia, such as tooth extraction, in susceptible patients.

- The most common bacterial isolates from blood cultures in patients with endocarditis are from the *Streptococcus oralis* group.

Key facts – (cont.)

- The clinical features of endocarditis are due largely to embolic phenomena produced by infected thrombi being released into the bloodstream.

- Prevention of endocarditis is essential. It involves the establishment and promotion of excellent oral health in at-risk patients and the provision of appropriate antibiotic cover for procedures likely to cause a bacteraemia.

- Treatment of endocarditis involves a long course of high-dose bactericidal antibiotics directed against the causative organism.

- Sepsis syndrome is a systemic response to infection mediated by a cascade of inflammatory cytokines such as tumour necrosis factor α and interleukin-1, which are commonly stimulated by microbial constituents or products.

- A collection of clinical signs has been grouped together into the systemic inflammatory response syndrome (SIRS). This may include hypotension, fever, rigors, oliguria, renal failure, disseminated intravascular coagulation, multiple organ failure, shock, and death.

- The most common causes of septicaemia are Gram-negative bacteria such as *Escherichia coli*. They are identified using blood culture techniques.

- Treatment consists of stabilizing the patient and providing 'best guess' broad-spectrum antibiotics until sensitivity test data are available.

Further reading

Dajani, AS, *et al.* (1993). Guidelines for the diagnosis of rheumatic fever: Jones criteria, updated 1992. *Circulation*, **87**, 302–7.

Dajani, AS *et al.* (1997). Prevention of bacterial endocarditis. Recommendations by the American Heart Association. *Journal of the American Medical Association*, **277**, 1794–801.

Durack, DT, *et al.* (1994). New criteria for the diagnosis of infective endocarditis. *American Journal of Medicine*, **96**, 200–9.

Editorial (1998). Sepsis. *Journal of Antimicrobial Chemotherapy*, Supplement A, Vol 41.

Shanson, DC (1989). Septicaemia; Infections of the heart. In *Microbiology in clinical practice* (2nd edn), Chapters 5 and 18. Butterworth–Heinemann, Oxford.

Working Party of the British Society for Antimicrobial Chemotherapy (1992). Antibiotic prophylaxis and infective endocarditis. *Lancet*; i, 1292–3.

18

Viral hepatitis

- Hepatitis A virus
- Hepatitis B virus
- Hepatitis C virus
- Hepatitis D virus
- Hepatitis E virus
- Hepatitis G virus

Viral hepatitis

A wide range of viruses may cause hepatitis. These agents include, for example, the two herpes group viruses – Epstein–Barr virus and cytomegalovirus – in addition to the recognized family of hepatitis viruses classified as hepatitis A to E. This chapter will concentrate on the true hepatitis viruses A to E, the cellular targets for which are the hepatocytes themselves, and will mention the newly described hepatitis G virus.

Hepatitis A virus

The important features of hepatitis A virus (HAV) are summarized in Fig. 18.1. It is classified as a member of the *Enteroviridae* and the particles have cubic symmetry. The virus is endemic world-wide and many infections are asymptomatic. HAV initially replicates in the gut, followed by a viraemic phase during which, it is believed, the virus enters the liver. The clinical disease is mild with few complications and no carrier state.

Prevention and control of hepatitis A are based on good hygiene measures and the sanitary disposal of excreta. Passive immunization with human immunoglobulin has been available for a long time and provides protection for 3–6 months. More recently, active vaccination has become available in the form of a formalin-inactivated vaccine made from HAV grown in human diploid cells. This provides a longer lasting, more solid protection.

The virus does not pose a major hazard in relation to cross-infection in dental surgery.

Hepatitis B virus

The virus

Hepatitis B virus is a member of the hepadnavirus family. Three different particles can be seen in the peripheral blood of patients with this infection (Figs 18.2 and 18.3). The largest particles, termed Dane particles, comprise the complete virion. These intact viral particles have a double-shelled structure, with the outer hepatitis B surface antigen (HBsAg) coat surrounding the central

HEPATITIS A VIRUS	
Biology	Spherical, non-enveloped virus of 27 nm Single-stranded RNA genome Exceptional stability
Transmission and epidemiology	Faecal—oral route Person-to-person, food-borne, and water-borne Developed countries: 20%—50% of adults have antibody Developing countries: >90% of adults have antibody
Clinical features	Incubation period: 2—7 weeks Many subclinical infections Illness usually brief and self limiting Mortality <0.2% No chronic disease
Diagnosis	Demonstration of HAV antigen in faeces Serology: detection of IgM anti-HAV

Fig. 18.1 Summary of the important biological and clinical features of hepatitis A virus.

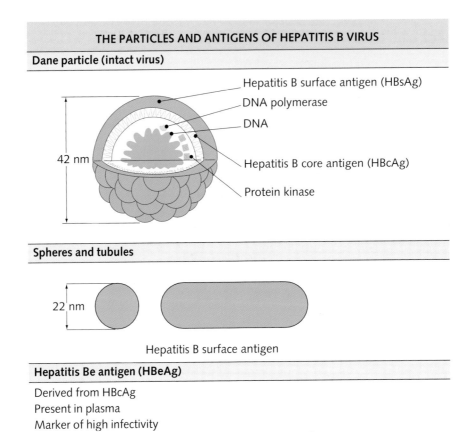

THE PARTICLES AND ANTIGENS OF HEPATITIS B VIRUS

Dane particle (intact virus)

Hepatitis B surface antigen (HBsAg)

DNA polymerase

DNA

42 nm

Hepatitis B core antigen (HBcAg)

Protein kinase

Spheres and tubules

22 nm

Hepatitis B surface antigen

Hepatitis Be antigen (HBeAg)

Derived from HBcAg
Present in plasma
Marker of high infectivity

Fig. 18.2 Diagram illustrating the particles and antigens of hepatitis B virus. Hepatitis Be antigen is a marker of high infectivity.

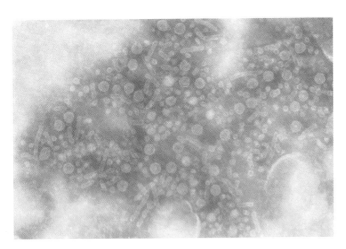

Fig. 18.3 Electron micrograph of serum from a patient with hepatitis B virus infection. The large spherical particles are the intact virions (Dane particles) and the smaller tubular and spherical forms comprise excess hepatitis B surface antigen. (Courtesy of Ian Miller.)

hepatitis B core antigen (HBcAg), the DNA and other components including the enzymes DNA polymerase and protein kinase. The DNA is circular and for most of its length is double-stranded, but one short section is single-stranded.

In addition to the Dane particles there are spherical particles with a diameter of 22 nm and filamentous forms of the same diameter. These smaller particles comprise surplus HBsAg and are non-infective.

Epidemiology and transmission

Hepatitis B virus is present in blood, cervical secretions, and semen. It may also be found in lower concentrations in a number of other body fluids including saliva. The virus is spread by the parenteral route, but transmission by intimate contact and sexual activity are also well documented. It is not transmitted by the respiratory route. There is a large reservoir of unidentified carriers within the population. Patients infected with HBV may have as many as 10^{10} Dane particles per millilitre of blood, with the result that as little as 0.0001 ml of blood may transmit the infection. Since infection can be transmitted by the inoculation of such minute amounts of infected blood there are significant risks of cross-infection between patients and staff in clinical practice, unless appropriate preventive measures are taken (Chapter 28).

Outcome of infection

There are a number of possible outcomes of exposure to HBV as summarized in Fig. 18.4. The incubation period varies widely but is long and often 2–3 months in duration.

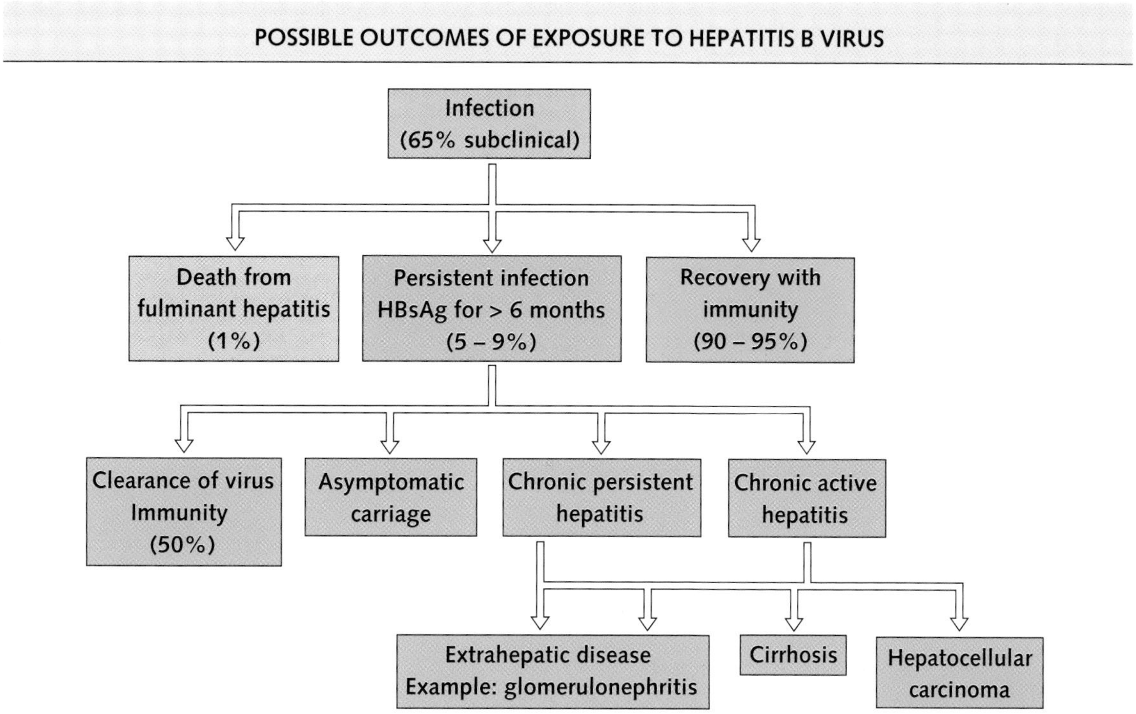

POSSIBLE OUTCOMES OF EXPOSURE TO HEPATITIS B VIRUS

Fig. 18.4 Flow diagram illustrating the possible clinical outcomes of infection with hepatitis B virus. Note the high proportion of subclinical infections (orange box).

Approximately 65% of individuals will have a subclinical infection, while a further 30% will have acute hepatitis B. Up to 9% of adults will become chronic carriers of the virus and a proportion of these will develop cirrhosis, liver failure, and hepatocellular carcinoma. Such patients also pose a risk of infection to health-care workers and other patients, particularly if they are hepatitis Be antigen (HBeAg) positive (Fig. 18.2).

Perinatal infection is an important problem in certain parts of the world, notably east and south-east Asia, the Pacific Islands, and tropical Africa. Infants born to mothers who are HBeAg-positive carriers have a 95% chance of becoming infected, and nearly all such infants become HBeAg carriers, often dying in later life of cirrhosis or liver cancer.

Diagnosis

Hepatitis B virus cannot be grown in the laboratory and diagnosis of this infection is serological. Laboratory tests can be undertaken for a wide range of antigens and antibodies but the initial screening investigation is for HBsAg. If this antigen is present in the serum it indicates that the patient is infected with hepatitis B virus.

The serological profile of markers seen in an individual making a normal recovery from hepatitis B virus infection is shown in Fig. 18.5, with loss of both HBsAg and HBeAg. The corresponding profile for a patient who is a carrier of the virus is shown in Fig. 18.6, with continuing production of HBsAg and, in a high-risk carrier, HBeAg for many years.

Prevention of infection

Control of HBV infection may take place on several fronts. Modifications to behaviour can reduce the risk of infection, and in the clinical setting this would include an adequate cross-infection control regimen.

Passive immunization is available in the form of hyperimmune hepatitis B immunoglobulin, which is used for dealing with a single acute exposure in an unprotected individual. This immunoglobulin must be given within 48 hours of a significant exposure if it is to be effective.

Active immunization with hepatitis B vaccine is now available. Current vaccines are produced by genetic engineering. The dosage is 20 μg of HBsAg given intramuscularly at 0, 1, and 6 months. Boosters are recommended at 5-year intervals in the UK. Protection is good in those who respond to the vaccine, but approximately 5% of individuals do not respond and do not develop a protective level of antibody. All vaccinees should, therefore, have blood taken at the end of a course of vaccination so that their antibody level can be assessed. Non-responders who are health-care workers should also undergo appropriate serological investigation to exclude high-risk carriage of HBV (HBeAg positive).

A number of antiviral agents have been assessed in the treatment of chronic HBV infection. Of these agents, interferon has proved to be the most effective.

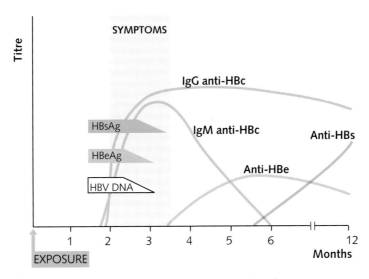

Fig. 18.5 The serological profile for a patient who recovers fully from hepatitis B virus infection.

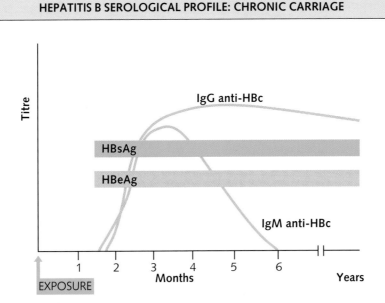

Fig. 18.6 The serological profile for a patient who becomes a high-risk (HBeAg-positive) carrier of hepatitis B virus.

Hepatitis C virus

Hepatitis C virus (HCV) is one of the agents responsible for the type of hepatitis known until recently as non-A, non-B hepatitis (Fig. 18.7). Its discovery was a remarkable feat of molecular biology and the virus has yet to be grown in tissue culture or visualized under the electron microscope. It is now known that there are at least six major genotypes of HCV, which show an interesting geographical distribution.

Epidemiology and transmission

Figure 18.8 illustrates our knowledge to date. The prevalence of HCV antibodies among blood donors in the United Kingdom is low (0.1–0.3%), although the epidemiology of this infection in

HEPATITIS C VIRUS

- Blood-borne virus discovered in 1989
- Enveloped RNA virus
- Diameter 30–38 nm
- Related to animal pestiviruses and human flaviviruses
- Multiple genotypes
- Morphology unknown
- Cannot be grown in tissue culture

Fig. 18.7 The biological characteristics of hepatitis C virus.

SPREAD OF HEPATITIS C VIRUS	
Seroepidemiology	Blood donors (UK): 0.1% – 0.3% Haemophiliacs given uninactivated factor VIII: 60% – 100% Intravenous drug users: 70% – 92%
Transmission	Intravenous drug use Blood and blood products Organ and tissue transplantation Sexual transmission Vertical transmission (mother to child) Occupational transmission Undefined routes (? saliva)

Fig. 18.8 Current knowledge of the epidemiology and transmission of hepatitis C virus.

the general population is unclear. The seroprevalence is high (>80%) in those who have received blood products and among intravenous drug users, indicating the importance of parenteral transmission.

The virus may be transmitted sexually, although this appears to be an inefficient route. Well-documented cases of occupational transmission through needlestick injuries to health-care workers have been reported, though the virus is less infectious than the hepatitis B virus. In up to 40% of individuals who are HCV antibody positive the route of infection is undefined, suggesting that the mechanisms of transmission are not fully known.

The clinical course of HCV infection is summarized in Fig. 18.9. There is a wide incubation period of up to 26 weeks and a long period for seroconversion, which may cause diagnostic difficulties. The acute disease is milder than acute hepatitis B and many cases are subclinical. However, the main problem is the high proportion of individuals who develop chronic HCV infection. These patients are at risk of long-term liver disease in the form of cirrhosis, autoimmune hepatitis, and hepatocellular carcinoma.

Diagnosis

The diagnosis of infection with HCV is serological (Fig. 18.10). The initial testing is for anti-HCV antibodies, but any positive specimens should be confirmed by the polymerase chain reaction assay for HCV RNA.

Prevention of infection

The prevention of infection with HCV is through changes in behaviour and through the recent introduction of screening donated blood. No vaccine is available, and because of the multiple genotypes, together with the rapid mutation of this virus, the development of a vaccine is proving extremely difficult. Hepatitis C virus is of potential relevance to dentistry because of the parenteral spread of this agent and also because it has been detected in saliva.

HEPATITIS C: CLINICAL COURSE	
Incubation	Mean incubation period: 6 – 12 weeks Mean seroconversion period: 15 weeks
Acute infection	Clinically mild — commonly subclinical Jaundice in 25% of patients
Chronic hepatitis C	High frequency: at least 60% of those infected Most cases preceded by clinically inapparent infection Most patients unaware of their disease and infectivity Indolent and slowly progressive over 20+ years Progression from mild hepatitis to cirrhosis Link with hepatocellular carcinoma

Fig. 18.9 The clinical outcomes of infection with hepatitis C virus. Note the high incidence of chronic disease.

HEPATITIS C: DIAGNOSIS

- **Detection of antibodies to HCV**
  Screening test:
  Enzyme-linked immunosorbent assay (ELISA)

  Supplementary test:
  Recombinant immunoblot assay (RIBA)
- **Detection of viral genome**
  Polymerase chain reaction (PCR) for HCV RNA
- **Histological features on liver biopsy**

Fig. 18.10 Methods available for diagnosing hepatitis C virus infection.

Hepatitis D virus

This virus is a defective but independently transmissible agent (Fig. 18.11) which requires hepatitis B virus for its replication. Its genome is single-stranded RNA. Transmission is primarily parenteral, and it may either infect at the time of first infection with HBV (co-infection) or during a subsequent exposure in a patient already infected with HBV (superinfection).

The possible outcomes of such infections are shown in Fig. 18.12. In general, hepatitis D virus appears to increase the severity of HBV infection and fulminant hepatitis is common, particularly following superinfection.

The virus has a world-wide distribution and is especially prevalent in Italy, parts of the Middle East and parts of Latin America. In the West it is mainly a problem among intravenous drug users. Hepatitis B vaccination is protective, since this agent cannot cause disease in the absence of HBV.

Hepatitis E virus

This is another recently discovered virus, responsible for the disease described previously as enterically transmitted non-A, non-B hepatitis. Details of the virus are given in Fig. 18.13.

HEPATITIS D (DELTA) VIRUS

Defective, small RNA virus

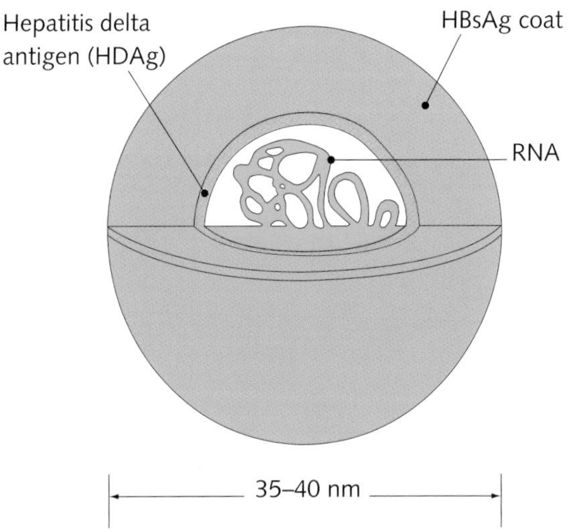

Hepatitis delta antigen (HDAg)

HBsAg coat

RNA

35–40 nm

Transmission

Blood-borne virus
Parenteral and sexual routes
Independently transmissible
Co-infection or superinfection with hepatitis B virus
Persistent infection common

Relationship with hepatitis B virus

Requires hepatitis B virus for replication
Outer coat of HBs Ag permits attachment to liver cells
Hepatitis B vaccination protects against hepatitis D virus infection

Fig. 18.11 Summary of the important features of hepatitis D virus (delta agent).

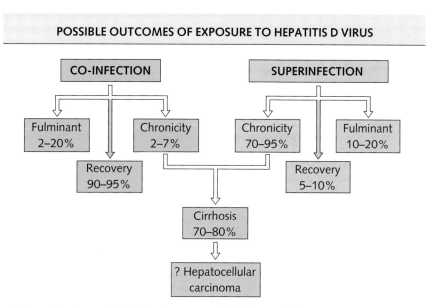

POSSIBLE OUTCOMES OF EXPOSURE TO HEPATITIS D VIRUS

Fig. 18.12 Flow diagram illustrating the possible clinical outcomes of infection with hepatitis D virus. The clinical features are generally more severe in the case of superinfection of a patient already infected with hepatitis B virus.

	HEPATITIS E
Biology	Spherical, non-enveloped virus (32–34 nm) Single-stranded RNA genome Calicivirus-like Cannot be grown in tissue culture
Transmission and epidemiology	Faecally contaminated drinking water Epidemic and sporadic forms Predominantly India, Asia, and Africa
Clinical features	Incubation period: 2–9 weeks Mainly young adults (15–40 years) Usually self-limiting acute disease High mortality (up to 20%) in pregnancy No chronic disease

Fig. 18.13 Summary of the important features of hepatitis E virus.

Clinically the disease is in many ways similar to hepatitis A virus infection, but the high mortality among pregnant women is notable. This virus does not pose a major risk of cross-infection in the dental surgery.

Hepatitis G virus

Hepatitis G virus is a flavivirus, first isolated in 1995 from the plasma of a patient with chronic hepatitis. Its genome shares 25% homology with hepatitis C virus. Seroprevalence studies have reported its presence in 1.7% of American blood donors and in over 3% of a similar cohort in the United Kingdom. In other studies, 18% of haemophiliac patients and 33% of intravenous drug users were infected. There is early evidence of transmission in haemodialysis units and of mother to infant spread. An understanding of the disease associations of this virus is presently unclear. It is known that both acute and chronic hepatitis may follow infection and that a normal carrier state probably exists, but in most cases hepatic damage appears to be mild or absent.

The importance of this virus in dentistry is not yet known, but in view of its apparent parenteral transmission the implementation of universal infection control measures is important.

Key facts

- Hepatitis A virus is transmitted by the faecal–oral route. Clinical disease is mild and there is no chronic carrier state.

- Hepatitis B virus (HBV) is a double-shelled DNA virus.

- HBV is transmitted by body fluids. Blood to blood contact, sexual transmission, and perinatal transmission are major routes. Very small volumes of blood may be infectious.

- During infection with HBV, blood contains intact virions (Dane particles) and smaller tubular and spherical forms of hepatitis B surface antigen (HBsAg).

- The outcomes of infection with HBV include subclinical infection (65%), acute hepatitis B (30%), and fatal fulminant hepatitis (1%). Between 5 and 10% of patients become chronic carriers.

- Chronic carriers of HBV are infectious and are at risk of cirrhosis and hepatocellular carcinoma.

- Diagnosis of HBV infection is serological, with initial screening for HBsAg.

- Prevention of HBV infection is based on blocking person-to-person transmission and on immunization.

- Hepatitis C virus (HCV) is a recently described, parenterally transmitted RNA virus, spread largely by blood-to-blood contact, for example intravenous drug users. No vaccine is available and prevention is based on blocking person-to-person transmission.

- A high proportion of those infected with HCV become chronic carriers and may develop liver disease in the long term.

- Diagnosis of HCV infection is serological.

- Hepatitis D virus (HDV) is an independently transmissible virus which can only cause disease in the presence of the hepatitis B virus.

- HDV increases the severity of hepatitis B virus infection, often resulting in fulminant hepatitis.

- Hepatitis E virus (HEV) is a recently identified enterically transmitted virus. The disease is clinically mild, but there is a high mortality among pregnant women.

- Hepatitis G virus is a newly described flavivirus, the disease associations of which are still to be defined.

Further reading

Cottone, JA and Puttaiah, R (1996). Hepatitis B virus infection. Current status in dentistry. *Dental Clinics of North America*, 40, 293–307.

Karaylannis, P and Thomas, H (1997). Hepatitis G virus: identification, prevalence and unanswered questions. *Gut*, 40, 294–6.

Mims, C, Playfair, J, Roitt, I, Wakelin, D, and Williams, R (1998). Gastrointestinal tract infections. In *Medical microbiology* (2nd edn), Chapter 20. Mosby, London.

Molinari, JA (1996). Hepatitis C virus infection. *Dental Clinics of North America*, 40, 309–25.

Zuckerman, AJ and Harrison, TJ (1994). Hepatitis viruses. In *Principles and practice of clinical virology* (3rd edn) (ed. AJ Zuckerman, JE Banatvala, and JR Pattison), Chapter 2. Wiley, Chichester.

19

Retroviruses and AIDS

- Introduction
- General properties of retroviruses
- HIV and AIDS

Retroviruses and AIDS

Introduction

The retrovirus family contains many viruses which infect a wide range of animal species. The first retrovirus, avian sarcoma virus, was discovered in 1910 by Peyton Rous, and in subsequent years other retroviruses, capable of causing tumours in animals, were described. The first human retrovirus, human T-lymphotropic virus type I (HTLV-I) was isolated in 1980 from a patient with T-cell leukaemia. In recent years it has become clear that another retrovirus, human immunodeficiency virus (HIV), is responsible for the acquired immune deficiency syndrome (AIDS).

The emergence of HIV infection and AIDS has made an immense impact on dentistry. The threat of cross-infection in the dental surgery has resulted in the adoption of much stricter infection control measures (Chapter 28). In addition, there are a number of oral manifestations of HIV infection (Fig. 19.9), some of which may be presenting features of the disease and to which practising dentists must always be alert.

General properties of retroviruses

The retroviruses comprise a single taxonomic group of RNA viruses. They all contain the enzyme reverse transcriptase, which is an RNA-dependent DNA polymerase. All retroviruses have an envelope composed of lipid and viral proteins. Each viral particle is about 100 nm in diameter. The important structural components are illustrated in Fig. 19.1.

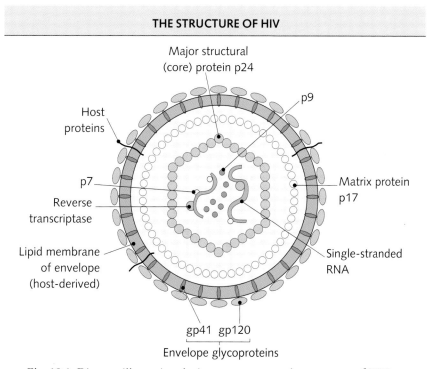

THE STRUCTURE OF HIV

Major structural (core) protein p24

p9

Host proteins

p7

Reverse transcriptase

Lipid membrane of envelope (host-derived)

Matrix protein p17

Single-stranded RNA

gp41 gp120

Envelope glycoproteins

Fig. 19.1 Diagram illustrating the important structural components of HIV.

RETROVIRUSES INFECTING HUMANS		
Subfamily	**Disease association**	**Natural hosts**
Oncoviruses		
Human T cell leukaemia virus I (HTLV-I)	Adult T cell leukaemia–lymphoma (ATLL)	Humans
Human T cell leukaemia virus II (HTLV-II)	Hairy cell leukaemia	Humans
Lentiviruses		
Human immunodeficiency virus-1 (HIV-1)	Immune deficiency, ultimately AIDS	Humans
Human immunodeficiency virus-2 (HIV-2)	Immune deficiency, ultimately AIDS	Humans and primates
Spumaviruses	Inapparent persistent infections	Humans and primates

Fig. 19.2 Classification of the retroviruses that may infect man.

Classification

The retroviruses are divided into three subfamilies: oncoviruses, lentiviruses, and spumaviruses (Fig. 19.2).

The oncoviruses include those retroviruses that cause tumours rather than immunosuppression. Lentiviruses are associated with diseases that are slowly progressive, and include HIV-1 and HIV-2. They are cytopathic, and destroy many of the cells they invade. The spumaviruses, so-called because of the foamy appearance of infected cells in culture, are not known to be pathogenic.

Replication

Retroviruses are different from other RNA viruses, since they replicate and produce viral RNA from a DNA copy of the virion RNA, through the action of reverse transcriptase.

The replication of HIV-1 will be used as an example (Fig 19.3). The HIV-1 envelope glycoprotein gp120 binds specifically to the CD4 molecule of T-helper lymphocytes. It may also bind to macrophages, dendritic cells, and brain cells which are believed to possess a few CD4 molecules. Following binding, the virus enters the host cell by membrane fusion and the RNA is released. Under the influence of reverse transcriptase, a double-stranded DNA copy is produced. This DNA is circularized, passes into the nucleus, and is spliced into the host-cell DNA as a provirus. From this point, infection with HIV is permanent. The virus may remain latent or enter a productive cycle. Host RNA polymerase enzymes can transcribe messenger RNA (mRNA) from the provirus to produce viral mRNA and RNA. New virions are then assembled at the cell membrane where envelope and core proteins are located. Release of the virions is by budding, and in the productive growth cycle the host cell is destroyed.

HIV and AIDS

Transmission

The main routes of transmission are summarized in Fig. 19.4. In the developed countries, homosexual men have been the group most at risk of HIV infection (Fig. 19.5). Intravenous drug users comprise a significant, though smaller, risk group and many haemophiliacs were infected with contaminated factor VIII.

Sexual transmission is primarily from male to male and from male to female. However, in Africa heterosexual transmission, including from female to male, is a common event, and in some parts of Central and East Africa as many as 40% of the population are infected, mainly young adults. This may result from the high prevalence of other sexually transmitted diseases, many of which result in genital ulceration.

Vertical transmission to infants from infected mothers occurs in about 20% of cases, and may occur *in utero*, either perinatally or postnatally. Transmission by close contact, aerosols, and kissing is not believed to occur.

Pathogenesis

The main determinant in both the pathogenesis and the disease caused by HIV is the tropism of this virus for CD4-expressing cells, namely the helper and delayed-type hypersensitivity T cells, together with macrophages and some brain cells.

HIV REPLICATION CYCLE

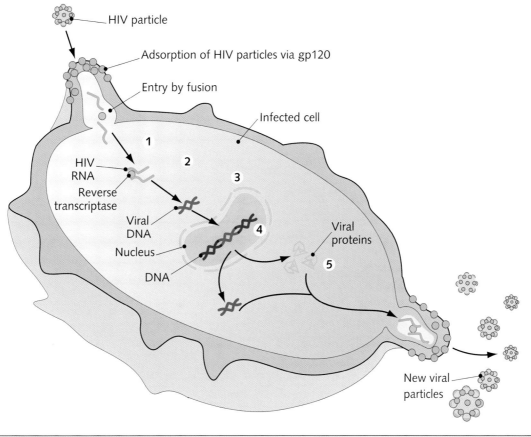

Key to stages in replicative cycle

1	HIV releases contents into target cell
2	Reverse transcriptase copies viral RNA into DNA
3	Viral DNA is inserted into cellular DNA
4	Many copies of viral RNA and proteins are made
5	New viral particles assemble and bud from cell, potentially killing it

Fig. 19.3 Summary of the HIV replication cycle. (Redrawn from Nowak and McMichael 1995; with permission.)

The interactions between HIV and the immune system are now known to be significantly more dynamic than scientists first thought. It was originally believed that after infecting CD4 cells the virus replicated and then established latency. Activation of the infected CD4 T cell at a later date, for example by contact with a foreign antigen, was then believed to result in viral killing of the cell. Recent evidence indicates that HIV replicates prodigiously and destroys many cells of the immune system every day. However, this growth is countered, usually for many years, by a vigorous host-defence response that prevents the virus from multiplying out of control. Destruction of CD4 T cells is achieved in several ways, including cytotoxic T-cell lysis, natural killer cells, and antibody-dependent cellular cytotoxicity. Ultimately, however, the balance of power shifts so that HIV gains the upper hand, resulting in the severe immunodeficiency characteristic of full-blown AIDS.

The CD4 T cells are central to the initiation of an immune response. They release lymphokines required for the activation of macrophages, other T cells, B cells, and natural killer cells. When the number of these cells is reduced substantially by HIV infection, antigen-specific immune responses, especially cellular responses, are incapacitated and humoral responses uncontrolled.

The abilities of HIV to disable the immune system and alter its antigenicity by repeated mutation allow the virus to escape complete immune clearance and prevent disease resolution.

HIV TRANSMISSION	
Inoculation of blood	Transfusion of blood and blood products
	Needle sharing by intravenous drug users
	Needlestick accidents and open-wound or mucous-membrane exposure in health-care workers
Sexual transmission	Male homosexuals
	Heterosexual contact
Perinatal transmission	Intrauterine
	Peripartum
	Breast milk

Fig. 19.4 Main routes of transmission of HIV.

HIV-1 INFECTED PERSONS IN THE UNITED KINGDOM			
Exposure category	**Male**	**Female**	**Total**
Male homosexual	17660	—	17660
Heterosexual contact			
'High-risk' partner	113	538	651
Exposure abroad	2116	2048	4164
Exposure UK	189	292	481
Under investigation	133	180	313
Heterosexual total	2551	3058	5609
Injection drug use	2075	957	3032
Blood factor (e.g. haemophiliac)	1249	11	1260
Blood/tissue transfer (e.g. transfusion)	101	107	208
Mother to child	203	212	415
Other/undetermined	737	171	908
TOTAL HIV-1 INFECTED	24576	4516	29092
TOTAL AIDS CASES	12614	1468	14082
TOTAL DEAD	9477	887	10364

Fig. 19.5 Table summarizing the total number of HIV-1 infected persons in the United Kingdom up to March 1997 in relation to exposure category. Male homosexuals comprise the largest subgroup. (Source: PHLS/CDSC, London and SCIEH, Glasgow.)

HIV infection also has effects on the nervous system. It is present in the brain, mainly in macrophages but also in microglial, oligodendroglial, and capillary endothelial cells. Most AIDS patients develop neurological disease and it has been suggested that macrophages carry the virus into the brain.

Clinical features

Time course

The classification of the various stages of HIV infection and AIDS proposed by the Centers for Disease Control in the USA is sum-marized in Fig. 19.6. The corresponding profiles for HIV antibody, CD4 cell count, and viral titre are illustrated in Fig. 19.7.

The acute seroconversion illness (Group I), which is recognized in up to 60% of those infected, has an incubation period of about 1 month and resembles mild glandular fever. Antibodies may take several months to develop (Fig. 19.7) and cytotoxic T cells are also formed. The disease then becomes quiescent (Group II). Persistent generalized lymphadenopathy (Group III) is present in up to 30% of those who are otherwise asymptomatic. As the disease progresses, patients develop other features including weight loss, fever, oral candidosis, and diarrhoea (Group IV). Viral replication

STAGES OF HIV INFECTION

- **Group I**
  Seroconversion illness
- **Group II**
  Asymptomatic
- **Group III**
  Persistent generalized lymphadenopathy
- **Group IV**
  A – constitutional disease
  B – neurological disease
  C – secondary infectious disease
  D – secondary cancers
  E – other conditions

Fig. 19.6 Classification of the various stages of HIV infection as proposed by the Centers for Disease Control, USA. Of the 27 specific diseases associated with Group IV, 19 are AIDS-defining diseases.

continues until the development of full-blown AIDS, which is defined as the presence of HIV and one or more AIDS-defining diseases. These include Kaposi's sarcoma and *Pneumocystis carinii* pneumonia, and are listed with the diseases associated with Group IV. Overall, more than half of those patients already diagnosed with AIDS have died (Fig. 19.5). If untreated, the median survival from the time of diagnosis is 1 year, and 95% are dead within 5 years of diagnosis.

Clinical features of late-stage infection

AIDS is an epidemic immunosuppressive viral disease. The clinical features are dominated by a susceptibility to life-threatening infections, the development of tumours, and neurological disease – typically a subacute encephalitis, often with dementia. These are summarized, with examples, in Fig. 19.8.

Oral manifestations of HIV infection

The oral manifestations have been classified by the strength of their association with HIV infection. Figure 19.9 lists the oral manifestations which are strongly associated with HIV infection.

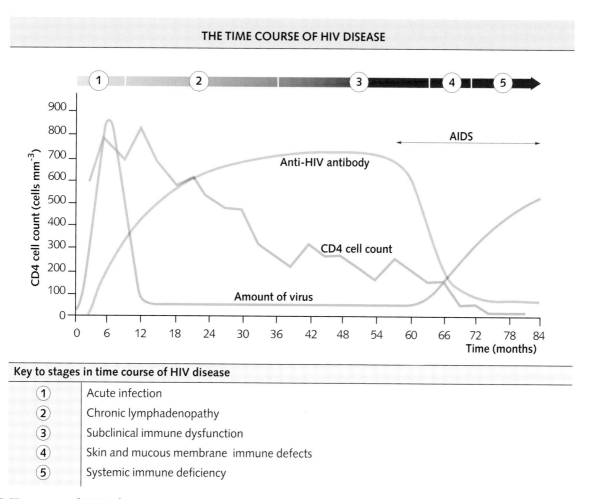

THE TIME COURSE OF HIV DISEASE

Key to stages in time course of HIV disease

①	Acute infection
②	Chronic lymphadenopathy
③	Subclinical immune dysfunction
④	Skin and mucous membrane immune defects
⑤	Systemic immune deficiency

Fig. 19.7 Time course of HIV infection showing elevated levels of virus at the beginning and end of infection, the gradual reduction in the CD4 cell count, and the anti-HIV antibody profile.

CLINICAL FEATURES OF AIDS

- **Lymphadenopathy and fever**
  Insidious onset
  May be accompanied by weight loss and malaise
- **Opportunistic infections**
  Pneumocystis carinii pneumonia
  Cerebral toxoplasmosis
  Cryptococcal meningitis
  Candidosis
  Herpesvirus infections
  Diarrhoeal disease
- **Malignancies**
  Kaposi's sarcoma
  Non-Hodgkin's lymphoma
- **Wasting**
  Common in Africa
- **AIDS-related dementia**
  Decrease in cognitive and/or motor functions

Fig. 19.8 Summary of the major clinical features of AIDS.

ORAL LESIONS STRONGLY ASSOCIATED WITH HIV INFECTION

Candidosis	Erythematous Pseudomembranous
Hairy leukoplakia	
Kaposi's sarcoma	
Non-Hodgkin's lymphoma	
Periodontal disease	Linear gingival erythema Necrotizing (ulcerative) gingivitis Necrotizing (ulcerative) periodontitis

Fig. 19.9 Oral lesions showing a strong association with HIV infection. These are important markers of HIV infection and disease progression.

Oral candidosis (Chapter 26) is a very common feature of HIV infection. Erythematous candidosis (Fig. 19.10) appears as red areas commonly found on the hard and soft palate, buccal mucosa, and tongue. Pseudomembranous candidosis (thrush) (see Fig. 26.10) presents as creamy white plaques that can be wiped off the mucosa to reveal a granular, erythematous base. Angular cheilitis (see Fig. 26.14) may also be seen and is often secondary to intraoral candidosis.

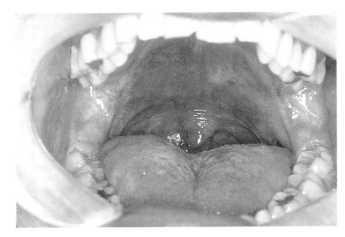

Fig. 19.10 Erythematous candidosis affecting the palatal mucosa in an HIV-positive patient. (Courtesy of Dr D. Felix.)

Oral hairy leukoplakia (Fig 19.11) is an asymptomatic, white, hyperkeratotic lesion, usually presenting on the lateral margins of the tongue. Classically it has vertical corrugations. Molecular biological investigations have shown that Epstein–Barr virus is invariably present in these lesions, and is believed to play a role in their aetiology.

Kaposi's sarcoma (Fig. 19.12) arises from endothelial cells of blood vessels and presents as purple/dark blue macules or nodules, most commonly on the palate. Kaposi's sarcoma is more common in homosexual men than in other groups with HIV infection, and the recently described human herpesvirus 8 (HHV-8) is now believed to play a role in its aetiology.

Non-Hodgkin's lymphoma appears as a rapidly growing swelling or intractable ulceration, which may occur anywhere in the mouth.

Periodontal manifestations of HIV infection are divided into three groups. Linear gingival erythema presents as a localized red

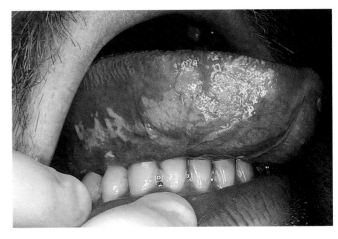

Fig. 19.11 Oral hairy leukoplakia in a patient with AIDS. (Courtesy of Dr D. Felix.)

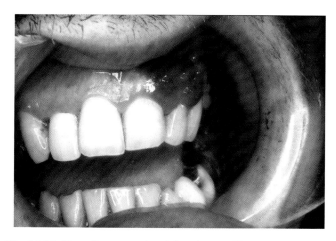

Fig. 19.12 Kaposi's sarcoma involving the maxillary gingivae in a patient with AIDS. (Courtesy of Prof. D. Wray.)

band on the marginal gingiva, often in the presence of good oral hygiene. Necrotizing ulcerative gingivitis involves localized ulcerative destruction of the gingiva with pain and spontaneous gingival bleeding. Finally, in necrotizing ulcerative periodontitis there is rapid, localized, ulcerative destruction of periodontal tissue, including bone.

Other miscellaneous oral lesions seen in HIV infection include recurrent intraoral herpes simplex infections, cytomegalovirus-associated oral ulceration, and parotid gland enlargement, the latter often in association with oral dryness (Chapter 25).

Laboratory diagnosis of HIV infection

A specific virological diagnosis of HIV infection can be achieved in several ways (Fig. 19.13) but, in practice, current laboratory tests depend on antibody detection. Patients must always be given appropriate counselling by a senior clinician or by a professionally trained counsellor, before blood is submitted for testing. An enzyme-linked immunosorbent assay (ELISA) test is initially performed for detection of HIV antibody. Positive results are always confirmed by examining a further blood sample from the same patient using a range of different test formats such as radioimmunoassay or immunofluorescence. This ensures that no false-positives are reported.

Prevention of HIV infection

The emphasis in controlling this infection must be on risk reduction. Public education programmes have concentrated on the need for changes in sexual behaviour, particularly the use of barrier contraceptives. The problem of spread among the intravenous drug-using population has been approached by the distribution of free sterile needles and syringes in some areas.

The risk of transmission to health-care workers is low (Chapter 28) and the use of protective workwear, together with measures to avoid needlestick accidents, will minimize the possibilities of infection.

Despite intense research efforts, the likelihood of a vaccine being developed in the near future seems remote. An attenuated virus vaccine is unlikely, because of the difficulty of assessing attenuation, whilst killed vaccines are poor inducers of a cytotoxic T-cell response. Vaccines containing viral envelope proteins (gp160, gp120, or gp41), or synthetic peptides identified as important epitopes for neutralizing antibodies offer the best prospects at present. However, the rapid rate of HIV mutation adds another layer of difficulty to the search for an effective vaccine.

LABORATORY DIAGNOSIS OF HIV INFECTION	
Serology	Demonstration of specific anti-HIV antibodies Mainstay of clinical diagnosis
Viral culture	Slow process (3–6 weeks) Not routinely available
Viral antigen (p24)	Present briefly at time of infection Reappears late in the infection Correlates with degree of viraemia Not routinely available
Viral nucleic acid	Polymerase chain reaction (PCR) useful in patients with indeterminate serological results May have role in confirming infection in babies born to carrier mothers

Fig. 19.13 Laboratory methods available for the diagnosis of HIV infection. At present, demonstration of anti-HIV antibodies is the only method routinely available for clinical diagnostic purposes.

MANAGEMENT OF AIDS

- **Treat opportunistic infections**
  Examples: Fluconazole for candidosis
  Pentamidine for *Pneumocystis carinii*
  Ganciclovir for cytomegalovirus

- **Treat Kaposi's sarcoma and other malignancy**
  Example: locally administered cytotoxic drugs

- **Antiretroviral therapy**
  Examples: Azidothymidine (AZT)
  Protease inhibitors

- **Supportive medicine**
  Psychosocial

Fig. 19.14 Summary of the main components in the management of patients with AIDS.

Key facts

- Retroviruses are enveloped RNA viruses containing the enzyme reverse transcriptase.

- Reverse transcriptase is an RNA-dependent DNA polymerase enzyme which transcribes viral RNA into DNA (provirus).

- HIV belongs to the cytopathic lentivirus subgroup of retroviruses.

- HIV may be transmitted by the inoculation of blood, sexual contact, and perinatally.

- HIV infects CD4-positive cells, notably T-helper lymphocytes, resulting in the eventual disablement of the immune system.

- Clinical features of AIDS are dominated by a susceptibility to life-threatening infections, the development of tumours, and neurological disease.

- Oral manifestations are common and important markers of HIV infection.

- Diagnosis of HIV infection is currently based on antibody detection.

- Management of HIV infection is with combinations of antiretroviral drugs together with prompt treatment of opportunistic infections and other complications.

Treatment

The management of patients with advanced HIV infection is complex, but the main aspects of treatment are outlined in Fig. 19.14.

In relation to specific antiretroviral drugs, azidothymidine (AZT) was the first anti-HIV drug licensed for treating AIDS. It reduced the symptoms and improved the survival of patients with AIDS, though some developed severe side-effects. However, other drugs, including nucleotide analogues such as 3TC and protease inhibitors such as ritonavir, have now been developed. Current evidence supports the use of combinations of these drugs, since dual or triple therapy is far more effective than AZT monotherapy. Such combination therapy has proved a major breakthrough, revolutionizing the outlook for AIDS patients. However, the drugs are very costly and the long term effectiveness of treatment is, as yet, unknown.

Further reading

BHIVA Guidelines Co-ordinating Committee. (1997). British HIV Association guidelines for antiretroviral treatment of HIV seropositive individuals. *Lancet*, 349, 1086–92.

Carpenter, CC, *et al.*(1997). Antiretroviral therapy for HIV infection in 1997. Updated recommendations of the International AIDS Society – USA panel. *Journal of the American Medical Association*, 277, 1962–9.

Dalgleish, AG and Weiss, RA (1994). Human retroviruses. In *Principles and practice of clinical virology* (3rd edn) (ed. AJ Zuckerman, JE Banatvala, and JR Pattison), Chapter 24. Wiley, Chichester.

EC Clearinghouse on Oral Problems Related to HIV Infection and WHO Collaborating Centre on Oral Manifestations of Immunodeficiency Virus (1993). Classification and diagnostic criteria for oral lesions in HIV infection. *Journal of Oral Pathology and Medicine*, 22, 289–91.

Fanning, MM (1997). *HIV infection: a clinical approach*. W.B. Saunders, Philadelphia.

Friedman-Kien, AE and Cockerell, CJ (1996). *Color atlas of AIDS* (2nd edn). W.B. Saunders, Philadelphia.

Kemeny, L, Gyulai, R, Kiss, M, Nagy, F, and Dobozy, A (1997). Kaposi's sarcoma-associated herpesvirus/human herpesvirus-8: a new virus in human pathology. *Journal of the American Academy of Dermatology*, 37, 107–13.

Lucht, E and Nord, CE (1996). Opportunistic oral infections in patients infected with HIV-1. *Reviews in Medical Microbiology*, 7, 151–63.

Nowak, MA and McMichael, AJ (1995). How HIV defeats the immune system. *Scientific American*, August, 42–9.

Section 3

20

The oral microflora and dental plaque

- Introduction

- Study of the oral microflora

- Composition of the oral microflora

- Acquisition of the oral flora

- Dental plaque formation

- Calculus

- Factors affecting the growth of oral micro-organisms

- Antiplaque agents

The oral microflora and dental plaque

Introduction

The oral flora is one of the most ecologically diverse microbial populations known to man. It contains at least 350 different cultivable species, with probably a further 50% that cannot be cultured using current laboratory techniques. Saliva contains up to 100 million organisms per millilitre. As long ago as 1674, Antonie van Leeuwenhoek, father of the modern-day microscope, observed 'little living animalcules very prettily amoving' in his own dental plaque (Fig. 20.1), and with remarkable foresight estimated that 'there are more animals in the scum on the teeth in a man's mouth than there are men in the whole kingdom'. In addition to this microbial complexity the oral cavity provides some unique habitats for bacterial colonization, including the teeth, mucosal surfaces, and gingival crevices.

Despite these distinctions the mouth is similar to other body sites in having a resident normal flora with a characteristic composition, including large numbers of anaerobes. Normally, the oral flora exists in a harmonious relationship with the host. This relationship can be disturbed by any changes to the habitat which affect the stability of the microflora, for example xerostomia or the use of broad-spectrum antibiotics. Some bacteria, including many oral micro-organisms, can exploit these lapses and behave as opportunistic pathogens (Chapter 4). Changes in the balance between the host and the microbial flora may lead to mucosal infections and increase the prevalence of both dental caries and periodontal disease. The latter pose large, essentially preventable, public health problems in both industrialized and non-industrialized nations, costing many millions of pounds per year to treat.

Study of the oral microflora

In order to understand the aetiology of many oral and dental diseases and to interpret the results of microbiological analyses of clinical specimens, a knowledge of the micro-organisms which comprise the resident flora within different ecological niches of the oral cavity is important. However, there are technical problems at all stages of analysing the oral microflora which potentially compromise the accuracy of studies. The various methods and associated problems involved in specimen collection and processing are shown in Fig. 20.2. The initial sample collection is often the most important step in a microbiological investigation and will significantly influence the results obtained.

Composition of the oral microflora

Most bacteria found in the oral cavity can be classified as Gram-positive (Fig. 20.3) or Gram-negative (Fig. 20.4). Streptococci comprise a major part of the oral flora and play an important role in dental caries, purulent oral infections, and infective endocarditis. Modern taxonomic methods have permitted their division into several major groups, as summarized in Fig. 20.5.

Some species of spirochaetes, protozoa, and mycoplasma are also members of the normal oral flora but are very difficult to cultivate. Spirochaetes are best demonstrated by the technique of dark-ground microscopy (Fig. 20.6). Other bacteria, such as the coliform *Escherichia coli*, are present only transiently in the healthy oral cavity but may become established in the elderly or immunocompromised. *Candida albicans* is the most common fungal isolate (Chapter 26) and an average carriage rate of 40% has been observed in asymptomatic adults. Candidal counts increase in the immunocompromised, denture wearers, and following some types of antibiotic treatment. Certain viruses, for example Epstein–Barr virus and human herpesvirus type 6, are also frequently shed in the saliva of healthy individuals.

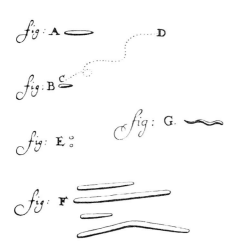

Fig. 20.1 The original drawings by Antonie van Leeuwenhoek of the microscopic appearance of bacteria from dental plaque.

ANALYSIS OF THE ORAL MICROFLORA			
Stage of study	**Examples**	**Comments**	**Problems**
Collect sample	Aspirate from dental abscess Paper point sample from periodontal pocket Oral rinse to assess *Candida* carriage	Each method will depend on the habitat sampled and the organism sought	Sampling methods should be standardized, reproducible, and prevent contamination of the specimen with organisms from the normal flora
Transport to laboratory	Use appropriate transport media, for example fastidious anaerobe broth for anaerobes	The shorter the transport time the better	A crucial stage since bacteria will not survive under adverse conditions
View sample	Dark-field microscopy	Allows visualization of organisms that are difficult to grow, such as spirochaetes	Difficult to obtain detailed specific information about the micro-organisms involved
	Gram stain	Provides 'rough guide' to micro-organisms in sample	Identification
	Specific fluorescence	May permit identification	
Treat sample	Disaggregate sample if necessary by adding small glass granules and shaking vigorously	An essential step to separate individual bacteria in specimens such as plaque	Difficult to disperse all the micro-organisms stuck together in plaque Delicate organisms may rupture and die
Culture sample	Semi-selective agars used, e.g. Sabouraud's agar for *Candida* spp., Mitis Salivarius Bacitracin (MSB) agar for mutans streptococci Anaerobic culture methods for growth of anaerobes	The method of culture will depend to a large extent on the organisms sought	Many organisms require special growth factors and atmospheric conditions Slow growing species overgrown by rapidly proliferating species
Identify organism	Enzyme profiles, sugar fermentation patterns, cellular lipids, antigen–antibody profiles, DNA probes, and PCR	Some are rapid and commercially available, such as API 32 Strep kit for identification of streptococci	Can be very time-consuming and expensive if large numbers of different species are investigated

Fig. 20.2 Stages in the collection and analysis of microbiological specimens from the oral cavity.

Acquisition of the oral flora

The oral cavity of the fetus is sterile and, although during birth the neonate comes into contact with the microflora of the mother's vagina, these organisms do not usually become established. The mouth is a highly selective environment for bacteria and only a few species are able to colonize the mouth of the newborn. From the first feeding, micro-organisms are transferred from the surrounding environment such as maternal saliva or the skin flora of the mother and nursing staff.

By 24 hours after birth the first (pioneer) species have become established. Streptococci, particularly *S. salivarius*, which bind to epithelial cells are usually the first to colonize. The early colonizers develop into a pioneer microbial community and begin to modify their environment by producing extracellular products which enhance conditions for the growth of other species. For example, *S. salivarius* produces extracellular polymers from sucrose to which other bacteria, for example *Actinomyces* spp., can attach. This process of microbial succession and increasing diversity will result in the eventual formation of a climax community.

GRAM-POSITIVE BACTERIA IN THE MOUTH			
Genus	Morphology	Atmospheric requirement	Comments and example
Streptococcus spp.	Cocci	Facultative anaerobe	These form the largest proportion of the oral flora. They comprise almost 50% of the total cultivable flora from saliva and the tongue but only 30% of the total flora from the gingival crevice and supragingival plaque. **Example:** *S. oralis*
		Obligate anaerobe	Anaerobic streptococci are present in the mouth and commonly isolated from purulent infections
Staphylococcus spp.	Cocci	Facultative anaerobe	Coagulase-negative staphylococci, for example *S. epidermidis*, are part of the normal flora. *S. aureus* is frequently isolated from children, the elderly, and those with systemic disease
Actinomyces spp.	Bacilli	Facultative anaerobe	Form a major proportion of bacteria found in dental plaque, especially at approximal sites. Numbers increase in gingivitis and in root surface caries **Example:** *A. naeslundii*
Lactobacillus spp.	Bacilli	Facultative anaerobe	Form a small percentage of the normal flora. Numbers increase at caries lesions **Example:** *L. acidophilus*
Eubacterium spp.	Bacilli	Obligate anaerobe	Found at periodontitis sites and in dental abscesses. **Example:** *E. brachy*

Fig. 20.3 Examples of important Gram-positive organisms found in the oral cavity.

By 1 year of age, when teeth have erupted, the predominant species isolated are *Streptococcus*, *Neisseria*, *Veillonella*, and *Staphylococcus*. Less frequently isolated species include *Lactobacillus*, *Actinomyces*, *Prevotella*, and *Fusobacterium*.

Tooth surfaces and gingival tissues provide new habitats for colonization with the resultant formation of dental plaque. Other shifts in the microbial flora take place during the lifetime of an individual, for example only 18–40% of 5-year-olds have spirochaetes and black pigmenting anaerobes, compared with 90% of 13–16-year-olds. The flora of adults remains relatively stable but denture wearers have an increased carriage rate of *Candida albicans*. From approximately 70 years of age there is an increased proportion of *Lactobacillus* and *Staphylococcus* species in the saliva of non-denture wearers, whilst after 80 years of age the number of yeasts increases.

Dental plaque formation

Adherence to a surface in the mouth is essential for the survival of oral bacteria. In the case of supragingival plaque formation,

organisms do not colonize clean enamel but interact with a layer of material on the tooth surface called the pellicle. The pellicle comprises mucins, salivary glycoproteins, minerals, and immunoglobulins. Pellicle formation occurs in seconds on cleaned enamel and reaches a maximum thickness in 90–120 minutes.

Bacterial attachment

The attachment of bacteria to surfaces is a complex process and can be divided into four main stages as shown below.

Stage I: transport

Bacteria must first approach the surface to which they will later bind. They can do this in several ways including liquid flow, diffusion through Brownian motion, or bacterial movement (chemotactic activity).

Stage II: initial adhesion

There are two types of forces involved at this stage. At distances of 10–100 nm, weak forces such as van der Waal's (Fig. 20.7) and electrostatic forces come into effect. These forces are highly

GRAM-NEGATIVE BACTERIA IN THE MOUTH			
Genus	**Morphology**	**Atmospheric requirement**	**Comments and example**
Neisseria spp.	Cocci	Aerobic	Early colonizers of teeth. Isolated in low numbers from most sites in the oral cavity. **Example:** *N. subflava*
Veillonella spp.	Cocci	Obligate anaerobe	Isolated from most surfaces in the oral cavity. High numbers on tongue and in dental plaque. **Example:** *V. parvula*
Haemophilus spp.	Bacilli	Facultative anaerobe	Commonly present in saliva, dental plaque and on epithelial surfaces **Example:** *H. aphrophilus*
Eikenella spp.	Bacilli	Facultative anaerobe	Found mainly in subgingival plaque Increased numbers in gingivitis **Example:** *E. corrodens*
Capnocytophaga spp.	Bacilli	Capnophilic	Often isolated in periodontal disease **Example:** *C. gingivalis*
Actinobacillus spp.	Bacilli	Capnophilic	Found in periodontal pockets and implicated in juvenile periodontitis **Example:** *A. actinomycetemcomitans*
Porphyromonas spp.	Bacilli	Obligate anaerobe	Found mainly in sub-gingival plaque Implicated in the aetiology of adult periodontitis. **Example:** *P. gingivalis*
Prevotella spp.	Bacilli	Obligate anaerobe	Found mainly in subgingival plaque Implicated in the aetiology of adult periodontitis. **Example:** *P. intermedia*
Fusobacterium spp.	Bacilli	Obligate anaerobe	Found mainly in subgingival plaque Implicated in the aetiology of adult periodontitis. **Example:** *F. nucleatum*
Spirochaetes	Spiral	Obligate anaerobe	Found mainly in periodontal pockets. Very difficult to culture or stain. Best visualized by dark-field microscopy. **Example:** *Treponema denticola*

Fig. 20.4 Examples of important Gram-negative organisms found in the oral cavity.

dynamic and are influenced by the ion content of surrounding saliva. As a result they are readily reversible.

As the bacterium approaches (2 nm), strong forces, such as hydrogen bonding between hydroxyl groups in the pellicle and phosphate groups in the bacterial cell wall, come into play (Fig. 20.7).

Stage III: attachment

Following initial adhesion, a more permanent attachment can occur by covalent, ionic, or electrostatic bonding (Fig. 20.8). These bonds form between specific receptors on the host surface termed ligands and components on the bacterium called adhesins. The latter are often situated on bacterial appendages such as fimbriae (Chapter 2). Oral bacterial attachment, and therefore plaque formation, is affected by a number of host and microbial factors and by saliva, as summarized in Fig. 20.9.

Stage IV: colonization

Once bound to a surface, the bacterium can divide and remain attached. Extracellular products are formed and microcolonies develop. Salivary glycoproteins and sugars such as glucose, sucrose, maltose, and lactose can be metabolized leading to the formation of bacterial cell-wall and intracellular polysaccharides. Sucrose may be the precursor of soluble and insoluble extracellular polysaccharides. The intracellular polysaccharide serves as a nutrient store for the organism and is degraded to release energy and organic acids. *Strep. sanguis* and *Strep. mutans* produce predominantly glucans (dextrans) from sucrose. Glucan is usually insoluble and produced by the enzyme glucosyl transferase.

Gradually the microcolonies coalesce to produce a biofilm. The picture now becomes even more complex, since inter- and intra-

CLASSIFICATION OF ORAL STREPTOCOCCI

Streptococcal group	Appearance on blood agar	Species found in humans	Comments
Mutans	Non-haemolytic	S. mutans	Most common species isolated and implicated in human caries. Colonizes teeth, especially in fissures
		S. sobrinus	Less commonly isolated
		S. cricetus	Rarely isolated
Salivarius	Alpha haemolytic	S. salivarius	Prefers keratinized surfaces. Commonly isolated from most areas but especially the tongue
		S. vestibularis	Commonly isolated from vestibular mucosa
Oralis	Alpha haemolytic	S. oralis	An early colonizer of smooth surfaces. Produces IgA protease and glucans (polymers of glucose)
		S. sanguis	Colonizes teeth and has been shown to cause caries. Produces IgA protease
		S. mitis	May occur in plaque but has a predilection for non-keratinized surfaces in the mouth
		S. gordonii S. parasanguis	Found in dental plaque

All members of the 'oralis group' may act as opportunistic pathogens and are frequently isolated from cases of infective endocarditis |
| Milleri | Most are beta haemolytic | S. anginosus S. intermedius S. constellatus | Are isolated readily from dental plaque. A common and important cause of purulent disease, for example dental and brain abscesses |

Fig. 20.5 Classification of the oral streptococci.

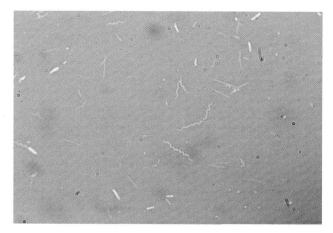

Fig. 20.6 Dark-field microscopy of spirochaetes from the oral cavity (1000 ×).

bacterial adhesion can occur, leading to the formation of dental plaque. This is a general term for the complex microbial community found on the tooth surface, embedded in a matrix of polymers of bacterial and salivary origin. The situation on oral mucosal cells is somewhat different because of a modified pellicle that covers their surface. The number of bacteria initially adhering to mucosal cells is small and regular desquamation ensures a light microbial load. Co-aggregation between similar species (intrageneric) can occur among streptococci. Aggregation between different bacterial species (intergeneric) can also occur, for example between *Strep. sanguis* and *A. naeslundii* or between *Streptococcus* spp. and *Porphyromonas* spp. This is known as co-aggregation (Fig. 20.10).

An equilibrium exists between the forces of retention and removal. Rough surfaces will allow more plaque to adhere because of the increased surface area and because they can shelter from the forces of removal. In addition, surfaces with a low surface free energy (water-repelling) such as Teflon® bind fewer microorganisms than those with a high surface free energy (water-attracting) such as enamel. Therefore in order to minimize plaque

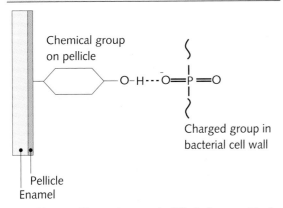

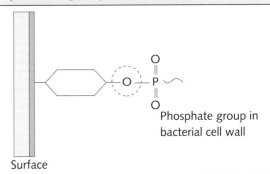

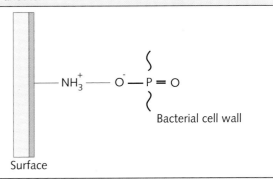

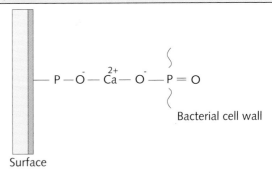

Fig. 20.7 Diagram illustrating van der Waal's forces and hydrogen bonds, types of weak bonds formed during initial bacterial adhesion. In the latter, a hydrogen atom acts as a bridge linking two electronegative atoms.

accumulation, intraoral devices should be designed with a smooth surface and possess a low surface free energy.

Plaque maturation is characterized by an increasing quantity and diversity of micro-organisms on the tooth surface. After 7 days streptococci are still the main organisms present, but after 14 days there is a shift to anaerobic rods and filaments, with streptococci comprising only 15% of the cultivable flora. The whole process of plaque development is summarized diagrammatically in Fig. 20.11.

Calculus

Dental plaque can become calcified – saliva is supersaturated with calcium and phosphate ions which may be deposited within the deeper layers of plaque. These ions accumulate within the plaque matrix together with organic débris from dead micro-organisms, while plaque phosphatases and proteases degrade some of the calcification inhibitors in saliva (statherin and proline-rich pro-

Fig. 20.8 Bonds involved in the later stages of bacterial adhesion (true attachment).

teins). These processes lead to the formation of insoluble calcium phosphate crystals which coalesce to form calculus. Many anti-calculus toothpastes contain pyrophosphate compounds designed to adsorb excess calcium thus reducing intraplaque mineral deposition. Mature calculus consists of about 80% (dry weight) mineralized material (mostly hydroxyapatite) and 20% organic compounds, although the actual composition will vary with the individual, age, site of the deposit, and the location of the tooth.

FACTORS INFLUENCING ADHERENCE		
Host factors (Ligands)	**Saliva (Suspending medium)**	**Bacterial factors (Adhesins)**
Mucosal cell surfaces contain **sialic acid** which binds to *Streptococcus mitis*	**Mechanical washing action** helps prevent microbial overgrowth	Adhesins are proteins associated with surface fibrils and fimbriae. Many are sugar-binding proteins called lectins
Enamel pellicle consists of albumin, lysozyme, immunoglobulins, proline-rich peptides, statherin, and mucins	Salivary **glycoproteins** contribute to enamel pellicle	**Lipoteichoic acid** in bacterial cell walls may help attachment to glycoproteins in tooth pellicle
Acidic proline-rich proteins can bind to *Actinomyces naeslundii* and some strains of *Streptococcus mutans*	**Salivary enzymes may inhibit bacteria.** **Examples:** lysozyme (destroys bacterial cell walls); lactoferrin (an iron-binding protein)	**Extracellular polymers** **Example:** glucosyl transferase enzymes produce glucans (polysaccharides) which may play a primary role in adhesion and support adherence of other microbial species
Minerals, such as calcium and phosphate, may influence the rate of calculus formation and provide larger surface areas for plaque to accumulate	**Buffering capacity** stabilizes pH to about 6.7. This prevents overgrowth of micro-organisms which require high or low pH for maximal growth	**Bacterial enzymes may expose binding sites.** **Example:** neuraminidase exposes a galactosyl ligand on host cell surfaces which allows Gram-negative bacteria to bind
Lectins on host cells or ingested in food bind bacteria to the host	**Salivary immunoglobulins,** especially secretory IgA, may obstruct microbial adherence	Some bacteria, for example *Streptococcus sanguis*, possess **IgA proteases** allowing them to overcome the blocking action of secretory IgA at mucosal surfaces

Fig. 20.9 Examples of factors influencing bacterial adherence in the oral cavity.

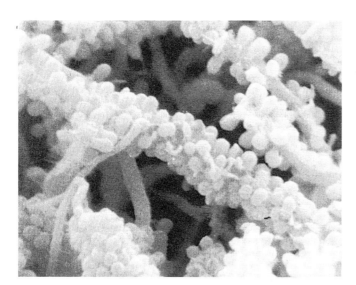

Fig. 20.10 Photomicrograph illustrating co-aggregation between *Corynebacterium matruchotii* and *Streptococcus sanguis*: the 'corn cob' appearance. (From Jones 1972; with permission.)

The bacterial flora associated with calculus is relatively non-specific and reflects the bacterial composition of the dental plaque with which it was associated. Thus early supragingival calculus (2 days) contains primarily Gram-positive cocci, whilst older and subgingival calculus will contain more Gram-negative rods. Calculus has a roughened surface and is porous, allowing bacteria and bacterial products such as toxins to be absorbed, thus providing an ideal reservoir for substances potentially harmful to the host. Calculus must therefore be removed from tooth surfaces to halt tissue damage and to promote healing from periodontal disease.

Factors affecting the growth of oral micro-organisms

As described in Chapter 2, maintenance of the microbial community requires a degree of symbiosis between the micro-organisms and the host. This will reflect a balance between factors that encourage growth and those that tend to inhibit growth. The oral flora, specifically, is influenced by a wide range of factors which may be associated with the diet, saliva, gingival crevicular fluid,

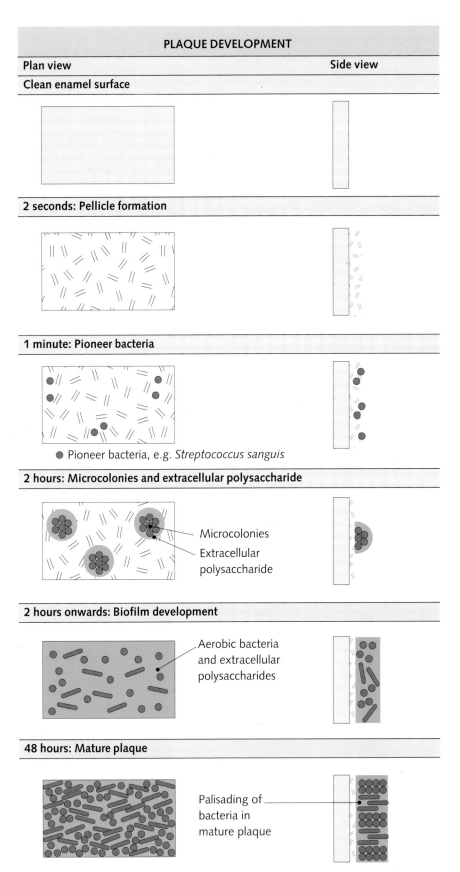

Fig. 20.11 Summary of dental plaque development on a clean enamel surface.

microbial products, the gaseous environment, and host factors (Fig. 20.12).

INFLUENCES ON THE ORAL MICROFLORA	
Factor	**Comments and examples**
Diet	Chemical composition, physical consistency, and frequency of intake
Saliva	Flow rate, pH balance, and antimicrobial factors, e.g. lysozyme
Gingival crevicular fluid	Contains many antimicrobial components, e.g. IgG
Microbial interactions	Some are beneficial (Fig. 20.13), others harmful
Gaseous environment	Relative oxygen concentrations help to determine species distribution
Host factors	Systemic disease, antibiotic use, and oral hygiene measures

Fig. 20.12 Important influences on the composition of the oral microflora.

Diet

The chemical composition of foods ingested will affect the availability of nutrients since large molecular weight dietary polysaccharides must first be broken down by salivary enzymes before they can be utilized. The presence of fermentable carbohydrates such as sucrose, maltose, lactose, and glucose will lead to increased plaque formation and the accumulation of microbial products such as organic acids and dextrans. Thus, the frequent ingestion of sucrose is associated with high caries activity. The physical consistency of large molecules such as starches and proteins restricts their availability to bacteria, since they may be removed from the mouth before they have been degraded. However, some foods are retained between the teeth or stick to fissures more easily, and the longer that bacteria have nutrients available, the more they can metabolize, grow, and release by-products such as lactic acid.

Saliva

One of the essential properties of saliva is its action as an efficient buffer that regulates the pH of most surfaces. The mean pH of unstimulated saliva is between 6.75 and 7.25. Many of the predominant bacterial components of healthy plaque can tolerate brief exposure to low pH but are killed or inhibited by prolonged exposure. A regular decrease in pH by frequent sugar intakes will lead to the proliferation of *Strep. mutans* and *Lactobacillus* species and an increase in dental caries. Changes in the flow rate will

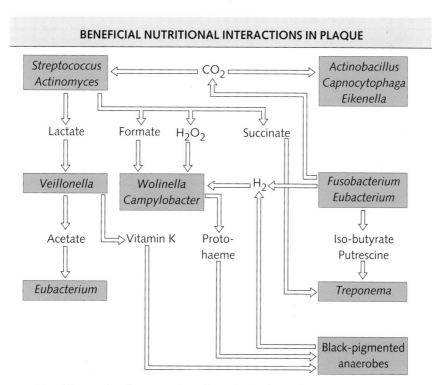

Fig. 20.13 Some nutritional interactions between plaque bacteria. (Redrawn from Marsh and Martin 1992; with permission.)

affect the concentrations of the bicarbonate, urea, ammonium, calcium, and phosphate ions which are of great importance to the balance of mineralization and demineralization.

Saliva contains many important growth factors, such as glycoproteins, proteins, and minerals, that may be utilized in bacterial adherence and metabolism. However, the microbial flora has to act synergistically to bring about the complete degradation of these compounds. Within the microbial community there are a multitude of possible interactions between the products produced by different species, some beneficial (Fig. 20.13) and some harmful. Extracellular end-products produced by one species may be essential for the growth of another species; for example isobutyrate, a cell-wall fatty acid produced by *Fusobacterium* spp. may be used by *Treponema microdentium*. Similarly, *Veillonella parvula* can produce vitamin K3 which, in turn, is essential for the growth of *Porphyromonas* spp. Conversely, metabolic products, such as hydrogen peroxide produced by the *Streptococcus oralis* group or butyrate produced by *Porphyromonas gingivalis*, may inhibit other bacteria.

Saliva also contains numerous antimicrobial factors such as salivary peroxidase, myeloperoxidase (peroxidases inhibit bacterial cell metabolism), lysozyme (lyses some bacterial cell walls), lactoferrin (binds iron which bacteria need for growth), histidine-rich peptides (inhibit *Candida albicans*), and immunoglobulins.

Gingival crevicular fluid (GCF)

This is a serum transudate which contains proteins such as albumin and immunoglobulins as well as amino acids, minerals, vitamins, and glucose. GCF has protective functions for the host by virtue of its flushing effect and high numbers of viable polymorphs, antibodies, and complement proteins (see Chapter 21).

The gaseous environment

Most oral micro-organisms are facultative anaerobes, although aerobic respiration is preferred if oxygen is present. However, some organisms are obligate anaerobes and are killed by oxygen.

The relative amounts of oxygen will help to determine the distribution of certain species within the oral cavity. Normal air contains 20% O_2, the anterior surface of the tongue 16%, the posterior surface of the tongue 12%, and the buccal folds 0.3%. This will be reflected in the number of anaerobic bacteria recovered from these sites. Sometimes the conditions available for the growth of bacteria are expressed as the oxidation–reduction level and are usually described as the redox potential (Eh) which is recorded in mV. A low Eh (negative value) is a highly reduced environment and favours the growth of anaerobes. Oxygen accepts electrons and raises the redox potential. Thus, a clean enamel surface has a redox potential of +200 mV, whilst after 7 days of plaque accumulation the Eh falls to −141 mV.

Early colonizers of plaque utilize O_2 and produce CO_2 thus allowing bacteria that are capnophilic (CO_2 requiring), such as milleri streptococci, to become established. Late colonizers of plaque will produce H_2 and other reducing agents, such as

sulphur-containing compounds, which will gradually lower the Eh, allowing more anaerobic bacteria, such as *Prevotella* spp., to colonize. Thus, periodontal pockets are more reduced (−48 mV) than healthy gingival crevices (+73 mV).

The host

In addition to host factors such as diet and salivary flow, others such as the presence of systemic disease, broad-spectrum antibiotic usage, or chemotherapy for cancer may disturb the host/microbial flora interactions. One of the easiest ways in which the host can influence the oral flora is by the use of oral hygiene methods, such as tooth brushing. This produces a persistently young plaque containing many facultative anaerobic Gram-positive bacteria with limited numbers of obligate anaerobes, a flora which is compatible with oral health. However, in an effort to make efficient plaque removal easier for patients, chemical agents have been introduced to reduce plaque build-up.

Antiplaque agents

There are three main approaches utilized for chemically interfering with the formation of dental plaque (Fig. 20.14).

Antimicrobial agents

These agents prevent bacterial proliferation on the tooth surface. Currently the most effective antiplaque agent is chlorhexidine. The molecule has a positive charge at either end and binds readily to negatively charged sites on the enamel pellicle, mucosal cells, and bacterial cell-wall structures. Once bound, the chlorhexidine can exert its antimicrobial effect by damaging the microbial cell membrane and precipitating the cell contents. Chlorhexidine also inhibits microbial adherence since it is able to adsorb onto a surface and is slowly released, maintaining its antimicrobial activity, a property known as substantivity.

ANTIPLAQUE AGENTS	
Mechanism of action	**Examples**
Antimicrobial	Chlorhexidine (also antiadherent action)
Plaque disruption	Sodium lauryl sulfate (detergent action) Delmopinol (plaque-loosening action) Plaque-degrading enzymes, such as dextranase
Antiadherent	Experimental compounds Fluoride-containing compounds

Fig. 20.14 Summary of the types of antiplaque agent available.

Other antimicrobial compounds such as topical or systemic antibiotics are often associated with the development of drug resistance and this precludes their use for the routine control of the oral flora.

Plaque disruption agents

Sodium lauryl sulphate is commonly used in toothpastes and mouthrinses as an anionic detergent which solubilizes plaque to reduce its accumulation. In addition, it has a moderate degree of substantivity and antimicrobial activity, although much less than chlorhexidine. Other attempts have been made to loosen plaque attached to teeth by using substituted amine alcohols such as delmopinol, which may form films on bacterial cells, blocking their attachment sites and causing plaque to fall away from the teeth. Novel attempts to reduce the plaque matrix using dextranase enzymes or amyloglucosidase enzymes have proved disappointing.

Antiadhesive compounds

Antiadhesive compounds are designed to alter the surface binding within the oral cavity, thus preventing or blocking interactions between bacteria and the oral environment. Many are still at the experimental stage and are currently unavailable as commercial oral hygiene products. Fluoride-containing compounds such as sodium fluoride and stannous fluoride are reported to have anti-adherent properties, although the mechanism of action is uncertain. The use of antiadhesive compounds shows great promise for the future development of oral hygiene agents.

References and further reading

Jones, S (1972). A special relationship between spherical and filamentous microorganisms in mature human dental plaque. *Archives of Oral Biology*, 17, 613–16.

Lang, NP, Mombelli, A, and Attström, R (1997). Dental plaque and calculus. In *Clinical periodontology and implant dentistry* (3rd edn) (ed. J Lindhe, T Karring, and NP Lang), Chapter 3. Munksgaard, Copenhagen.

Marsh, PD and Martin, MV (1999). *Oral microbiology* (4th edn). Butterworth–Heinemann, London.

Key facts

- Study of the oral flora is complicated by the large number of species, their fastidious nutritional requirements, and slow growth together with the complexities of species identification.

- Dental plaque is a general term for the complex microbial community found on the tooth surface, embedded in a matrix of polymers derived from bacteria and saliva.

- Streptococci comprise the largest proportion of the oral flora.

- There are four main species groups of oral streptococci: mutans, oralis, milleri, and salivarius groups.

- In subgingival plaque, *Actinomyces*, *Porphyromonas*, *Prevotella*, *Fusobacterium*, and *Veillonella* spp. are the predominant cultivable anaerobes.

- For successful colonization, organisms must first adhere to a surface. This involves interaction between adhesins on the microbial cell surface and ligands on the host surface.

- There are four stages in plaque formation: transport, initial adhesion, irreversible attachment, and colonization.

- In plaque formation, pioneer bacteria form microcolonies which become embedded in bacterial products, e.g. polysaccharides and salivary proteins and glycoproteins to form a confluent biofilm.

- The bacterial species present in plaque change with time, becoming increasingly anaerobic and Gram-negative as the plaque matures.

- Factors affecting the growth of oral micro-organisms include the diet, host defences, salivary components, and oxygen tension.

Defence mechanisms of the mouth

Defence mechanisms of the mouth

Introduction

The general aspects of host defences have already been described in Chapter 7. In this short chapter, attention will be drawn to some of the specific aspects relating to immunity in the mouth. The key factors responsible for maintaining oral health are listed in Fig. 21.1.

Oral mucosa

Oral health is dependent on the integrity of the oral mucosa, which normally functions as an effective barrier against micro-

CONTRIBUTORS TO ORAL HEALTH
• Integrity of oral mucosa
• Lymphoid tissue
• Saliva
• Gingival crevicular fluid
• Humoral and cellular immunity

Fig. 21.1 The major biological factors contributing to the maintenance of oral health.

organisms. If this barrier becomes compromised, for example in cancer patients with mucositis following chemotherapy, then infectious complications may ensue, including the risk of systemic infection. In addition, the oral mucosa is in continuity with a number of anatomical structures, such as the pharynx, which are vulnerable if the oral defences break down. A major area of risk is the junction between the gingiva and the tooth – the various forms of periodontal disease encountered at this site are described in Chapter 23.

There are several factors which may prevent the penetration of intact oral mucosa by micro-organisms (Fig. 21.2). These include keratinization in certain areas of the mouth, the discharge of membrane-coating granules in the granular layer, the formation of immune complexes through antigen–antibody interactions, and the barrier function of the basement membrane. The small numbers of lymphoid cells adjacent to the basement membrane may help to deal with any organisms which pass through the overlying barriers.

Oral lymphoid tissues

Both extraoral lymph nodes and intraoral lymphoid aggregations are associated with the mouth.

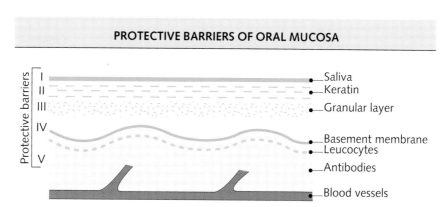

Fig. 21.2 Diagram illustrating the main protective barriers of the oral mucosa. (Redrawn from Lehner, T. (1992) *Immunology of Oral Diseases*; with permission from Blackwell Scientific Publications.)

Extraoral lymph nodes

Lymph capillaries originating superficially in the oral mucosa, gingivae, and pulps of the teeth join to form larger lymphatics which later join lymph vessels from a deep network in the other facial structures, such as muscle of the tongue. These vessels drain into the submandibular, submental, upper deep cervical, and retropharyngeal lymph nodes in an ordered fashion. Microbes which have passed through oral epithelium into the lamina propria may enter the lymphatics directly or be transported to them by phagocytic cells. The antigen will thereby reach the anatomically neighbouring lymph nodes where an immune response may be elicited (Chapter 7).

Intraoral lymphoid tissue

There are four types of lymphoid aggregations in the mouth (Fig. 21.3). While the functions of the intraoral lymphoid tissue are not fully understood, the tonsils are believed to guard the entry into the digestive and respiratory tracts, whilst the gingival lymphoid tissue responds to dental plaque. Secretory IgA, produced in the salivary glands, not only helps to prevent infection within the glands themselves but also protects the oral mucosa and tooth surfaces from microbial colonization.

Saliva

Saliva is a very important component of the oral defences, both through its mechanical washing activity and because of the antimicrobial factors it contains. The important antimicrobial activities and components of saliva are summarized in Fig. 21.4. Secretory IgA is by far the most important immunoglobulin in saliva. The salivary gland plasma cells secrete IgA, two molecules of which are combined by means of a J (joining) chain (see Fig. 7.10); IgA is also secreted by local plasma cells. The resultant dimeric IgA is then complexed to the secretory component, synthesized by epithelial cells of the salivary acini, and the complete secretory IgA is transported into the duct lumen and thence into the mouth. Secretory IgA is more resistant to proteolytic degradation than other immunoglobulins. It probably functions by combining with micro-organisms and preventing their adherence to host surfaces.

Gingival crevicular fluid

Blood components, including leucocytes, are able to reach the oral cavity via the flow of fluid through the junctional epithelium of the gingiva. The flow of this so-called gingival crevicular fluid (GCF) increases greatly with the inflammation accompanying periodontal disease (Chapter 23). Experiments using radiolabelled IgG, IgM, IgA, and neutrophils have shown that both humoral and cellular components from blood can reach the oral cavity in GCF.

In addition to immunoglobulins, complement components have been detected in GCF, suggesting that both the classical and alternative complement pathways (Chapter 7) may be activated in the gingival crevice. Other components include enzymes such as lysozyme, proteases, and collagenases released by cells of both the host and bacteria. Specific proteases which inactivate IgA have been described.

The cellular component of GCF comprises mainly neutrophils, with small numbers of macrophages and B and T lymphocytes. These cells migrate continuously from the blood through the junctional epithelium into the gingival crevice. Over 80% of neutrophils in the gingival crevice itself are functional and can phagocytose micro-organisms.

INTRAORAL LYMPHOID TISSUE	
Palatine and lingual tonsils	Classical structure of lymphoid follicles
	B cells and perifollicular T cells
	Antigen penetrates through covering epithelium (no afferent lymphatics)
Salivary gland lymphoid tissue	Concerned mainly with synthesis of secretory IgA
Gingival lymphoid tissue	Plasma cells, lymphocytes, macrophages, and polymorphs
	Important in immunological response to dental plaque
Scattered submucosal lymphoid cells	

Fig. 21.3 Summary of the collections of intraoral lymphoid tissue.

ANTIMICROBIAL ACTIONS OF SALIVA	
Mechanical cleansing	Muscular movements, in conjunction with saliva, maintain hygiene in accessible areas of mouth
	Swallowed microbes are inactivated in the stomach
Lysozyme	Bactericidal, by splitting the bond between *N*-acetyl glucosamine and *N*-acetyl muramic acid in the cell wall
Peroxidase	Heat-labile, antibacterial enzyme
Lactoferrin	Heat-stable protein, bacteriostatic to many micro-organisms
Leucocytes	Saliva contains many leucocytes (99% polymorphs)
	Migrate from blood via the gingival crevice
Secretory IgA	IgA is the predominant immunoglobulin in saliva
	Produced by plasma cells within salivary glands
	Mainly in dimeric form, complexed with secretory component
	Functionally, secretory IgA prevents microbial adherence to host surfaces

Fig. 21.4 Summary of the major antimicrobial actions of saliva.

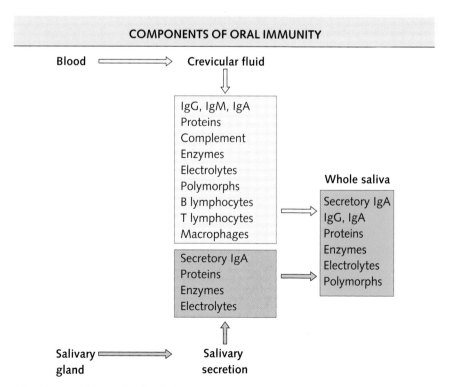

COMPONENTS OF ORAL IMMUNITY

Fig. 21.5 Diagram illustrating the main humoral and cellular components in gingival crevicular fluid, salivary gland secretion, and whole saliva. (Adapted from Lehner, T. (1992) *Immunology of Oral Diseases*; with permission from Blackwell Scientific Publications.)

It is clear, therefore, that the tooth surface is influenced by both local salivary immune mechanisms, mediated largely through secretory IgA, and by systemic immunity involving all the varied immune components present in blood. The way in which these contributing factors interact to provide immunity within the oral cavity is illustrated in Fig. 21.5.

References and further reading

Edgar, WM and O'Mullane, DM (ed.). (1996). *Saliva and oral health* (2nd edn). British Dental Association, London.

Lehner, T (1992). *Immunology of oral diseases* (3rd edn). Blackwell, Oxford.

Marsh, PD and Martin, MV (1999). *Oral microbiology* (4th edn). Butterworth–Heinemann, London.

Slots, J and Taubman, MA (ed.). (1992). Oral immunology. In *Contemporary oral microbiology and immunology*, Section V. Mosby Year Book, St Louis.

Key facts

- Integrity of the oral mucosa is a key factor in the maintenance of oral health.

- Both extraoral lymph nodes and intraoral lymphoid aggregations are associated with the mouth.

- Saliva has many important antimicrobial activities.

- Secretory IgA is the most important immunoglobulin in saliva.

- Secretory IgA probably functions by combining with micro-organisms and preventing their adherence to host surfaces.

- Antibodies, leucocytes, complement components, and enzymes are present in gingival crevicular fluid.

- The tooth surface is influenced by both local salivary and systemic immune mechanisms.

22

Dental caries

Dental caries

Introduction

Dental caries can be thought of as a chronic infection of enamel or dentine in which the microbial agents are members of the normal commensal flora. Lesions result from the demineralization of enamel or dentine by acids produced by plaque micro-organisms as they metabolize dietary carbohydrates. Once the surface layer of enamel has been lost, the infection invariably progresses via dentine, with the pulp first becoming inflamed and later necrotic. Dental caries is ubiquitous, and while its prevalence is falling overall in Western countries, there is an uneven distribution of decay. For example, in Scotland during 1995/96, all of the decayed teeth reported were found in 54% of children and more than half of the untreated caries was present in just 10% of children. In less developed countries where changes in diet, especially with respect to carbohydrate content have occurred, the prevalence is rising.

There is a vast literature about the aetiology, diagnosis, management, and prevention of dental caries. In this chapter only the main factors are discussed.

Clinical presentation and diagnosis

Dental caries can be classified with respect to the site of the lesion, examples of which are shown in Fig. 22.1. The main stages and factors involved in enamel caries are shown diagrammatically in Fig. 22.2. The earliest clinical appearance of the disease is a well-

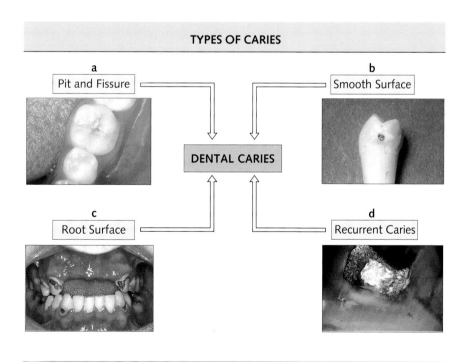

TYPES OF CARIES

a Pit and Fissure

b Smooth Surface

DENTAL CARIES

c Root Surface

d Recurrent Caries

a Molars, premolars, and lingual surface of maxillary incisors
b Mainly approximal tooth surfaces just below the contact point
c On cementum and/or dentine when the root is exposed to the oral environment
d Associated with an existing restoration

Fig. 22.1 Composite clinical photograph of different types of caries. (The clinical photographs are courtesy of Dr S. Creanor.)

PROGRESSION OF DENTAL CARIES

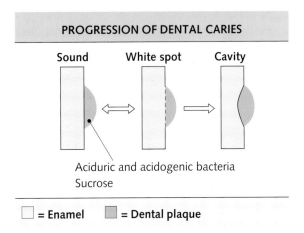

Sound   **White spot**   **Cavity**

Aciduric and acidogenic bacteria
Sucrose

☐ = Enamel   ▨ = Dental plaque

Fig. 22.2 Diagram showing the initiation and progression of dental caries. Note that the white spot lesion may be reversible if sugar intake is reduced and fluoride therapy employed.

AETIOLOGICAL FACTORS IN DENTAL CARIES

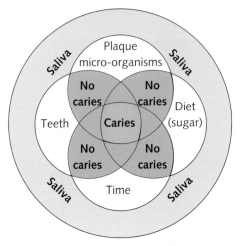

Fig. 22.4 Diagrammatic representation of the interaction of the aetiological factors in dental caries.

demarcated chalky-white lesion (Fig. 22.3) in which the surface continuity of enamel is still intact. This so-called 'white spot' lesion can heal or remineralize, with the result that this stage of the disease is reversible. However, as the lesion develops the surface becomes roughened and cavitation occurs. Depending on the rate of tissue destruction, caries can be described as rampant, slowly progressive, or arrested. If the lesion is untreated, micro-organisms extend the disease into dentine, the pulp may become infected and die, and there is a risk of subsequent periapical abscess formation (Chapter 24).

Diagnosis is traditionally by a combination of direct observation and radiographs, but early white spot lesions may easily be missed using these techniques alone. It is also possible for large carious lesions to develop in pits and fissures with very little clinical evidence of disease. Recent research has identified a number of innovative methods for detecting caries, including laser fluorescence (buccal/lingual caries) and electrical resistance techniques (occlusal caries), both of which show promise. However, neither can be used routinely at present.

Aetiology

The main factors involved in dental caries are the tooth, saliva, supragingival plaque, the diet (especially sucrose intake), and the time necessary for caries development (Fig. 22.4). These complex factors can interact in numerous different ways, but certain patterns of interrelationships are more likely than others to result in the initiation and progression of carious lesions or healing of an early white spot lesion.

Host factors

The two main host factors are the structures of enamel or dentine (root surface caries) and the composition and flow of saliva.

Enamel

The susceptibility of different areas of enamel on the same tooth to a standard acid attack *in vitro* can vary markedly. This and other information strongly suggests that some areas of the same tooth are more susceptible to carious attack than others. Similarly, a microbial challenge to a susceptible surface may produce an early carious lesion, whilst one on a more mineralized area may fail to initiate disease. Such interactions are often ignored when the role of micro-organisms in caries is studied *in vivo* or *in vitro*. Susceptibility to demineralization by acid is probably related to many factors including the mineral and fluoride content, together with the structure of particular areas of enamel. The typical

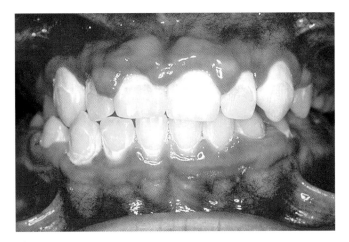

Fig. 22.3 Clinical photograph of white spot lesions. In this instance they have followed orthodontic treatment with a fixed appliance. (Courtesy of Dr S. Creanor.)

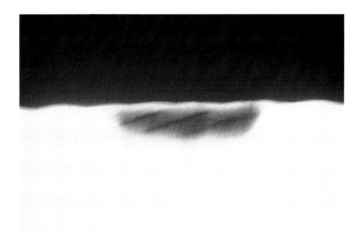

Fig. 22.5 Microradiographic appearance of an early carious lesion in enamel. The subsurface position and striae of Retzius are seen clearly. (Courtesy of Dr S. Creanor.)

appearance of a carious lesion in enamel after microradiography is shown in Fig. 22.5.

Saliva

Mixed or whole saliva consists of secretions from the major (parotid, submandibular, and sublingual) and minor salivary glands, with a variable input from the gingival crevicular fluid. Also present are exfoliated epithelial cells, oral micro-organisms and their products, and food residues. The rate of secretion and the composition of mixed saliva can be affected by a wide range of variables including age, sex, time of day, and possibly genetic differences. Some of the constituents of mixed saliva are shown in Fig. 22.6. The pH and buffering capacity of saliva are determined by the bicarbonate and phosphate concentrations, the normal pH of mixed saliva ranging from 5.6 to 7.8 with a mean of 6.7. Saliva should be regarded as a slow moving, thin film about 0.1 mm thick with a variable velocity related to site (0.8 mm/min in the upper labial area and 5.0–8.0 mm/min on the lingual surfaces of the lower incisors and molars when the salivary flow is unstimu-

MAIN CONSTITUENTS OF MIXED SALIVA	
Antimicrobial factors	IgA, histidine-rich proteins, lysozyme, peroxidase systems
Minerals	Sodium, chloride, fluoride, calcium, phosphate, bicarbonate
Other constituents	Amylase, glucose, urea, albumin

Fig. 22.6 Constituents of mixed saliva.

lated). The complex constituents of saliva are not well mixed *in vivo* and the thin mobile film both removes substances from, and deposits them in, dental plaque. Recent research suggests that saliva provides a series of distinctly different fluid environments, some of which interact with dental plaque to produce dental caries, while others favour calculus formation and the remineralization of early carious lesions.

Saliva plays a number of important roles in maintaining oral and dental health, some of which are related to dental caries. For example, the mechanical washing action of saliva is a very effective mechanism for removing food debris and unattached oral micro-organisms from the mouth. The protective role of saliva is highlighted in patients with severe Sjögren's syndrome (a degenerative disease of salivary glands) who have a very low salivary flow rate, retain food debris in their mouth for long periods, and suffer from rampant dental caries. Saliva has a high buffering capacity which tends to neutralize acids produced by plaque bacteria on tooth surfaces. It is also supersaturated with calcium and phosphorus which, together with fluoride, are important in the remineralization of white spot lesions. The precise roles of some of the other salivary antimicrobial factors in dental caries, for example lysozyme, the lactoperoxidase system, and immunoglobulins, are not clear.

Diet

A number of epidemiological studies have demonstrated clearly a direct relationship between dental caries and the intake of carbohydrate. The most cariogenic sugar is sucrose and the evidence for its central role in the initiation of dental caries includes the following:

* an increase in the prevalence of caries in isolated populations with the introduction of sucrose-rich diets;
* clinical association studies;
* short-term experiments in human volunteers using sucrose rinses;
* experimental animal studies.

In addition, sucrose is highly soluble and diffuses easily into dental plaque, acting as a substrate for the production of extracellular polysaccharide and acids. *Streptococcus mutans* produces water-insoluble glucans from sucrose and although this polysaccharide could be involved in its primary adherence to surfaces, it is more likely to be important in consolidating the attachment of bacterial cells already on the surface and assisting in the development of plaque. The direct relationship between sucrose and dental caries is more complex than can be simply explained by the total amount of sugar consumed. There is good evidence that the frequency of sugar intake, rather than the total sugar consumption, is of decisive importance in caries development. Also important are the stickiness and concentration of the sucrose consumed, both factors influencing the period for which sugar is retained in the mouth in close contact with the tooth surface.

Carbohydrates other than sucrose are also cariogenic, for example glucose and fructose, but to a lesser degree. Carbohydrates with low cariogenicity also exist, for example xylitol, a sugar alcohol.

Micro-organisms

Dental caries does not occur *in vivo* if micro-organisms in the form of dental plaque are absent, therefore it is clear that dental caries is a plaque-associated disease. However, over the years there has been debate about whether one or more specific bacteria are principally involved in the initiation of caries (specific plaque hypothesis) or if the disease is caused by a non-specific mixture of bacteria (non-specific plaque hypothesis). In the former hypothesis, *S. mutans* is believed to initiate virtually all carious lesions in enamel, while in the latter, caries is not dependent on the presence of *S. mutans*. A synthesis of these two views is that *S. mutans* is important, but not essential, in the aetiology of the disease. Whilst the evidence advanced to support or disprove these different hypotheses is incomplete, there are sufficient data to indicate that it is likely that all three can occur in specific circumstances. The microbial composition of supragingival plaque collected from the same site in the same mouth with respect to time varies substantially, and, in view of the wide variability in plaque microbiology, it is unreasonable to expect that the initiation and progression of all carious lesions are associated with identical or even similar plaques either from a qualitative or quantitative point of view. However, there is good evidence that overall some bacteria (*S. mutans*, *Lactobacillus* spp., and perhaps *Actinomyces* spp.) are more important than others in enamel and root surface caries.

Streptococcus mutans

Most of the research performed in recent years into the role of micro-organisms in caries has concentrated on mutans streptococci, especially *S. mutans*.

The term mutans streptococci refers to a group of seven different species (*S. cricetus*, *S. downei*, *S. ferus*, *S. macacae*, *S. mutans*, *S. rattus*, and *S. sobrinus*) and eight serotypes (a–h). *S. mutans* (serotypes c/e/f) and *S. sobrinus* (serotypes d/g) are the species most commonly found in humans, with serotype c strains being most frequently isolated, followed by d and e. The others are rarely encountered. The evidence for the aetiological role of *S. mutans* in dental caries is shown in Fig. 22.7.

The strongest correlation between *S. mutans* and human caries is for fissure caries, but its relationship to all other forms of caries is also very substantial. Early studies implicated *Actinomyces* species in the aetiology of root surface caries, but more recent work has implicated *S. mutans* and possibly lactobacilli. The role of *S. sobrinus* in human caries is less certain, and this is due mainly to the use of a selective culture medium in clinical studies which inhibits the growth of *S. sobrinus* but not *S. mutans*. However, it is

---

FACTORS RELATED TO CARIOGENICITY OF *STREPTOCOCCUS MUTANS*

- Significant correlations in humans between *S. mutans* counts in saliva and plaque with the prevalence and incidence of caries
- *S. mutans* can be isolated from precise sites on the tooth surface before the development of caries
- Correlation between the progression of carious lesions and *S. mutans* counts
- Produces water-soluble and insoluble extracellular polysaccharides from sucrose which help in the colonization of tooth surfaces by consolidating microbial attachment
- Most effective streptococcus in experimental caries in animals (rodents and non-human primates)
- Ability to initiate and maintain microbial growth and to continue acid production in sites with a low pH
- Rapid metabolism of sugars to lactic and other organic acids
- Can attain the critical pH for enamel demineralization more rapidly than other common plaque bacteria
- Produces intracellular polysaccharide which can act as a food store for use when dietary carbohydrate is low
- Immunization of animals with *S. mutans* significantly reduces the incidence of caries

Fig. 22.7 Factors related to the cariogenicity of mutans streptococci, especially *Streptococcus mutans*.

commonly isolated from dental plaque, though usually at a lower frequency than *S. mutans*, and possesses the pathogenic determinants believed to be necessary to cause caries.

Not all strains of *S. mutans* possess the complete range of properties described in Fig. 22.7 and, therefore, strains of *S. mutans* may well vary in their potential to produce dental caries. It is possible that certain strains of *S. mutans* are more pathogenic than others and that in a small number of individuals caries may be an infectious disease, with a highly pathogenic strain being transmitted from one individual to another, for example during kissing. While there is little evidence to support this hypothesis, molecular typing techniques have indicated that strains of *S. mutans* are transmitted between mothers and children during the first 6 months of life and that some adults vary in the number of genotypes they carry in their oral microflora.

Not all evidence supports the apparently strong relationship between *S. mutans* and the initiation and progression of caries. However, there are many problems involved in clinical studies, for example difficulty in diagnosing approximal 'white spot' lesions accurately at an early stage, problems in obtaining plaque samples directly from the surface of a developing lesion free of surrounding plaque, and technical difficulties in the microbiological identification and enumeration of the plaque microflora. A combination of the new methods of diagnosing caries and innovative molecular biology techniques should enable important new knowledge about the natural history of caries to emerge.

Lactobacillus species

Lactobacilli can be divided into two groups: the homo-fermentative species which produce mainly lactic acid (>65%) from glucose fermentation (for example *L. acidophilus* and *L. casei*); and the heterofermentative species which produce lactic acid as well as significant amounts of acetate, ethanol, and carbon dioxide (for example *L. fermentum*). The most commonly isolated species from oral samples appear to be *L. casei* and *L. fermentum*, although characterization of isolates to species level is rarely performed since existing tests are expensive with doubtful specificity.

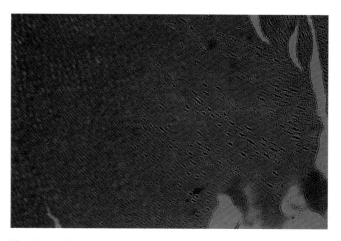

Fig. 22.9 Photomicrograph of a Giemsa-stained section of carious dentine, showing bacteria in the tubules. (Courtesy of Dr S. Creanor.)

For many years lactobacilli were believed to be the causative agents of dental caries. Although they possess some properties which would be valuable to a cariogenic organism (Fig. 22.8), their affinity for the tooth surface and their numbers in dental plaque associated with healthy sites or early carious lesions are usually low. At present, the general opinion supports the concept that lactobacilli are not involved in the initiation of dental caries, but more in the progression of the lesion deep into enamel and dentine where they are the main pioneer organisms in the advancing carious process (Fig. 22.9).

There is evidence from *in vivo* human studies that, on a group basis, salivary lactobacillus counts are related statistically to caries activity. However, when the counts for individuals are examined and used to predict activity, overall the level of statistical significance is relatively low and the results of such tests are difficult to interpret. However, the characterization of oral lactobacilli is poor and no in-depth laboratory investigations of clinical isolates have been performed in recent years. Until much more information is available, the precise role of lactobacilli in the initiation and progression of dental caries cannot be defined clearly.

FACTORS RELATED TO CARIOGENICITY OF LACTOBACILLUS SPECIES

- Present in increased numbers in most carious cavities affecting enamel and root surfaces
- Numbers in saliva correlate positively with caries activity
- A few strains produce caries in gnotobiotic rats
- Able to initiate and maintain growth at low pH levels (aciduric)
- Produce lactic acid in conditions below pH 5.0 (acidogenic)
- Some strains synthesize extracellular polysaccharides

Fig. 22.8 Factors related to the cariogenicity of *Lactobacillus* species.

Actinomyces species

Actinomyces spp. form a major part of the microflora of dental plaque, particularly at approximal sites. Since difficulties occur in the characterization and identification of actinomyces their precise role, especially at species level, in dental caries is uncertain. *Actinomyces viscosus* has been associated with the development of root surface caries, which is a disease of middle-aged and older adults. Gingival recession exposes the root surface to the mouth and microbial colonization follows, with subsequent attack by acid. This disease is becoming more common, as an increasing number of individuals retain their teeth with advancing age. The lesions are clinically different from enamel caries, in that the calcified tissues are often softened without obvious cavitation. They tend to form on the buccal and lingual surfaces close to the gingival margin and slowly progress laterally round the neck of the tooth. Human isolates of *A. naesludii* have been shown to cause root surface caries in gnotobiotic rats and hamsters. Although *Actinomyces* spp., especially *A. naeslundii*, are the predominant organisms isolated, their role in the initiation and development of the disease has been uncertain. Recent studies have tended to show strong associations between root surface caries and mutans streptococci and lactobacilli rather than with *Actinomyces* species. Furthermore, the sites from which *S. mutans* and lactobacilli were isolated appear to have a higher risk of developing root surface caries than other sites. The microflora of advanced lesions seems to be non-specific with a variable and diverse range of micro-organisms. Factors such as the role of diet, as well as salivary flow rate and constituents, have received little or no detailed study in this form of dental decay, and the role of specific micro-organisms is not yet entirely clear.

Veillonella species

There is some evidence which suggests that *Veillonella* spp., which are present in significant numbers in most supragingival plaque samples, may have a protective effect on dental caries. *Veillonella* spp. require lactate for growth, but are unable to metabolize carbohydrates. They therefore utilize lactate and other intermediate metabolites formed by plaque bacteria as energy sources and convert them into a range of weaker and probably less cariogenic organic acids, predominantly acetic and propionic. This protective effect has been demonstrated *in vitro* and in animal experiments, but has not been described clinically.

Plaque metabolism

Saliva is the main source of nutrition for oral micro-organisms. Carbohydrate is present in saliva as glycoproteins (for example mucin), but since no single bacterial species possesses the full complement of enzymes to utilize these substrates, synergistic activity is necessary. However, the rate and production of acid is slow and is unlikely to cause significant demineralization. Following a meal, salivary carbohydrate increases dramatically and, in order to avoid possible toxic effects and to gain maximum benefit from these high levels of carbohydrate, oral bacteria have developed a number of regulatory mechanisms which act at three main levels:

- transport of sugar into the organisms;
- the glycolytic pathway;
- the conversion of pyruvate into metabolic end-products.

The bacterial metabolism of carbohydrate, especially sucrose which is consumed at levels of about 50 kg/person/year in many industrial countries, is important in the aetiology of caries since the acid end-products are responsible for enamel demineralization. The metabolic fate of dietary sucrose and other carbohydrates in the mouth is complex. Initially, sucrose is broken down by various bacterial extracellular enzymes (glucosyl- and fructosyl-transferases), with the release of glucose and fructose, some of which are polymerized into water-soluble or water-insoluble polysaccharides (glucans or fructans). The insoluble polysaccharides are important in plaque formation, the consolidation of bacterial attachment to the teeth, and as extracellular storage compounds. Some sucrose is transported intact into plaque bacteria as the disaccharide or disaccharide phosphate and is cleaved intracellularly by invertase or sucrose phosphate hydrolase to glucose and fructose. Most plaque bacteria catabolize these sugars internally by glycolysis to pyruvate for immediate energy needs, but they can also store excess carbohydrate as intracellular polysaccharides (IPS). Sugars are also utilized in anabolic pathways to generate biomass. In glycolysis, most oral bacteria metabolize pyruvate anaerobically to organic acids. In the case of *S. mutans* this involves the conversion of pyruvate to lactate by lactate dehydrogenase when sugar is in excess – formate and acetate are also produced. As mentioned earlier, *S. mutans* is probably the most aciduric and acidogenic organism in plaque and can create environmental conditions that are lethal for other bacteria. When carbohydrate is scarce, bacteria that form IPS can utilize these stores with the production of acid which is sufficient to cause dissolution of enamel and dentine. Thus, overall, the interaction of plaque bacteria and carbohydrate results in a rapid fall in plaque pH, which is usually followed by a slow return to the original pH value in about 1 hour.

Management of dental caries

The clinical management and prevention of dental caries is based on an understanding and practical application of the scientific information presented so far. In the past, the general approach in the treatment of dental caries was to remove diseased tissue and replace it with an inert restoration. This form of management made no attempt to cure the disease, and the patient often returned some 1–3 years later requiring further fillings due to new or recurrent caries.

The modern philosophy in dental caries management highlights the importance of accurate early diagnosis, encouraging remineralization where appropriate, minimal cavity preparation techniques, and active prevention. The end result of such measures should be that, with the passage of time, less restorative work will be required by an individual patient.

Evaluation of patients

In patients with a low incidence of caries, a case history, together with clinical and radiographic examination, are probably sufficient for treatment planning. However, for patients with rampant or recurrent caries, or where extensive crown and bridge work is planned, additional investigations are necessary. These include the assessment of dietary habits, determination of salivary flow rate and buffering capacity, and microbiological tests. It is outside the scope of this book to describe how these different factors are used to assess caries risk and subsequently incorporated into the treatment plan. However, the microbiological tests are described briefly below.

Microbiological tests in caries assessment

The standard microbiological method is to enumerate the numbers of *S. mutans* and *Lactobacillus* spp. in mixed saliva from patients. Briefly, a paraffin wax-stimulated sample of mixed saliva is collected and sent to the laboratory, where it is vortex-mixed, diluted, and cultured on selective media for *S. mutans* (Mitis Salivarius Bacitracin (MSB) agar) and *Lactobacillus* spp. (Rogosa SL agar). The number of typical colonies at a suitable dilution is recorded and the count per millilitre of saliva calculated using simple arithmetic. The salivary counts per millilitre which are accepted as high and low are as follows:

High value >1 million *S. mutans* >100 000 *Lactobacillus* spp.
Low value <100 000 *S. mutans* <1000 *Lactobacillus* spp.

Tests in very young children who have difficulty in producing a stimulated salivary sample, or in patients with severe xerostomia, require alternative methods of sample collection, for example a wooden spatula pressed on the tongue or a scraping of plaque or tongue debris obtained using a bacteriological wire loop. Commercially available dip-slide kits (Fig. 22.10) are available for lactobacillus and mutans streptococcus counts which correlate well with laboratory plate counts. They can be performed in dental practice without the need for special facilities.

While there are good statistical correlations between caries prevalence and increment and laboratory counts of lactobacilli and mutans streptococci when data are analysed on a group basis, the correlations are less convincing when analysis involves the diagnosis or prediction of disease on an individual basis. The apparent success of these tests is surprising since many of the underlying assumptions are doubtful. For example, it is unlikely that the target bacteria are removed from teeth in a controlled and reproducible fashion by chewing wax, and also it does not discriminate between a few teeth with high counts of target bacteria and a full dentition with an overall low count. Another way to assess carious activity by microbiological means is to collect a number of minute samples of plaque accurately from specific sites – such as white spot lesions, margins of crowns, and fillings – and, using similar laboratory methods as for salivary samples, to express the percentage of mutans streptococci in the plaque sample. The presence of high salivary levels of *S. mutans* or lactobacilli does not necessarily mean that the patient has a high incidence or risk of developing dental caries because other factors, such as diet, buffering capacity, fluoride content of enamel, and degree of oral hygiene, may combine to produce a protective effect, and thus tip the host–parasite balance from disease towards health. Microbiological assessment of caries risk differs from conventional tests in medical microbiology where the presence or absence of a pathogen indicates a positive or negative diagnosis, for example in tuberculosis. However, the identification of a patient who has an abnormally high oral count of lactobacilli or mutans streptococci allows this fact to be taken into account when assessing all the factors which may contribute to the caries experience of the individual and when deciding short- and long-term treatment. The tests can also be used subsequently to monitor the efficacy of preventive techniques, such as dietary and oral hygiene advice and chlorhexidine therapy.

Prevention of dental caries

The most common approaches used in caries prevention are shown in Fig. 22.11. The rationale for the use of the different procedures is detailed below.

Sugar substitutes

The use of artificial sweeteners is based on the premise that they cannot be absorbed and metabolized by plaque bacteria to produce acid. There are two types of sugar substitutes available: those which have a calorific value (nutritive sweeteners), for example the sugar alcohols and lycasin, prepared from corn-starch syrup; and non-nutritive sweeteners such as xylitol and saccharin.

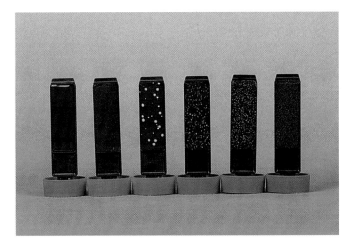

Fig. 22.10 Salivary lactobacillus counts can be performed on dip slides. (Courtesy of Prof. K.W. Stephen.)

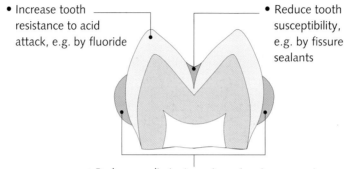

Fig. 22.11 Methods of preventing dental caries.

Both xylitol and lycasin are effective in reducing caries by stimulating salivary flow and encouraging remineralization. Xylitol also interferes with acid production by *S. sobrinus*.

Fluoride and tooth solubility

The various ways in which fluoride protects human teeth from carious attack are summarized in Fig. 22.12. Mutans streptococci are particularly sensitive to low levels of fluoride at moderately low pH values. However, in these circumstances mutans streptococci are not eliminated from the mouth but bacterial growth appears to be suppressed in plaques under conditions in which it would otherwise be expected to be stimulated.

Mechanical cleansing techniques

Conventional toothbrushing with a fluoridated toothpaste, even although it depends very much on the motivation and skill of the patient, is related to an overall reduction in the incidence of caries. Other aids for plaque removal, for example interdental brushes, wood sticks, and dental floss, may achieve some reduction in interdental caries, but there is no good evidence for this. Certainly it is unlikely that mechanical cleansing methods alone will significantly reduce or prevent caries in fissures or pits.

Antimicrobial agents

Chlorhexidine as a 0.12% to 0.2% mouthwash is by far the most effective agent in controlling dental plaque formation and has activity against many Gram-positive and Gram-negative oral bacteria. The antiseptic can also be applied to teeth in gel-form contained in special trays. At high concentrations the antiseptic is bactericidal by damaging cell membranes. Chlorhexidine also binds to oral surfaces (especially teeth), and is then slowly released into saliva over many hours at bacteriostatic concentrations that can reduce acid production in plaque by abolishing the activity of certain bacterial sugar transport systems. It is also possible that the presence of chlorhexidine on enamel surfaces and in saliva interferes with the adherence of plaque-forming bacteria, thus reducing the rate of plaque accumulation. Mutans streptococci tend to be more sensitive to chlorhexidine than other streptococci commonly involved in plaque development, for example *S. sanguis*. This fact is convenient, in that the antiseptic not only reduces the numbers and effectively the metabolic end-products of the major group of cariogenic bacteria, but also tends to favour the growth of streptococci which are associated with health. However, due to the dual problems of tooth staining and unpleasant taste, chlorhexidine is normally used only for short-term therapy.

Vaccination

It is well established that immunization, with either cell-wall associated antigens or glucosyltransferases from *S. mutans*, is effective in reducing experimental dental caries in rats and monkeys. It is not entirely clear how the vaccine produces its protective effect, although the following mechanisms have been suggested:

- inhibition of bacterial colonization of enamel by secretory IgA;
- interference with bacterial metabolism;
- enhancement of phagocytic activity in the gingival crevice area due to the opsonization of *S. mutans* with IgA or IgG antibodies.

However, convincing proof that any of these mechanisms prevent the development of dental caries *in vivo* is lacking. A number of cell-wall associated vaccines have been tested and all have produced good protection against caries in monkeys. Although

ANTICARIES ACTIVITIES OF FLUORIDE

1. Systemic effect
Incorporation of ingested fluoride into developing enamel as fluorapatite which reduces its solubility in acid and promotes remineralization

2. Topical effect
The surface layer of enamel is converted into fluorapatite which reduces its solubility in acid and promotes remineralizaton

3. Antimicrobial effect
Fluoride inhibits plaque metabolism and is concentrated within plaque. Activity increases at pH values <5, especially in the case of *Streptococcus mutans*

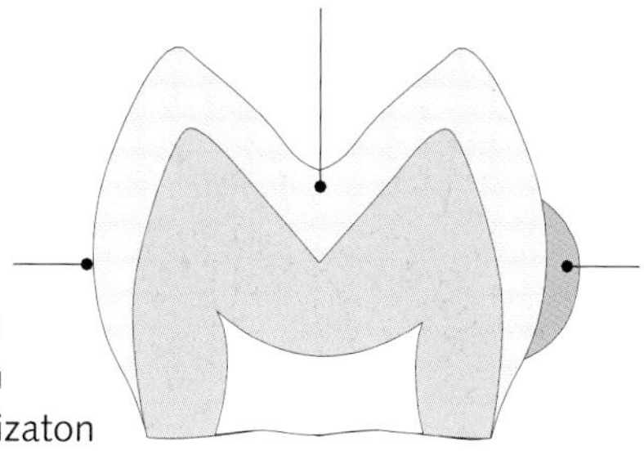

KEY
1. Fluoride present in water (naturally or artificially at 1 part per million), certain foods, tablets, or added to milk
2. Fluoride-containing toothpastes, gel and certain filling materials, e.g. glass ionomers
3. Inhibiting mechanisms include reducing glycolysis, indirectly inhibiting sugar transport, interfering with bacterial permeability, and inhibiting the synthesis of glycogen for intracellular storage

Fig. 22.12 Simplified diagram of the anticaries activities of fluoride.

potential vaccines against *S. mutans* have been manufactured to legally acceptable standards, no major field trials have been performed on humans. Some of the antigens tested elicited antibodies that cross-reacted with heart tissue, although this potential and undesirable problem has been eliminated through the careful selection of antigens. However, theoretically, other side-effects could emerge, and this raises the question of balancing the risk of using a potentially hazardous vaccine in the prevention of a non life-threatening disease.

Another problem in instituting a vaccination programme is the fact that the incidence of dental caries has fallen dramatically in most industrialized countries, probably as a result of fluoride, and vaccination is deemed unnecessary. However, it can be argued that a vaccine could be regarded as a benefit to particular high-risk groups in the population. Until immunization has been tested *in vivo* it can only be regarded as a potential method of preventing dental caries.

Fissure sealants

Fissure sealants prevent caries in pits and fissures by eliminating stagnation areas and blocking potential routes of infection by oral bacteria deep within the tooth. Early carious lesions in fissures that are sealed tend not to progress, probably because the source of microbial nutrition has been blocked. However, more extensive lesions will probably extend into the pulp, since the bacteria will obtain sufficient nutrients from the carious dentine.

Key facts

- Dental caries is a multifactorial, ubiquitous, plaque-related chronic infection of enamel or cementum/dentine.

- The main factors involved in the development of dental caries are a susceptible tooth surface, dietary carbohydrate (especially sucrose), saliva, and the oral microflora.

- The earliest clinical evidence of dental caries is the 'white spot' lesion which is reversible; cavitation represents irreversible disease.

- Some areas of the same enamel surface are more susceptible to demineralization than others.

- Severe xerostomia predisposes to rapid widespread dental caries.

- The frequency of sugar intake is more decisive than total consumption in the development of dental caries.

- Mutans streptococci, especially *S. mutans* and *S. sobrinus*, are implicated in the initiation of a high proportion of enamel and root surface carious lesions (Specific Plaque Hypothesis).

- Dental caries can occur in relation to dental plaque that is free from *S. mutans* (Non-specific Plaque Hypothesis).

Key facts – (*cont.*)

- *Lactobacillus* species are associated with the extension of the carious process into dentine rather than in the initiation phase of the disease.

- Dental treatment of a carious lesion should aim at permanent cure and eradication of the disease from the individual's mouth. Recurrent caries represents treatment failure.

- Patients with extensive or recurrent caries should be evaluated to identify relevant risk factors prior to treatment. These should include microbiological tests.

- High salivary or plaque counts of *Lactobacillus* species or mutans streptococci are related in many cases to a high risk of disease.

Further reading

Bowen, WH and Tabak, LA (ed.). (1993). *Cariology for the nineties*. University of Rochester Press, New York.

Fejerskov, O, Ekstrand, J, and Burt, BA (ed.). (1996). *Fluoride in dentistry* (2nd edn). Munksgaard, Copenhagen.

Kidd, EAM and Joyston-Bechal, S (1996). *Essentials of dental caries* (2nd edn). Oxford University Press, Oxford.

Marsh, PD and Martin, MV (1999). *Oral microbiology* (4th edn). Butterworth–Heinemann, London.

Tanzer, JM (1992). Microbiology of dental caries. In *Contemporary oral microbiology and immunology* (ed. J Slots and MA Taubman), Chapter 22. Mosby Year Book, St Louis.

Periodontal diseases

23

Periodontal diseases

Introduction

Periodontal disease in its widest sense includes all disorders of the supporting structures of the teeth, namely the gingiva, periodontal ligament, and supporting alveolar bone. This may vary from inflammation of the gingiva alone, termed gingivitis (Fig. 23.1), to the severe inflammation of the periodontal ligament called periodontitis (Fig. 23.2), in which there is destruction of alveolar bone and eventual tooth loss.

Unlike many medical infections, periodontal diseases are not caused by pathogens that have their primary habitat outside the host. Instead, they are associated with a shift in the balance of the resident microflora, a similar situation to dental caries (Chapter 22). The micro-organisms may produce disease directly, by invasion of the tissues, or indirectly via bacterial toxins. The host response to these challenges may be protective, for example phagocytosis of invading bacteria, or destructive, for example immune-complex activation of osteoclasts. Frequently it is a combination of both, and the interaction between these components determines the wide spectrum of disease that is seen clinically.

Gingivitis

As shown in Fig. 23.3, there are several types of gingivitis. The most common of these is plaque-associated chronic marginal gingivitis.

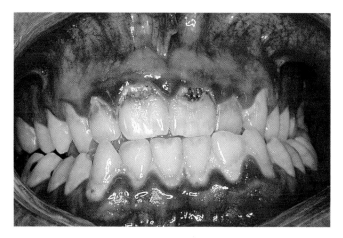

Fig. 23.1 Clinical photograph of plaque-associated gingivitis. (Courtesy of Dr M. Kjeldsen.)

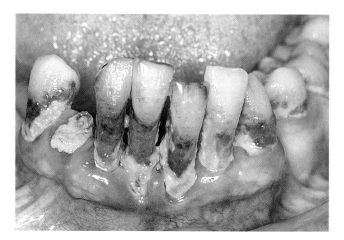

Fig. 23.2 Clinical photograph of periodontitis.

Plaque-associated gingivitis

The microflora of the healthy gingival crevice is relatively sparse and composed mainly of Gram-positive cocci, especially *Streptococcus* spp. The crevice has a lower redox potential (Chapter 20) than most sites within the oral cavity, which initially encourages the growth of *Actinomyces* spp. and an increase in capnophilic (carbon dioxide-requiring) bacteria such as *Capnocytophaga* species. Toxins released by these bacteria induce an inflammatory response in the gingival tissues, with a resultant increase in gingival crevicular fluid flow and the provision of nutrients essential to the changing needs of the plaque flora. The environment ultimately changes to one which can support the growth of obligately anaerobic bacteria and spirochaetes. The inflammatory reaction in the gingiva progresses, with resultant chronic marginal gingivitis. Clinically, gingivitis is characterized by redness, gingival bleeding, and oedema.

There is strong evidence for a bacterial aetiology of gingivitis. Both cross-sectional and longitudinal oral hygiene studies, in particular the experimental gingivitis studies of Löe in the 1960s, demonstrated that the development and accumulation of dental plaque can be correlated with clinically demonstrable gingivitis. However, it is the presence of dental plaque *per se* that correlates with gingivitis and there is no evidence to suggest that any particular bacterial species is responsible.

CLASSIFICATION OF GINGIVITIS	
Type of gingivitis	**Comments and examples**
Chronic marginal gingivitis	Non-specific inflammatory response to dental plaque involving the gingival margins. Early gingivitis associated with *Streptococcus* spp. and *Actinomyces* spp. Long-standing gingivitis has more Gram-negative anaerobes and spirochaetes
Acute ulcerative gingivitis (AUG)	An acute gingival infection characterized by necrosis of tips of the gingival papillae, spontaneous bleeding, pain, and halitosis. Predisposing factors include stress and cigarette smoking. Micro-organisms can be seen invading the gingival tissues and studies have identified large numbers of spirochaetes and fusiform bacteria. Other bacteria cultured are *Prevotella intermedia*, *Veillonella* spp., and *Fusobacterium* spp.
Steroid hormone induced gingivitis	Characterized clinically by an exaggerated response to plaque, leading to intense inflammation, redness, oedema, and enlargement. May occur during puberty, pregnancy, and with steroid therapy. Subgingival growth of *Porphyromonas gingivalis* may be enhanced when steroid hormones are elevated
Medication influenced gingivitis	Begins as small spherical enlargements of the gingival margin and papillae. May progress until most of the tooth surface is covered, forming false periodontal pockets. Induced by phenytoin, cyclosporin, and nifedipine
Gingivitis associated with systemic disease	Acute leukaemia may present clinically with intense gingival redness, swelling, and bleeding
Acute herpetic gingivostomatitis	One of the commonest causes of acute gingivitis is herpes simplex virus. Presents clinically with well-defined vesicles succeeded by ulcers
Desquamative gingivitis	Characterized by desquamation of the gingival epithelium, leaving an intensely red surface. Most cases represent oral manifestations of dermatological diseases, such as lichen planus, pemphigus vulgaris, and pemphigoid

Fig. 23.3 A summary of the common forms of gingivitis.

Acute ulcerative gingivitis is a specific form of gingivitis in which there is necrosis of the tips of the gingival papillae, spontaneous bleeding, pain, and halitosis (Fig. 23.4). Diagnosis is based on the demonstration of the characteristic fusospirochaetal complex in a deep gingival smear (Fig. 23.4).

Gingivitis often presents as clinically atypical forms among the immunocompromised. Thus, patients with acute leukaemia may develop sudden-onset gingival swelling, ulceration, and bleeding in conjunction with other oral manifestations such as petechial haemorrhages. HIV-associated gingivitis is an atypical gingivitis characterized by a band-like marginal erythema, usually accompanied by diffuse redness which extends onto the vestibular mucosa.

Stages in the development of gingivitis

Plaque-associated gingivitis has been separated into three stages based on the sequence of histopathological events that occur when plaque is allowed to accumulate at the gingival margin (Fig. 23.5).

STAGE 1: THE INITIAL LESION

This develops within 4 days of plaque accumulation. The microflora consists mostly of Gram-positive cocci (*Streptococcus*

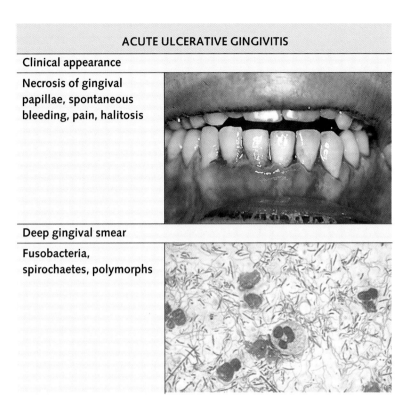

Fig. 23.4 Acute ulcerative gingivitis. Clinical photograph and the microscopic appearance of a Gram-stained deep gingival smear. The fusobacteria, spirochaetes, and polymorphs are clearly visible.

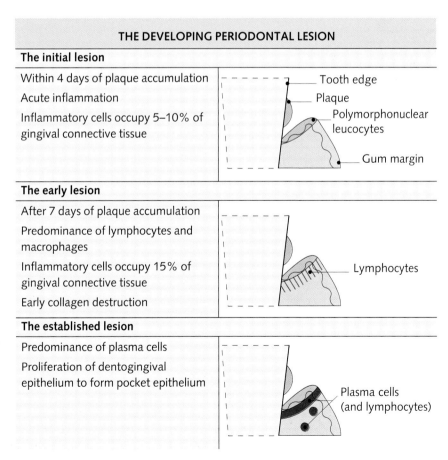

Fig. 23.5 Summary of the histological features of the developing periodontal lesion.

CLASSIFICATION OF PERIODONTITIS		
Classification	**Clinical findings**	**Laboratory findings**
Early-onset periodontitis	Includes prepubertal, juvenile, and rapidly progressive forms of the disease. Characterized by rapid loss of connective tissue attachment and severe loss of alveolar bone especially around the first permanent molars and lower incisors	Cellular immune defects may be present. *A. actinomycetemcomitans*, *Prev. intermedia, E. corrodens*, and *C. sputigena* are frequently isolated. These diseases may be associated with a genetic defect
Adult periodontitis	Between 8 and 10% of the population have significant destructive disease, exhibiting at least one site with an attachment loss of 6 mm or greater. Prevalence and severity increase with age	A wide range of bacteria have been associated (Fig. 23.11) depending on the rate of periodontal destruction, disease activity, and host resistance
Refractory periodontitis	Refers to disease in multiple sites which continue to demonstrate attachment loss following treatment	Residual infection by *B. forsythus, F. nucleatum, Prev. intermedia, E. corrodens*, and *P. gingivalis*
HIV-associated periodontitis	Characterized by its severity and rapidity. It is often painful with cratered gingival papillae, ulceration, bone loss, and bleeding	Bacteria associated include *Streptococcus* spp., *P. gingivalis, Prev. intermedia, A. actinomycetemcomitans*, and *F. nucleatum*
Lateral periodontal abscess	Acute inflammation within the periodontium as a result of invasion of bacteria into the tissues. It may be associated with pain and swelling of the affected area	The microflora consists of mixed anaerobes, mostly Gram-negative rods such as *P. gingivalis* and *F. nucleatum*
Periodontitis and systemic disease	Conditions such as diabetes mellitus, Down s syndrome, and neutropenia may present with rapidly progressive and severe periodontitis	The microflora is similar to other forms of periodontal diseases

Fig. 23.6 A summary of the classification of various forms of periodontitis.

spp.). Histologically, there is an acute inflammatory reaction. The lesion is characterized by an increased flow of gingival crevicular fluid (Fig. 23.5) and migration of polymorphonuclear leucocytes into the gingival sulcus from the local vasculature. Adjacent to the junctional and sulcular epithelia, the inflammatory infiltrate occupies approximately 5–10% of the gingival connective tissue. This initial lesion is not visible clinically.

STAGE 2: THE EARLY LESION
The early lesion appears after approximately 7 days of plaque accumulation and is detectable clinically as gingivitis. The environment now has a lower oxygen tension and the plaque flora shifts to contain more *Actinomyces* spp., spirochaetes, and capnophilic organisms. Histologically, the gingival infiltrate in the early lesion is dominated by lymphocytes (75%) and macrophages, with some plasma cells located at the periphery of the lesion (Fig. 23.5). The infiltrated area occupies approximately

15% of the marginal gingival connective tissue, with some local destruction of collagen. Migration of polymorphonuclear leucocytes into the gingival sulcus and crevicular fluid peaks at 6 to 12 days following the onset of clinically detectable gingivitis.

STAGE 3: THE ESTABLISHED LESION
After a variable period of time the subgingival microflora develops into an environment that can support the growth of obligate anaerobes such as *Porphyromonas gingivalis* and *Prevotella intermedia*. Histologically, there is a further increase in the size of the inflammatory lesion within the affected gingiva, with a shift to a predominance of plasma cells and B lymphocytes. A periodontal pocket lined with pocket epithelium may be present (Fig. 23.5). The junctional and pocket epithelia are heavily infiltrated with neutrophils. Plasma cells are found at the periphery of the lesion, while macrophages and

lymphocytes are present in the lamina propria of the pocket wall. Established lesions may persist for months or years without progression to periodontitis.

Periodontitis

Periodontitis may be defined clinically as inflammation of the supporting tissues of the teeth. It can be subdivided clinically into several groups (Fig. 23.6), the commonest of which is adult periodontitis.

The lesion of adult periodontitis maintains all the features of the established lesion of gingivitis, with additional migration of the junctional epithelium down the root surface, alveolar bone resorption, and subsequent pocket formation (Fig. 23.7). In addition, it is characterized by progressively destructive changes which lead to the loss of alveolar bone and periodontal ligament, with an attachment loss >3 mm. Histologically, the conversion of the established lesion of gingivitis into periodontitis is characterized by destruction of the connective tissue attachment to the root surface and by alveolar bone loss. The exact mechanism(s) for the transition from gingivitis to periodontitis is unknown.

Formation of a periodontal pocket creates an environment that is highly anaerobic. The pH shifts from 6.9 to approximately 7.4–7.8, and the pocket is continually bathed by a protein-rich solution of gingival crevicular fluid which encourages the growth of proteolytic bacteria. Subgingival plaque appears to have a dense zone of mostly Gram-positive bacteria attached to the tooth surface and a less densely packed zone of mainly Gram-negative organisms next to the gingival surface.

Subgingival plaque may undergo calcification to form subgingival calculus (Chapter 20). Clinically, subgingival calculus is darker in colour and more firmly attached to the root surface than its supragingival counterpart. Subgingival calculus is covered by a layer of micro-organisms and its porous nature serves as a reservoir for bacterial antigens, toxins, and enzymes.

The aetiology of periodontal disease

The search for the causative agent(s) of periodontal disease has been dogged by considerable difficulties. These have included:

(1) technical difficulties, for example obtaining uncontaminated plaque samples during the active stages of periodontal disease and the problem of culturing and discriminating between the 300 or more candidate species;

(2) an inadequate understanding of the progression of periodontal diseases;

(3) an inability to apply Koch's postulates (Chapter 1) since the causative organisms are likely to be part of the normal flora;

(4) the lack of an adequate animal model for periodontal disease.

In this section, a summary will be given of the present state of knowledge, though it must be recognized that this is currently incomplete.

Host and microbial factors

The search for the aetiology of periodontal disease must consider both host and microbial factors. The exact roles of each remain unclear but, as with most infections, it seems likely that the clinical outcome in periodontal disease is a result of the complex interactions between a wide range of host and microbial factors.

Host factors

For infectious disease to occur, the host must be susceptible to the relevant pathogen. Some of the factors which may increase host susceptibility to infection include an inadequate or unregulated host immune response, diabetes mellitus, stress, and tobacco use. Many of these are relevant to periodontal diseases, as summarized in Fig. 23.8.

Microbial factors

The important bacterial factors relevant to the role of micro-organisms in periodontal disease are summarized in Fig. 23.9.

The role of micro-organisms in periodontal disease

Studies on dogs have shown that chronic plaque-associated gingivitis can progress to periodontitis. However, epidemiological studies in humans have demonstrated that while 85–96% of the population have gingivitis, only a small proportion (12%) suffer from severe periodontitis. It remains unclear whether gingivitis is a necessary prerequisite for the development of periodontitis in humans.

Adult periodontitis may have its onset in adolescence and continue throughout the life of the individual, the severity increasing

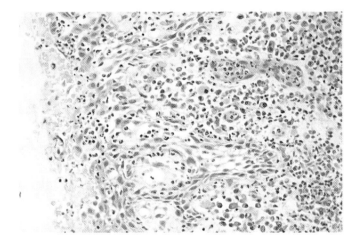

Fig. 23.7 Histological appearance in advanced periodontitis. Pocket epithelium is seen within connective tissue which is densely infiltrated with inflammatory cells, many of which are plasma cells.

HOST FACTORS IN PERIODONTAL DISEASE

Host factor	Beneficial effects	Harmful effects
Immunoglobulins	IgG enhances phagocytosis by opsonization of bacteria IgA decreases bacterial adherence	Antibody/antigen complexes may lead to type 3 hypersensitivity reactions. The attracted leucocytes release proteolytic enzymes resulting in tissue damage
Complement proteins	Endotoxin or antigen–antibody complexes can activate complement proteins. This initiates inflammatory reactions leading to lysis of bacteria, chemotaxis and activation of neutrophils and macrophage degranulation	Type 2 hypersensitivity reactions may follow activation of complement
Cytokines	Have a multitude of activities. For example, IL-2 recruits other members of the immune system	Cell-mediated tissue destruction may occur via the release of cytokines such as osteoclast-activating factor
Polymorphs and macrophages	Phagocytose bacteria	Release of neutral proteases and reactive oxygen metabolites may lead to tissue damage
T cells	T-helper cells co-operate with B cells in antibody production	
B cells	Produce antibodies against a wide range of periodontal pathogens	

Fig. 23.8 Table summarizing the host factors involved in the aetiology of periodontal disease.

with age. Early work suggested that the course of the disease was a slow, constant, and progressive destruction of the tissues. However, more recently it has been proposed that the disease occurs in short periods (bursts) of destruction followed by periods of inactivity, these occurring randomly with respect to time and site within an individual. There is currently much interest in developing methods to detect exactly when periodontal disease is active. The efficiency of periodontal disease prevention could be greatly increased and treatment better focused if the clinician or public health administrator were able to identify, in advance, those sites, subjects, or groups who will experience periodontal disease activity. Periodontal disease activity refers specifically to the dynamic stage of the disease characterized clinically by a loss of supporting bone and connective tissue attachment.

Specific and non-specific plaque hypotheses

Periodontal disease occurs in sites normally inhabited by numerous bacteria, where 300–400 different species have been

described. Even this figure is thought to be an underestimate, since an unknown number of species have not yet been cultured. However, since there is disagreement over the precise role of plaque bacteria in periodontal disease, several hypotheses have evolved to explain the part played by micro-organisms.

The specific plaque hypothesis

Cross-sectional and longitudinal studies of the predominant cultivable microflora have revealed that of the 300–400 bacterial species that can inhabit the oral cavity, only a small number are regularly associated with periodontal diseases. According to the specific plaque hypothesis, particular species of micro-organism are responsible for causing each type of periodontal disease. For example, early workers observed large numbers of a spirochaete in sections of tissue from acute necrotizing ulcerative gingivitis, and believed that this organism played a major role. Later, studies on localized juvenile periodontitis implicated *Actinobacillus actinomycetemcomitans* as a possible pathogen in this disease, while, more

BACTERIAL FACTORS IN PERIODONTAL DISEASE

Bacterial factor	Examples and comments
Attachment to host tissues	Mediated by fimbriae and capsules
Multiplication at a susceptible site	Inhibitor production, for example bacteriocins
Evasion of host defences	Capsules and slimes inhibit phagocytosis
Enzymes	Microbial collagenases have been implicated in destruction of collagen in periodontal ligament *Porphyromonas gingivalis* produces a wide range of proteases including trypsin-like protease (gingivain), collagenase, fibrinolysin, hyaluronidase, and heparitinase
Endotoxin (lipopolysaccharide)	Produced by Gram-negative bacteria. May initiate an inflammatory response via complement activation, mediate bone resorption, and kill macrophages
Leukotoxins	Kill polymorphs. Produced by some strains of *Actinobacillus actinomycetemcomitans*
IgA and IgG proteases	Degrade IgA and IgG. Produced by *Streptococcus oralis*, *Porphyromonas gingivalis*, and *Capnocytophaga* spp.
Cytotoxins	Butyric and propionic acids produced by *Porphyromonas gingivalis*
Indirect effects	The induction of an inflammatory response and IL-1 production in response to plaque antigens may cause indirect activation of host collagenases and stromolysins which degrade connective tissues
Superoxide dismutase	Protects aerobic bacteria from harmful oxygen products such as hydroxyl radicals

Fig. 23.9 Table summarizing the bacterial factors involved in the aetiology of periodontal disease.

recently, *Porphyromonas gingivalis* has been suggested as an important agent in adult periodontitis. Owing to the difficulties in identifying aetiological organisms in periodontal disease, a modified set of criteria has been developed for a specific micro-organism to be considered as a periodontal pathogen (Fig. 23.10). The species that have been implicated in periodontal disease by various workers are summarized in Fig. 23.11, though *Porphyromonas gingivalis*, *Prevotella intermedia*, and *Actinobacillus actinomycetemcomitans* are currently viewed as the mainstream periodontal pathogens.

The non-specific plaque hypothesis

The non-specific plaque hypothesis proposes that bacteria 'collectively' have the total complement of virulence factors required to cause destruction of the periodontal tissues, and that some micro-organisms can substitute for others which are not present in the pathogenic consortia. It implies that plaque will cause disease regardless of its composition. The wide range of species that have been associated with periodontal disease (Fig. 23.11) may reflect this view.

The plaque ecology hypothesis

This hypothesis suggests that conditions within the periodontal pocket allow the overgrowth of certain organisms already present in low numbers, and that this shift in balance predisposes the site to disease. This theory may be viewed as a combination of the specific and non-specific plaque hypotheses, but the plaque ecology hypothesis also helps to explain some of the current findings relating to periodontal disease activity. Thus, if the right ecological conditions developed within a site and allowed the production of virulence factors sufficient to overwhelm the host defences for a period of time, then this would result in a period of tissue destruction or disease activity. These conditions are continually changing *in vivo* and the pattern of disease progression would reflect changes in the ecosystem in the periodontal pocket.

PERIODONTAL PATHOGEN
• The organism is present in high numbers in periodontal disease compared with either the absence of the micro-organism or its presence in much smaller numbers (carrier state) in periodontally normal subjects
• Patients infected with the periodontal pathogen demonstrate specific antibodies in serum, saliva, and gingival crevicular fluid and may also develop a cell-mediated immune response to the putative pathogen
• The organism demonstrates *in vitro* production of virulence factors that can be correlated with clinical histopathology
• Experimental implantation of the organism into the gingival crevice of an appropriate animal model leads to the development of at least some characteristics of the naturally occurring disease, for example, inflammation, connective tissue disruption, and bone loss
• Clinical treatment that eliminates the organism from periodontal lesions should result in clinical improvement

Fig. 23.10 A modified set of criteria, based upon Koch's postulates, for the categorization of an organism as a periodontal pathogen.

BACTERIA ISOLATED FROM DESTRUCTIVE PERIODONTAL DISEASE	
Gram-positive	*Eubacterium* spp.
	Peptostreptococcus micros
Gram-negative	*Actinobacillus actinomycetemcomitans*
	Porphyromonas gingivalis
	Bacteroides forsythus
	Fusobacterium nucleatum
	Prevotella intermedia
	Capnocytophaga spp.
	Selenomonas spp.
	Spirochaetes

Fig. 23.11 Table listing the bacteria commonly isolated from periodontal pockets of patients with destructive periodontal disease.

The validity, or otherwise, of these hypotheses is very significant for the appropriate treatment of periodontal disease. The non-specific plaque hypothesis and the plaque ecology hypothesis imply that the appropriate treatment for periodontal disease may be either to reduce plaque to an acceptable level, maintain a 'healthy plaque', or achieve total plaque control. The specific plaque hypothesis suggests that treatment should be directed towards elimination of the specific pathogen(s). Furthermore, microbiological tests to detect specific pathogens or their products (Fig. 23.12) may be of additional use to assess disease activity in treatment planning, monitor the effects of treatment, identify sites or patients that are refractory to treatment, and identify antibiotic sensitivity patterns of organisms that prove difficult to eradicate by conventional means.

Whichever hypothesis turns out to be correct, recent data suggest that periodontitis results from the activity of mixtures of interacting bacteria. All studies agree that the disease can vary in degree from person-to-person and site-to-site, and that there is a progressive change in the composition of the flora from health to gingivitis to periodontitis. This is reflected by a switch from aerobic, non-motile, Gram-positive cocci (gingivitis) to anaerobic, motile, Gram-negative bacilli (periodontitis).

Treatment of periodontal disease

Whilst the exact aetiology of the various forms of periodontal disease has not been fully identified there is still a need to provide

ANALYSIS OF PERIODONTAL MICROFLORA	
Detection of:	**Examples and comments**
Viable bacteria	The reference method for determining microbial composition of plaque is bacterial culture. Disadvantages: potential errors in sampling, plaque dispersion, culture, and counting. Time-consuming, labour-intensive, and requires immediate access to laboratories
Microbial enzymes	*Treponema denticola, Porphyromonas gingivalis, Bacteroides forsythus,* and some *Capnocytophaga* strains possess an enzyme which hydrolyses the synthetic peptide benzoyl-DL-arginine-naphthylamide (BANA) from a colour-less substrate to a blue/black colour. This enzyme activity is detectable in subgingival plaque samples and has been associated with the levels and proportions of spirochaetes and anaerobes in the plaque and with pocket probing depth
Microbial antigens	Entails use of antibodies directed against specific bacterial antigens. The antigen–antibody complex may then be detected by, for example, a fluorescent labelling technique. These methods rely on recognition of specific antigen(s) which may be blocked or missing in certain strains and are therefore open to error. In addition, cross-reaction with other similar antigens may also occur giving rise to false-negative or positive results
Microbial DNA/RNA	DNA/RNA probes are sequences of DNA or RNA with a known specificity, labelled with a chemiluminescent marker. They are used to probe plaque samples for the presence of a specific organism. If the organism is present, the DNA probe will be retained and detected. These probes can be species-specific and the technique does not depend on bacteria remaining viable. PCR techniques are being applied to analysis of the periodontal microflora

Fig. 23.12 Summary of the laboratory methods available for the detection of specific micro-organisms in dental plaque.

treatment. The main methods for preventing and treating periodontal disease can be summarized as follows:

- supragingival plaque control (Chapter 20);
- root surface debridement;
- surgery, if improved access is required;
- consideration of adjunctive antimicrobial agents.

Antibiotics may be required for the management of acute periodontal conditions, such as metronidazole for the treatment of acute ulcerative gingivitis and penicillin for an acute periodontal abscess. However, the use of systemic antibiotics has no place in the routine treatment of chronic periodontitis. Systemic antibiotic therapy is occasionally indicated for the management of some forms of periodontal disease, for example juvenile or rapidly progressive periodontitis. Thus, *A. actinomycetem-comitans*, which can be difficult to eradicate from the periodontal tissues, may respond to tetracycline, an antibiotic to which it is usually very sensitive. Locally delivered antibiotics (usually tetracycline or metronidazole) inserted into pockets, may occasionally have a role to play in the treatment of refractory periodontitis in the presence of adequate supragingival plaque control.

Key facts

- Plaque-related gingivitis is a non-specific response to plaque which is characterized clinically by gingival redness, bleeding, and oedema.

- In plaque-associated gingivitis the microflora becomes progressively more diverse, with an increase in plaque mass and a shift from the streptococcal domination of gingival health to one in which *Actinomyces* species, capnophilic organisms, and obligate anaerobic Gram-negative organisms predominate.

- Gingivitis does not lead inevitably to periodontitis.

- Periodontitis is defined clinically as inflammation of the supporting tissues of the teeth, commonly presenting as a progressively destructive change leading to loss of bone and periodontal ligament, with an attachment loss greater than 3 mm.

- Periodontitis may be the result of infection with specific bacteria ('the specific plaque hypothesis'), a non-specific response to plaque bacteria ('the non-specific plaque hypothesis'), or the establishment of the right ecological conditions for the expression of sufficient virulence factors to result in tissue destruction ('the plaque ecology hypothesis').

- In periodontitis there is a progressive change in the composition of the microflora from aerobic, non-motile, Gram-positive cocci to anaerobic, motile, Gram-negative bacilli.

- Some Gram-negative bacteria implicated in the aetiology of periodontal disease include *Actinobacillus actinomycetemcomitans*, *Porphyromonas gingivalis*, *Prevotella intermedia*, *Bacteroides forsythus*, *Fusobacterium nucleatum*, and *Capnocytophaga* spp.

- Bacteria present in periodontal pockets may be detected by microbial culture techniques, detection of certain microbial enzymes, immunological methods, and DNA/RNA probes.

- Clinical outcome in periodontal disease is likely to be a result of the complex interactions between a wide range of individual host and microbial factors.

- Methods for the treatment of periodontal disease include supragingival plaque control, root surface debridement, periodontal surgery, and the use of antimicrobial agents.

- Systemic antibiotics should not be used routinely for the management of chronic periodontal disease.

Further reading

Marsh, PD and Martin, MV (1999). *Oral microbiology* (4th edn). Butterworth–Heinemann, London.

Socransky, SS and Haffajee, AD (1997). Microbiology of periodontal disease. In *Clinical periodontology and implant dentistry* (3rd edn) (ed. J Lindhe, T Karring, and NP Lang), Chapter 4. Munksgaard, Copenhagen.

Zambon, JJ (1996). Periodontal diseases: microbial factors. *Annals of Periodontology*, 1, 879–925

24

Infections of the pulp, periapical tissues, and bone of the jaw

- Pulpitis

- Dentoalveolar abscess

- Periodontal abscess

- Ludwig's angina

- Osteomyelitis of the jaws

- Actinomycosis

Infections of the pulp, periapical tissues, and bone of the jaw

As discussed in previous chapters, bacteria are responsible for both dental caries and periodontal diseases. Extension of these diseases commonly causes infection in the adjacent tissues, notably the pulp, periapical area, and orofacial soft tissues. More rarely, infection may become established in the bone of the jaw to cause osteomyelitis. These infections, which are usually acute, are among the commonest seen by dentists, and will be covered in this chapter.

Pulpitis

Inflammation of the pulp (pulpitis) may follow exposure to a range of irritants. These include thermal, mechanical, or chemical stimuli, in addition to micro-organisms which are the focus of this chapter. Since the pulp is enclosed within the hard tissues of the tooth, it is unable to expand during the acute inflammatory

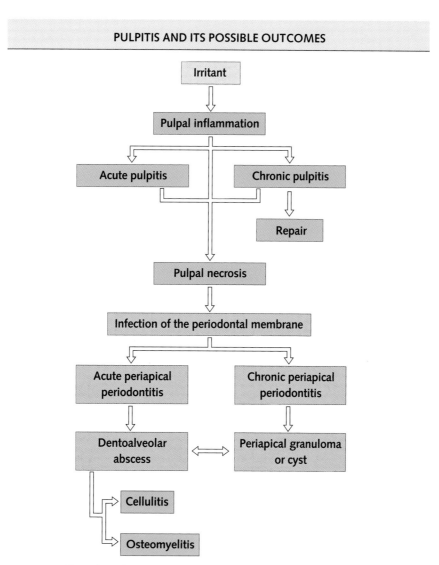

PULPITIS AND ITS POSSIBLE OUTCOMES

Irritant → Pulpal inflammation → Acute pulpitis / Chronic pulpitis → Repair → Pulpal necrosis → Infection of the periodontal membrane → Acute periapical periodontitis / Chronic periapical periodontitis → Dentoalveolar abscess ⇄ Periapical granuloma or cyst → Cellulitis, Osteomyelitis

Fig. 24.1 Flow chart illustrating the possible outcomes of pulpitis.

phase of pulpitis, with a resultant rise in internal pressure. This not only results in severe pain but also impairs the circulation within the inflamed pulp, which may cause pulpal necrosis and subsequent periapical disease. The possible outcomes are illustrated in Fig. 24.1. Whilst the commonest cause of pulpal necrosis is dental caries, others include accidental trauma to the tooth, exposure of the pulp during instrumentation, and spread of infection from a deep periodontal pocket.

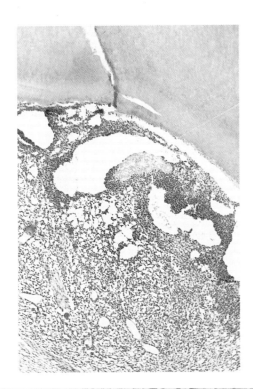

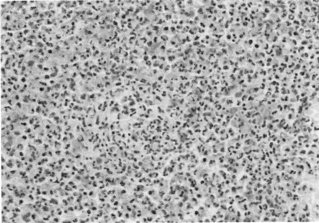

Fig. 24.2 Low- and high-power photomicrographs illustrating a pulp abscess. This decalcified section of a fractured tooth has been stained with haematoxylin and eosin. Note the dense infiltration of polymorphonuclear leucocytes and the hyperaemia. (Courtesy of Prof. D.G. MacDonald.)

Pulpitis following dental caries

Gram-positive bacteria, especially lactobacilli and certain streptococci, predominate in the advancing front of a carious lesion. Whilst bacterial penetration of the tubules is slow, acids and other toxic products of the organisms diffuse quickly, causing damage to the odontoblasts and local pulp tissue. Providing the bacteria have not actually infected the pulp, these effects may be transient.

Once the pulp tissue becomes invaded by bacteria (initially lactobacilli and streptococci, but later mixed species (Fig. 24.3)) the organisms multiply and large numbers of polymorphonuclear leucocytes appear. Microabscesses will develop and enlarge (Fig. 24.2), with ultimate death and liquefaction of pulp tissue.

Pulpitis through an open cavity

If the pulp becomes exposed to the mouth, either through dental decay, instrumentation, or other trauma, several types of bacteria establish themselves and produce even higher concentrations of toxic products which diffuse throughout the pulp. Bacteria themselves may spread through the entire tissue, resulting in rapid disintegration and liquefaction of the pulp. A mixed, mainly anaerobic flora, is often identified in such cases (Fig. 24.3).

Pulpitis through the apical foramen

The pulp may become infected via the apical foramen. This can occur from a lateral canal in communication with a deep periodontal pocket (a 'perio-endo' lesion), from an adjacent periapical lesion, or through haematological spread. An impaired state of

BACTERIA ISOLATED FROM NECROTIC PULPS	
Category	**Genus**
Obligate anaerobes:	
Gram-positive cocci	*Peptostreptococcus*
Gram-negative cocci	*Veillonella*
Gram-positive rods	*Eubacterium*
	Propionibacterium
	Arachnia
Gram-negative rods	*Porphyromonas*
	Prevotella
	Fusobacterium
	Campylobacter
	Wolinella
Facultative anaerobes:	
Gram-positive cocci	*Streptococcus*
Gram-positive rods	*Lactobacillus*
Gram-negative rods	*Eikenella*
	Capnocytophaga

Fig. 24.3 The most common genera of bacteria isolated from necrotic dental pulps. Obligate anaerobes predominate.

the pulp is a prerequisite for this type of infection to establish, and rapid pulpal necrosis often follows.

Pulpal necrosis

A necrotic pulp may remain sterile for varying periods of time, but it can become infected very readily with rapid bacterial spread, because of the lack of host defences in such tissue. The possible routes of infection are the same as those for a vital pulp. A necrotic pulp in contact with the mouth microflora usually becomes infected with several bacterial species, with obligate anaerobes playing an important role. The main genera commonly isolated from infected necrotic pulps are shown in Fig. 24.3.

Dentoalveolar abscess

This common infection develops typically at the apices of the roots of teeth, following necrosis of the pulp (Fig. 24.4). The clinical presentation is largely dependent on the local anatomy, but is also influenced by the pathogenicity of the infecting organisms and by the adequacy of treatment.

Abscesses may arise *de novo* or may develop within a preexisting granuloma (Figs 24.1 and 24.5). The abscess may remain localized within the alveolar bone, in which case the tooth is usually very tender to pressure. Alternatively, the infection may burst through the alveolar bone and into the soft tissues. This may result in intra- or extraoral swelling (Fig. 24.6) or in a potentially dangerous spread of infection through fascial planes, as described later.

Microbiology

The microbiology of dentoalveolar abscesses (Fig. 24.7) has become better understood in recent years through the application of improved sampling methods and anaerobic culture techniques. Overall the related microflora is similar to that isolated from necrotic pulps (see Fig. 24.3). Lesions are typically caused by organisms which comprise part of the normal oral flora (endogenous infections). A mixture of bacteria is usually isolated, often including obligate anaerobes. Facultative anaerobes, particularly those of the *Streptococcus milleri* group, are also frequently found.

Specimen collection

Collection of the correct specimen is critical if a microbiological analysis of pus from dentoalveolar infections is to be attempted. Swabs have often been employed in the past, but this is entirely

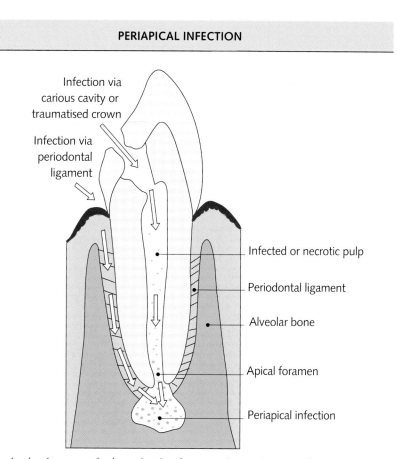

PERIAPICAL INFECTION

Infection via carious cavity or traumatised crown

Infection via periodontal ligament

Infected or necrotic pulp

Periodontal ligament

Alveolar bone

Apical foramen

Periapical infection

Fig. 24.4 Diagram illustrating the development of a dentoalveolar abscess at the tooth apex. Infection arises most commonly via the pulp chamber. (Courtesy of Dr M.A.O. Lewis.)

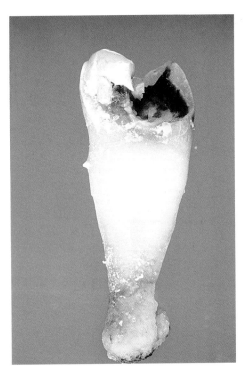

Fig. 24.5 A premolar tooth extracted because of gross dental caries and a periapical granuloma.

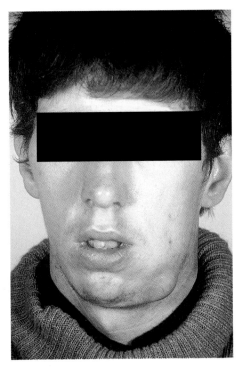

Fig. 24.6 Obvious facial swelling in a patient with a dentoalveolar abscess.

MICROBIOLOGY OF DENTAL ABSCESSES

- Endogenous infections
- Often mixed infections
- Strict anaerobes important

Ideal specimen: aspirated pus

Fig. 24.7 Key features in the microbiology of dentoalveolar abscesses.

---

inappropriate for two reasons. First, since these infections are typically endogenous, contamination of the swab with salivary organisms confuses the interpretation of culture results. Second, obligate anaerobes are very sensitive to the effects of oxygen and die rapidly on the surface of a swab.

The specimen of choice, which overcomes these problems of contamination and oxygen contact, is an aspirate of pus (see Fig. 12.7) collected by means of a needle and syringe. The syringe and its contents are then submitted to the laboratory. The needle may either be carefully removed and a cap placed on the hub, or the needle resheathed using a safety device and the needle cover taped to the syringe barrel for safe transportation.

Treatment

The essential element of treatment is to establish drainage of the pus. This can be achieved in several ways, depending on the clinical circumstances. If the tooth is expendable, then extraction will allow drainage. For teeth which are to be retained, drainage should be established through the root canal and by incision of any residual fluctuant collections of pus, for example in the buccal sulcus.

Antimicrobial agents are not required in every case. They are useful as an initial approach to treating patients with gross facial swelling for whom drainage cannot be established immediately, and they are useful adjuncts to drainage in patients who are febrile. Penicillin V or amoxycillin are suitable agents, whilst erythromycin is appropriate for those with penicillin hypersensitivity. Since many of these infections have an anaerobic component, metronidazole may also be used, although it is ineffective against facultative organisms such as the *Streptococcus milleri* group.

Periodontal abscess

Clinical features

Periodontal abscesses usually occur in patients with established periodontal pockets. The associated tooth may be vital or non-vital. It is believed that occlusion of the opening of the pocket prevents normal drainage and results in an acute episode. Impaction of foreign bodies in the periodontium may also play a role in the aetiology. The periodontal abscess is of sudden onset.

There is usually swelling, redness, and tenderness of the overlying gingiva. These abscesses frequently drain themselves along the root surface to the pocket opening, but if occlusion of the pocket is complete there may be local spread of infection with destruction of bone and soft tissue.

Microbiology

It is extremely difficult to collect an uncontaminated specimen of pus from a periodontal abscess. The related microflora is not, therefore, well characterized and routine microbiological examination is not undertaken. Subgingival plaque is the source of the organisms in periodontal abscesses and those believed to play a role include anaerobic Gram-negative rods, alpha haemolytic and anaerobic streptococci, together with others such as spirochaetes.

Treatment

This should form part of an overall clinical assessment of the patient's dentition. The options include extraction of the tooth or drainage of the abscess followed by appropriate periodontal treatment. Antibiotics may be considered as an adjunct to treatment, as described earlier in the management of dentoalveolar abscesses.

Ludwig's angina

Clinical features

Ludwig's angina is a bilateral infection of the sublingual and submandibular spaces. The infection often represents cellulitis of the fascial spaces, rather than true abscess formation. The key clinical features are a brawny oedema with elevation of the tongue, airway obstruction, and very little pus. Although uncommon, the mortality is close to 100% in patients who do not receive treatment.

Dental infection is the causative factor in up to 90% of cases, though Ludwig's angina may be secondary to other infections, for example submandibular sialadenitis.

Microbiology

A wide range of organisms has been reported from these infections, including staphylococci, streptococci, and enterobacteria. However, oral commensal bacteria, especially anaerobic Gram-negative bacilli and anaerobic streptococci, are most commonly isolated. Like dentoalveolar abscesses, the infections are usually mixed.

Treatment

Ludwig's angina is a life-threatening infection, requiring urgent treatment. The key elements of management are early diagnosis, maintenance of the airway, high-dose antibiotic treatment, removal of the source of infection (usually tooth extraction), parenteral hydration, and early surgical drainage. A pus sample should be collected if possible for microbiological examination. Intravenous penicillin is the empirical antibiotic of choice, but may be changed in the light of the microbiological results.

Osteomyelitis of the jaws

Though once a fairly common disease, osteomyelitis of the jaws is now encountered only rarely. Osteomyelitis is defined as inflammation of the medullary cavity of bone, but it usually spreads to involve the cortical bone and periosteum as well. Following ischaemia, the infected bone becomes necrotic. Osteomyelitis may present as an acute or chronic infection and is much commoner in the mandible than the maxilla.

Aetiology and predisposing factors

Odontogenic infections are common, and in view of the close relationship of the teeth to the medullary cavity it is surprising that osteomyelitis of the jaws is so rare. This is thought to relate to host resistance and it is well recognized that systemic diseases which reduce host defences, for example diabetes or agranulocytosis, predispose to the infection. The vascularity of bone is an essential part of the defence system and any conditions which reduce this vascularity, for example radiotherapy or Paget's disease, will increase the risk of osteomyelitis.

When the organisms reach the medullary cavity they proliferate and stimulate an acute inflammatory response. There is hyperaemia, increased capillary permeability, infiltration by granulocytes, and tissue necrosis. Pus accumulates, increasing the intramedullary pressure, with resultant venous stasis and ischaemia. Pus may then travel through the haversian and nutrient canals and accumulate beneath the periosteum, further compromising the blood supply. Eventually the periosteum is penetrated and mucosal or cutaneous abscesses and fistulae often develop. If left untreated the infection may proceed to chronic osteomyelitis with, for example, new bone formation and loss of dead bone by sequestration.

Clinical features

In early, acute, suppurative osteomyelitis of the mandible the four key features are intense pain, high and intermittent fever, paraesthesia or anaesthesia of the mental nerve and, finally, a clearly defined aetiology. At this point there is minimal swelling.

If untreated the condition will progress to established suppurative osteomyelitis. Patients complain of deep pain, malaise, fever, and anorexia. Teeth in the involved area become loose and tender to percussion and pus may exude from the gingival sulcus or through fistulae. The patient is febrile, regional lymph nodes are enlarged, and there may be cellulitis of the cheek and trismus.

Radiographs show no significant abnormalities in the early stages of acute osteomyelitis. The full extent of bone destruction is seen radiographically about 3 weeks after osteomyelitis develops, and is described as having a 'moth eaten' appearance (Fig. 24.8).

Microbiology

Historically, staphylococci were implicated as important organisms in osteomyelitis of the jaws. More modern studies indicate that members of the normal oral flora, particularly anaerobic

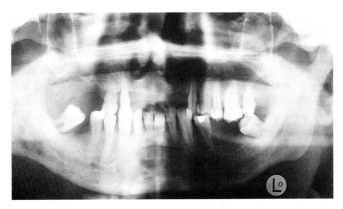

Fig. 24.8 A radiograph of the mandible illustrating the 'moth eaten' appearance caused by the bone destruction of osteomyelitis. (Courtesy of Mrs L. Brocklebank.)

Gram-negative rods and anaerobic streptococci, are usually the organisms of importance. The infections are typically mixed.

Since a wide range of organisms may be isolated, culture and sensitivity tests are an important part of the management of acute osteomyelitis, although it may be difficult to obtain a specimen in the early stages. In the later stages, pus can be collected, but great care must be taken to avoid contamination with organisms of the normal skin and oral flora.

Treatment

Both medical and surgical treatment are usually required in the management of osteomyelitis of the jaws. Successful treatment is based on early diagnosis, drainage of pus, bacterial culture and sensitivity testing, antibiotic therapy, supportive treatment, debridement, and, if necessary, surgical reconstruction. Attention must also be paid to any predisposing factors.

Antibiotics of value in the management of osteomyelitis include penicillin, penicillinase-resistant penicillins (e.g. flucloxacillin), clindamycin, cephalosporins, and erythromycin. In the early stages, before a pus sample can be collected, empirical treatment is usually provided with both a penicillin and a penicillinase-resistant penicillin. Thereafter, the antibiotic regimen should be based on the results of microbiological examination.

Actinomycosis

The cervicofacial region is the commonest site for actinomycosis (Fig. 24.9), accounting for approximately 90% of the recorded cases. Most of the remaining cases are abdominal. The disease is usually a chronic, long-standing infection, sometimes with a history of a mild preceding trauma such as a tooth extraction. It is a good example of an endogenous infection.

It presents typically as a swelling, often at the angle of the lower jaw (Fig. 24.10) and is commoner in young people, particularly males. If left untreated, multiple draining sinuses will develop. The exudate from these sinuses contains visible, yellow particles known as sulphur granules, which are aggregates of actinomyces filaments that may have a calcified centre (Fig. 24.11). The slow growing *Actinomyces* species induce a granulomatous type reaction at the periphery of the lesions, resulting in the formation of fibrous walls in and around the swellings. These must be broken down if treatment is to be effective.

Microbiology

The most frequent isolate is *Actinomyces israelii*, though *A. naeslundii* and *A. bovis* may also be detected. Other organisms are commonly present in addition to *Actinomyces* species, including *Actinobacillus actinomycetemcomitans*, *Haemophilus* species, and obligate anaerobes.

CERVICOFACIAL ACTINOMYCOSIS	
Aetiology	*Actinomyces israelii* ± other organisms, e.g. *Actinobacillus actinomycetemcomitans* Trauma
Clinical features	Younger patients, more commonly male Swelling, typically at angle of jaw Discharging sinuses Dental focus of infection
Laboratory diagnosis	Gram-stained film of sulfur granules in pus: Gram-positive branching filaments Anaerobic culture
Treatment	Extraction of dental focus of infection Surgical drainage Extended course of penicillin

Fig. 24.9 Summary table of the important features of cervicofacial actinomycosis.

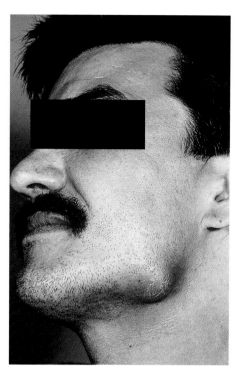

Fig. 24.10 Actinomycosis presenting as a swelling at the angle of the mandible in a young, male patient.

Diagnosis

The ideal specimen for diagnosis is an uncontaminated sample of pus collected by needle aspiration. This is examined macroscopically in the laboratory for the presence of sulphur granules. If granules are detected they can be squashed between two glass microscope slides and Gram-stained (Fig. 24.11). This will reveal a mass of Gram-positive branching filaments, allowing a pre-

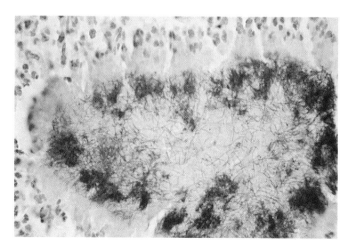

Fig. 24.11 A Gram-stained film of a squashed sulfur granule. Note the branching Gram-positive filaments.

sumptive diagnosis of actinomycosis. The diagnosis can be confirmed by anaerobic culture of the pus. *A. israelii* is usually a strict anaerobe whilst the remaining *Actinomyces* species are facultative anaerobes. On agar plates the colonies, which take several days to appear, have a morphology similar to 'molar teeth'. Antibiotic sensitivity tests can also be undertaken once the organism has been isolated.

Treatment

Whilst *Actinomyces* species are sensitive *in vitro* to a wide range of antibiotics, the bacterial cells within sulphur granules and in locules of pus surrounded by fibrous septa may be protected from and survive antibiotic treatment *in vivo*. The treatment of actinomycosis therefore includes thorough surgical drainage and removal of dead tissue in addition to long-term administration of an antibiotic, typically a penicillin or erythromycin.

Key facts

- Dental caries is the commonest cause of pulpal necrosis.

- Bacterial infections of the pulp are often mixed and largely anaerobic.

- Dentoalveolar abscesses are endogenous infections usually caused by a mixture of bacteria including obligate anaerobes.

- Pus specimens from the head and neck region for microbiological examination should be collected by needle aspiration.

- Drainage of pus is the essential element of treatment for a dentoalveolar or periodontal abscess.

- Ludwig's angina is a life-threatening infection involving the sublingual and submandibular spaces.

- Maintenance of the airway is paramount in the management of Ludwig's angina.

- Osteomyelitis of the jaws is uncommon, but typically occurs in patients with deficient host defences or reduced vascularity of the bone.

- Osteomyelitis of the jaws is usually a mixed infection, requiring both medical and surgical treatment.

- Actinomycosis is an endogenous infection, associated with *Actinomyces israelii*, which presents as a swelling, often at the angle of the mandible.

- 'Sulphur granules' are particles seen in pus from actinomycotic lesions and which contain aggregates of actinomyces filaments.

- Actinomycosis is treated by surgical drainage and long-term administration of antibiotics, ideally penicillin.

Further reading

Dahlén, G and Möller, AJR (1992). Microbiology of endodontic infections. In *Contemporary oral microbiology and immunology*. (ed. J Slots and MA Taubman) Chapter 24. Mosby Year Book, St Louis.

Lewis, MAO, MacFarlane, TW, and McGowan, DA (1990). A microbiological and clinical review of the acute dentoalveolar abscess. *British Journal of Oral and Maxillofacial Surgery*, 28, 359–66.

Marsh, PD and Martin, MV (1999). *Oral microbiology* (4th edn). Butterworth–Heinemann London.

25

Salivary gland infections

- Viral infections of salivary glands
- Bacterial infections of salivary glands

Salivary gland infections

Salivary gland infections may be viral or bacterial. There are several ways of classifying salivary gland infections, including acute or chronic, bacterial or viral, and obstructive or non-obstructive (Fig. 25.1). The most common salivary gland infection is that caused by the mumps virus. Acute sialadenitis is usually bacterial in origin.

SALIVARY GLAND INFECTIONS	
Bacterial	Acute parotitis
	Chronic parotitis
	Recurrent parotitis of childhood
	Submandibular sialadenitis
	Tuberculosis
	Actinomycosis
Viral	Mumps

Fig. 25.1 Classification of salivary gland infections.

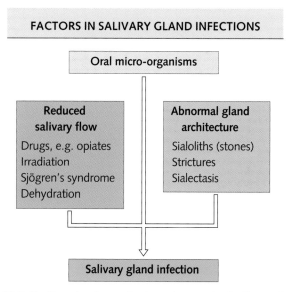

Fig. 25.2 Predisposing factors in the pathogenesis of salivary gland infections.

A number of factors are involved in the pathogenesis of salivary gland infections (Fig. 25.2). Decrease in host resistance is of particular importance and may relate to general factors, such as dehydration or previous radiotherapy, or to local factors including sialolithiasis, ductal strictures, and other salivary gland pathology.

Viral infections of salivary glands

A number of viruses, in addition to mumps virus, may infect salivary glands and cause clinical disease. Cytomegalovirus causes cytomegalic inclusion disease, whilst others such as echo and coxsackieviruses have been implicated in non-suppurative sialadenitis. These, however, are rare disorders and will not be discussed further.

Mumps

Mumps virus is an RNA paramyxovirus. The saliva of patients who are incubating mumps is infectious for several days before parotitis develops and for up to 2 weeks after the onset of clinical symptoms. The disease is highly infectious and is transmitted by direct contact with saliva and by droplet spread.

Clinical presentation

Mumps is characterized by inflammation and enlargement of the salivary glands, 15–18 days after exposure (Figs 25.3 (a), (b)). There is a prodromal phase of pyrexia, sore throat, and sometimes a complaint of pain on chewing. Reddening of the opening of the parotid duct and pain or tenderness on upward pressure beneath the angle of the lower jaw may be early signs of mumps. Painful swelling of one or both parotid glands follows, often displacing the earlobe. Swelling of the submandibular glands may also occur, typically a few days after the parotids.

The clinical course of mumps is variable, ranging from subclinical or mild infection to a severe, febrile illness lasting 10–14 days. Symptomatic relief of pain and fever is necessary together with prevention of dehydration. Complete recovery within 5–10 days is normal but complications include pancreatitis, orchitis (inflammation of the testes; about 20% of young men), and mumps meningitis.

Diagnosis

The diagnosis is usually made on clinical grounds. In patients with an unusual clinical presentation, such as unilateral swelling,

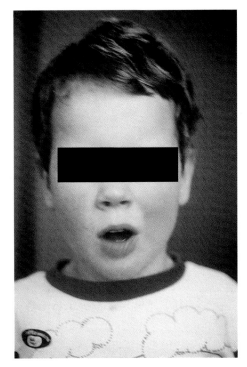

(a)

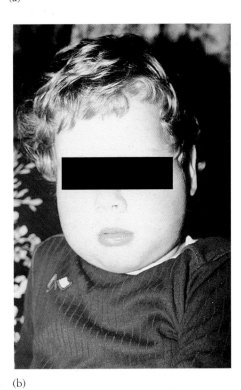

(b)

Fig. 25.3 Photographs illustrating (a) a child in health and (b) the same child with enlargement of the parotid and submandibular glands as a result of mumps.

the diagnosis is normally confirmed by serological tests, typically to detect specific IgM class antibodies.

Human immunodeficiency virus

Salivary gland disease has been reported as a feature of HIV infection (Chapter 19) in some patients. The two categories of disease presentation are xerostomia and enlargement of the major salivary glands.

Approximately 10% of patients with AIDS complain of xerostomia. The enlargement of the parotid and/or submandibular glands is usually bilateral and may accompany a Sjögren's syndrome-like disease. The histological appearance is extremely variable and, in addition to lymphocytic sialadenitis, may show other pathologies such as hyperplasia of parotid nodes, Kaposi's sarcoma, or lymphoma. The aetiology of the swelling is often unclear but there is a suggestion that in some cases it may follow infection with other viruses such as cytomegalovirus or Epstein–Barr virus.

Bacterial infections of salivary glands

Acute bacterial parotitis

In health, oral bacteria are prevented from ascending the parotid duct and invading the salivary gland tissue by the natural flushing activity of saliva. If this flow is significantly reduced, a retrograde infection up the duct is possible. Thus, bacterial parotitis normally occurs in patients with reduced salivary flow or local abnormalities in the salivary gland architecture (see Fig. 25.2).

Clinical presentation

There is a sudden onset of firm, erythematous swelling of the pre- and postauricular areas, extending to the angle of the mandible (Fig. 25.4). The swelling is associated with extreme local pain and tenderness. Milking of the parotid duct produces a thick, puru-

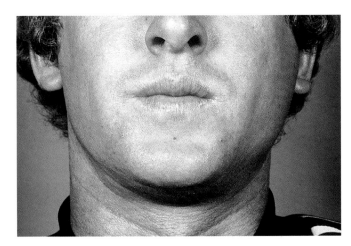

Fig. 25.4 Swelling in the left preauricular region in a patient with bacterial parotitis.

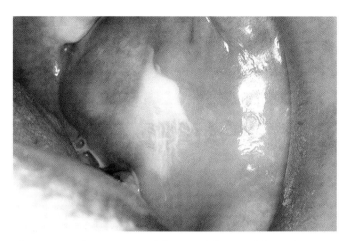

Fig. 25.5 Pus being expressed from the left parotid duct of the patient with bacterial parotitis shown in Fig. 25.4.

lent discharge at the duct orifice (Fig. 25.5). Patients may be febrile, experience chills, and have a leucocytosis.

Specimen collection and microbiology

Collection of an uncontaminated specimen of pus from this type of infection is difficult. Ideally, pus should be aspirated through a small-bore catheter attached to a syringe, but in view of the pain and associated trismus often experienced by patients with parotitis this is rarely feasible. An alternative is to isolate the duct orifice and collect a bead of pus onto a swab for immediate transportation to the laboratory.

As a result of the sampling difficulties, the causative microorganisms have not been well defined. *Staphylococcus aureus* and alpha haemolytic streptococci have been most commonly reported, but *Haemophilus* species and anaerobes are also implicated.

Management

Treatment relies on appropriate antimicrobial therapy, ideally guided by the results of culture and sensitivity tests on a pus specimen. Until such results are available, a penicillinase-resistant penicillin, for example flucloxacillin, should be administered. Erythromycin is suitable for patients with penicillin hypersensitivity. Increased fluid intake is important. In severe cases, antibiotic treatment may need to be supplemented with surgical drainage.

Following resolution of the acute infection, patients should be examined for factors which may have predisposed them to infection. This typically entails sialography or a related imaging technique to identify any correctable salivary gland abnormalities such as calculi or strictures. Sialography should never be performed during the acute infection.

Chronic bacterial parotitis

Some adults suffer recurrent episodes of parotitis. These are often a result of persistence of the aetiological agent and are seen in damaged glands, for example in patients with Sjögren's syndrome. Unilateral or bilateral swelling of the parotid gland can occur, lasting from a few days to months. The clinical course is of intermittent exacerbations and remissions. This chronic, low-grade infection can functionally destroy the gland.

Conservative therapy with antibiotics is recommended initially, but parotidectomy may be appropriate for long-term chronic parotitis.

Recurrent parotitis of childhood

This infection is observed prior to puberty. The child experiences repeated acute episodes of painful enlargement of one or both parotid glands. The aetiology is unclear, but suggested predisposing factors include congenital abnormalities of the ductal system, preceding mumps, foreign bodies in the parotid duct, and trauma from orthodontic appliances.

Removal of any identified predisposing factor is an important element of treatment. For idiopathic cases, antibiotic administration and symptomatic therapy are recommended, since most will resolve spontaneously at puberty. Rarely, surgical drainage may be required.

Submandibular sialadenitis

Bacterial sialadenitis can affect salivary glands other than the parotids. Although submandibular sialadenitis is less common than parotitis, the submandibular glands usually become infected with similar organisms, resulting in glandular swelling and pain. In most cases, however, it follows ductal obstruction, for example calculi or strictures.

Treatment, therefore, depends on the removal of such obstructions in addition to hydration and provision of an appropriate antibiotic.

Other uncommon salivary gland infections

Tuberculosis

Very rarely, the salivary glands themselves may be involved in tuberculosis or there may be infection of lymph nodes associated with the glands. Tuberculosis of the salivary glands develops secondary to pulmonary tuberculosis, an important consideration in relation to diagnosis (Chapter 16). The parotids are affected most commonly, the infection presenting as a firm, non-tender swelling. Rarely, facial paralysis may be a presenting feature.

The major salivary glands and associated lymph nodes may also become infected with atypical mycobacteria (Chapter 16). This is seen most commonly in children, usually presenting as facial or cervical masses which may drain spontaneously (Fig. 25.6). Skin testing can distinguish between true tuberculosis caused by *Mycobacterium tuberculosis* and infections with atypical mycobacteria. The latter are fairly resistant to antituberculous medication and are best treated by excision.

Actinomycosis

This infection is dealt with in detail in Chapter 24. *Actinomyces israelii* may cause infection of salivary glands that is clinically

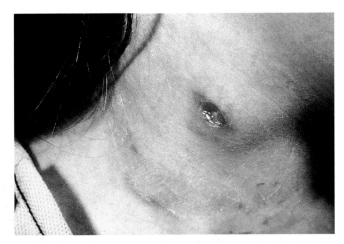

Fig. 25.6 A draining cervical swelling caused, in a young girl, by a lymph node infection with *Mycobacterium intracellulare*, an atypical mycobacterium.

indistinguishable from other types of sialadenitis. Indeed, salivary glands may be involved in up to 10 per cent of cases of cervico-facial actinomycosis.

Further reading

Van Cauwenberge, PB (1991). Microbiology of salivary gland infections. In *Diagnosis of salivary gland disorders* (ed. K Graamans and HP van den Akker). Kluwer, Dordrecht.

Key facts

- The commonest salivary gland infection is with mumps virus.

- Mumps virus is transmitted by direct contact with saliva and droplet spread.

- Mumps is characterized by inflammation and enlargement of the salivary glands.

- A clinical diagnosis of mumps can be confirmed by the detection of specific IgM.

- HIV infection may cause xerostomia and enlargement of the major salivary glands.

- Bacterial parotitis normally occurs in patients with reduced salivary flow or abnormalities in gland architecture.

- The swelling of bacterial parotitis is exquisitely painful and pus may be expressed from the duct opening.

- Treatment of acute bacterial parotitis is by hydration, antibiotics and, if necessary, surgical drainage.

- Following resolution of acute parotitis, sialography should be undertaken to identify correctable salivary gland abnormalities.

- Recurrent parotitis of childhood should be treated conservatively, since most cases resolve spontaneously at puberty.

- Submandibular sialadenitis usually follows ductal obstruction.

- Tuberculosis and actinomycosis are less common bacterial causes of salivary gland infection.

26

Oral fungal infections

Oral fungal infections

Introduction

Fungi are eukaryotic, and possess a nucleus enclosed by a membrane that contains multiple chromosomes. Within the cytoplasm there are also mitochondria, ribosomes, and other inclusion bodies. Fungi are ubiquitous in the environment as decomposers and have great commercial importance in baking, brewing, and in the pharmaceutical industry. There are an estimated 500 000 species of fungi but only about 200 or so are pathogenic to humans.

Fungal infections in the oral and perioral regions occur either as primary localized lesions or as manifestations of systemic mycoses. By far the commonest group of fungal infections that dental practitioners diagnose and treat is caused by *Candida* spp. Some of the rarer mycoses which have oral manifestations, such as histoplasmosis, are found almost exclusively in the United States of America, while others, such as mucormycosis, are found particularly in immunocompromised individuals. As a result, this chapter will deal mainly with candida infections, with brief notes about a selection of other rarer fungal diseases.

Fungal structure and growth

Typically, fungi grow either as ovoid yeast cells or as thin filamentous hyphal elements. A mass of hyphal filaments is called a mycelium.

Yeasts are round to oval unicellular fungi which reproduce by budding. Some species exhibit dimorphism (i.e. grow as either yeast or hyphal cells) or polymorphism (i.e. grow in a number of different cellular forms). The structure of *Candida albicans* and the different cellular forms it takes are shown in Fig. 26.1. The conversion of a yeast cell (blastospore) to a hyphal cell occurs via germ-tube formation, which consists of a smooth tube-like protuberance with no constriction at its junction with the mother cell. Candida also produce pseudohyphae, both *in vivo* and *in vitro*; these have the appearance of branching filaments of elongated yeast cells but with constrictions where they join one another. Under certain conditions, chlamydospores develop from the hyphae; these are round, thick-walled structures, larger than the hypha but of uncertain function.

Yeasts are aerobic and derive their nutrition for growth from the environment. The majority grow on simple media containing a carbon source (glucose) with either ammonium or nitrate as a nitrogen source, while some species require essential growth factors, for example *C. albicans* needs biotin. *Candida* species can grow over a temperature range of 20 to 40°C and within a pH range of 2 to 8.

Candidal carriage in the oral cavity

The carriage rate of *Candida* species in the oral cavity is relatively high but only a few individuals develop oral candidosis. The transition from carrier state to infection appears to depend on changes in the host defences and on environmental factors that allow the yeast to express virulence factors which are normally repressed. The oral carriage rate of *Candida* spp. in healthy volunteers is about 35%, but this rises to around 55% when hospitalized patients or individuals with oral prostheses are studied. Yeasts are also members of the commensal flora in the throat, vagina, and anorectal region. The dorsum of the tongue is the primary oral reservoir of the organism in carriers, although candida can also be found in dental plaque and on intraoral appliances. There are seven medically important *Candida* species, of which *C. albicans*, *C. tropicalis*, *C. glabrata*, *C. parapsilosis*, and *C. krusei* are the most frequently isolated. *C. albicans* is better adapted for growth in the mouth than other species (Fig. 26.2) and is by far the commonest species present in health and disease.

Factors that affect the carriage of candida and predispose to infection

The main factors that predispose to infection with *Candida* spp. are listed in Fig. 26.3. While each factor will tend to increase the risk of candidal carriage and/or proliferation, a combination of factors will increase the chances of infection substantially. The complex way in which different factors interact to produce oral candidosis is shown diagrammatically in Fig. 26.4, with reference to a patient with severe xerostomia.

Pathogenicity factors of *Candida* species

The factors involved in the pathogenicity of *C. albicans* are presented in Fig. 26.5. It is not possible to rank these in order of importance at present, and it seems likely that the potential to cause disease is related to the possession of a mixture of these factors.

STRUCTURE OF *CANDIDA ALBICANS*

Structure

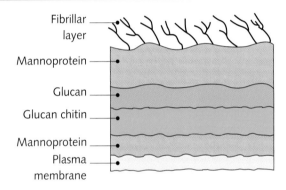

Cell-wall components

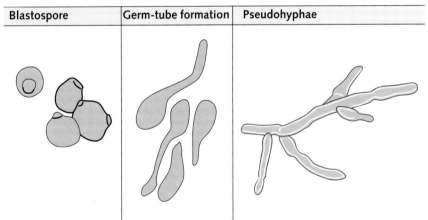

Blastospore	Germ-tube formation	Pseudohyphae

Fig. 26.1 Structural components of *C. albicans*.

Adherence

The ability of *Candida* spp. to adhere to an oral surface is crucial in pathogenesis, for if a yeast cell is unable to attach to a surface it will be removed by the mechanical washing action of saliva, swallowed, and destroyed by the gastric acid. Adherence to an oral surface gives the yeast cell the chance to proliferate and colonize the host, with or without signs or symptoms of infection. There is a large literature on the adherence of *C. albicans* and other *Candida* spp. to mucosal and plastic surfaces. Species and strains vary in their ability to adhere to buccal epithelial cells and denture acrylic, with *C. albicans* being most adherent (see Fig. 26.2). The extracellular polymeric material that coats the surface of

CANDIDA SPECIES IN THE HUMAN MOUTH

	Prevalence	Mucosal adherence	Proteinase production	Fluconazole sensitivity
C. albicans	+ + + +	+ + + +	+ + +	+ + + *
C. tropicalis	+ +	+ +	+ + +	+ + +
C. glabrata	+ +	+	+	±
C. parapsilosis	+	+	+	+ + +
C. krusei	+	±	-	-

* Resistant strains emerging

Fig. 26.2 *Candida* species in the human mouth.

FACTORS THAT PREDISPOSE TO ORAL CANDIDOSIS

Predisposing factor	Effects on host defences	Possible host changes
Prosthesis	Epithelial shedding and mechanical washing action of saliva compromised	Mucosal atrophy, hyperplasia and inflammation
Sjögren's syndrome Radiotherapy Cytotoxic drugs	Washing action of saliva and associated defence mechanisms depressed	Xerostomia Mucosal atrophy, e.g. tongue Mucositis
High sugar intake Diabetes	Loss of competitive inhibition between yeasts and bacteria due to nutrient limitation	Increased numbers of candida within more acidic environment
Antibiotics	Inhibition of commensal bacteria antagonistic to candida	Increased numbers of candida
Malignant disease, cytotoxic drugs	Phagocytosis by neutrophils and macrophages impaired	Neutropenia and oral ulceration

Fig. 26.3 Factors that predispose patients to the development of oral candidosis.

C. albicans, especially the mannoprotein component, appears to be important in adherence.

Proteinases and phospholipase

C. albicans produces a range of proteinases which can degrade salivary proteins, including secretory IgA, lactoferrin, mucin, and keratin, and which are cytotoxic to a range of host cells. They are pH-dependent and while limited hydrolysis can occur at pH 6.0, indiscriminate hydrolysis takes place at pH 3.0–3.5. Since non-proteolytic strains of *C. albicans* are less virulent in animal models, there is a strong suspicion that this complex group of enzymes is involved in the pathogenesis of candidosis.

The production of phospholipase by *C. albicans* appears to be limited to acidic growth conditions (pH 3.5–5.0) and is particularly concentrated at the tips of fungal hyphae. The enzyme disrupts cell membranes and may be important, therefore, in the invasion of candida into host tissues.

Switching mechanisms

Careful examination of *C. albicans* cultures often reveals a variety of colonial morphologies, especially in samples from patients with AIDS. Differences include 'rough' and 'smooth' colony surfaces and 'white' and 'opaque' cells. It seems likely that these switches are triggered by environmental factors that are antagonistic to the

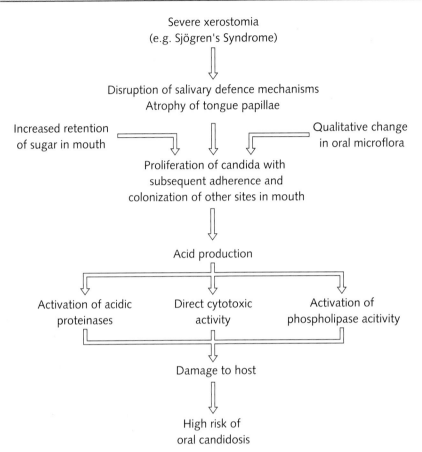

ORAL CANDIDOSIS IN XEROSTOMIA

Severe xerostomia
(e.g. Sjögren's Syndrome)

Disruption of salivary defence mechanisms
Atrophy of tongue papillae

Increased retention
of sugar in mouth

Qualitative change
in oral microflora

Proliferation of candida with
subsequent adherence and
colonization of other sites in mouth

Acid production

Activation of acidic
proteinases

Direct cytotoxic
activity

Activation of
phospholipase acitivity

Damage to host

High risk of
oral candidosis

Fig. 26.4 The role of xerostomia in the development of oral candidosis.

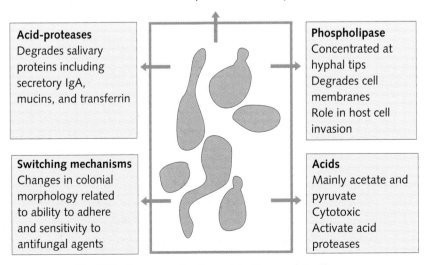

PATHOGENICITY FACTORS OF *CANDIDA ALBICANS*

Extracellular polymeric material (mannoprotein)
Adherence to epithelial cells and plastics

Acid-proteases
Degrades salivary
proteins including
secretory IgA,
mucins, and transferrin

Phospholipase
Concentrated at
hyphal tips
Degrades cell
membranes
Role in host cell
invasion

Switching mechanisms
Changes in colonial
morphology related
to ability to adhere
and sensitivity to
antifungal agents

Acids
Mainly acetate and
pyruvate
Cytotoxic
Activate acid
proteases

Fig. 26.5 The range of pathogenicity factors of *C. albicans*.

SPECIFIC DEFENCE MECHANISMS AGAINST *CANDIDA*	
Defence mechanism	**Effect on *Candida***
Humoral immunity Serum antibody Secretory IgA	Opsonization: phagocytosis Inhibition of adherence to surfaces
Cell-mediated immunity Activation of macrophages Activation of cytotoxic cells	Phagocytosis: intracellular killing of *Candida* Direct killing of *Candida*

Fig. 26.6 Specific defence mechanisms against *Candida* species.

yeasts, for example the presence of antifungal agents *in vivo*. Switching affects the functional activity of yeasts, for example 'white' cells are more adhesive than 'opaque' cells. Therefore, the switching mechanisms of candida may assist in pathogenesis by permitting the yeast to, first, escape the action of antifungals; second, elude the immune system by altering surface antigens; and, third, to maximize the attachment, colonization, and invasion of a variety of body surfaces.

Host defence mechanisms

The host has specific (Fig. 26.6) and non-specific defences against *Candida* spp., infection developing only when the host–parasite balance is disrupted.

Antifungal drugs

Antifungal drugs active against *Candida* spp. are discussed in Chapter 9. Additional information relevant to the treatment and prophylaxis of oral candidosis is presented in Fig. 26.7. In den-

tistry, nystatin, amphotericin B, and miconazole are prescribed as topical drugs which are non-absorbable and available in a number of different formulations that deliver and release the active agent to the oral mucosa. Fluconazole and itraconazole are newer triazole antifungal drugs which can be administered systemically. Itraconazole is available as a lozenge and also, more recently, as a cyclodextrin solution which is believed to have both a topical and systemic effect, since the preparation is absorbed once it has been swallowed. Fluconazole is not available in a topical form and is used systemically. There are reports indicating that resistance to fluconazole among strains of *Candida albicans* may develop following prolonged use in the immunocompromised patient and that in some cases this has been related to clinical failure. *Candida glabrata* and *C. krusei* are naturally resistant to fluconazole and may be selected as pathogens in patients on long-term fluconazole. The antiseptic chlorhexidine has anticandidal activity and can be used topically to help control and prevent oral candidal infections.

ANTIFUNGAL DRUGS		
Drug	**Preparations**	**Activity**
Nystatin Amphotericin B	**Topical:** suspension, pastilles, lozenges, and ointment	All *Candida* spp. sensitive Resistance rare and no antibacterial activity Patient compliance often poor
Miconazole	**Topical:** oral gel or cream	*Candida* spp.: variable sensitivity Possesses antistaphylococcal activity
Fluconazole	**Systemic:** capsules	*C. albicans* generally sensitive but resistant strains can develop *C. krusei* and *C. glabrata* naturally resistant
Itraconazole	**Systemic:** capsules **Systemic and topical:** cyclodextrin solution	*Candida* spp. generally sensitive Little sign of resistance developing to date
Chlorhexidine	**Topical:** solution	Antibacterial and anticandidal

Fig. 26.7 Topical and systemic antifungal drugs.

CLASSIFICATION OF ORAL CANDIDOSIS

Confined to mouth and commissure

Pseudomembranous	– thrush
Erythematous	– atrophic (e.g. HIV-related)
	– denture-related
Hyperplastic	– candidal leukoplakia
Angular cheilitis	

Generalized candidosis with oral manifestations
Chronic mucocutaneous

Fig. 26.8 Classification of oral candidosis.

Oral candidosis

Candida infections confined to the mouth are relatively common and can be classified as shown in Fig. 26.8.

Pseudomembranous candidosis (PMC)

This form of candidosis, also known as thrush, is prevalent in infants, the elderly, and debilitated patients and may occur as an acute or chronic infection. Between the extremes of age it is an important marker of underlying disease. Predisposing factors include malignancy, AIDS, diabetes mellitus, radiation therapy of the head and neck, and the use of aerosol steroid inhalers. The disease is also common in AIDS patients where the signs and symptoms may persist for some months. Probably all patients who die from AIDS will have suffered from PMC at some time during the course of their disease. PMC is characterized by the presence of creamy-white plaques (pseudomembranes), consisting of superficial mucosal cells, neutrophils, and yeasts (Fig. 26.9); these are found on the surface of the tongue, soft palate, cheek, gingivae, or pharynx and are easily rubbed off to leave red, raw,

and bleeding areas underneath. The lesions vary in size from small discrete areas to confluent white patches covering a wide area (Fig. 26.10). Symptoms are uncommon but sometimes patients complain of dryness or roughness of the mucosa and pain, especially if the lesions extend onto the pharynx and oesophagus.

The specimens and techniques for the laboratory diagnosis of PMC are shown in Fig. 26.9.

Systemic or topical antifungals can be prescribed (see Fig. 26.7). In severe cases of infection in immunocompromised patients, for example those with AIDS, a systemic antifungal agent such as fluconazole is preferred. Resolution usually occurs quickly with treatment, but patients who fail to respond should be investigated further by clinical and laboratory means for unsuspected underlying disease or other predisposing factors.

Erythematous candidosis and denture-related candidosis

Erythematous candidosis

This form of candidosis may arise as a consequence of a number of different factors and local conditions:

- following acute pseudomembranous candidosis after the white plaques are shed and infection persists;
- *de novo* in patients with AIDS;
- in patients receiving prolonged drug therapy, for example topical steroids or broad-spectrum antibiotics;
- most commonly related to denture wearing.

The lesions of erythematous candidosis consist of red areas of varying sizes and can appear on any part of the oral mucosa (Fig. 26.11). The dorsum of the tongue is commonly affected in non denture-related infections and lesions may be painful, fiery-red, and shiny with evidence of marked depapillation. While atrophic changes characterize some of these erythematous lesions this is not a constant feature and, therefore, the use of the term

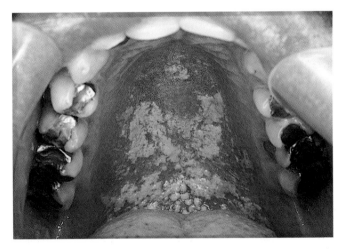

Fig. 26.10 Acute pseudomembranous oral candidosis. (Courtesy of Prof. D. Wray.)

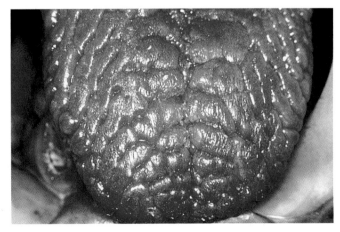

Fig. 26.11 Erythematous oral candidosis affecting the tongue in a patient with Sjögren's syndrome.

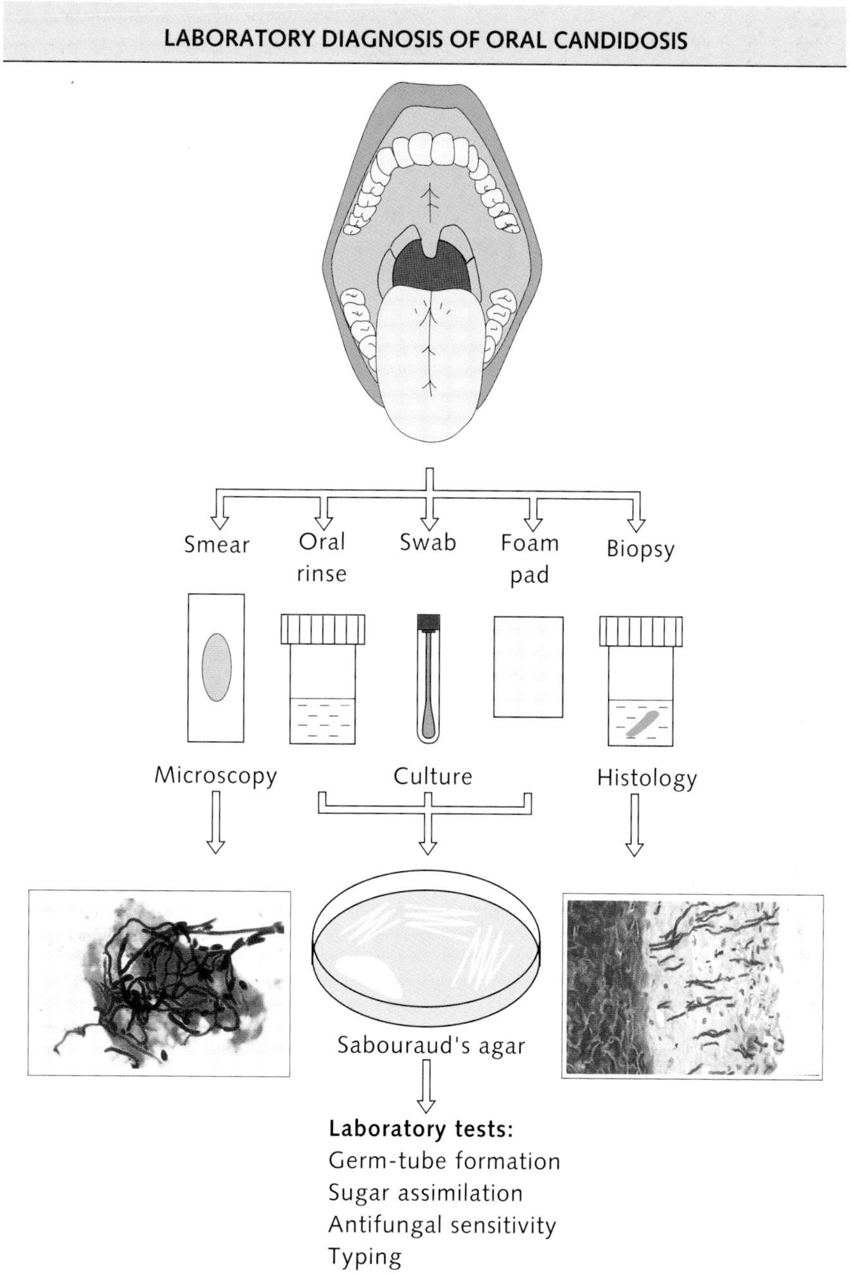

LABORATORY DIAGNOSIS OF ORAL CANDIDOSIS

Smear   Oral rinse   Swab   Foam pad   Biopsy

Microscopy   Culture   Histology

Sabouraud's agar

Laboratory tests:
Germ-tube formation
Sugar assimilation
Antifungal sensitivity
Typing

Disease	Smear	Swab	Biopsy
Pseudomembranous candidosis	+	+	−
Erythematous candidosis	±	+	−
Denture stomatitis:			
palate	+	+	−
denture	+	+	−
Angular cheilitis	+	+	−
Hyperplastic candidosis	+	±	+

+ = Useful   ± = May be useful   − = Inappropriate

Fig. 26.9 Summary of the methods for the laboratory diagnosis of oral candidosis. Note the hyphae and spores in the Gram-stained smear from a patient with pseudomembranous candidosis and the candidal hyphae in the mucosal biopsy of a patient with hyperplastic candidosis. (Biopsy courtesy of Prof. D.G. MacDonald.)

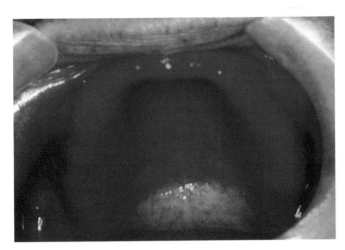

Fig. 26.12 Denture-related erythematous candidosis involving the entire denture-bearing area of the palatal mucosa.

'atrophic' in the classification of this form of candidosis has not been used here. The duration and severity of erythematous candidosis is very variable and there seems little value in diagnosing lesions as either acute or chronic when they can persist for many weeks or months, if untreated.

Erythematous candidosis related to dentures is the commonest form of oral candidosis and is present in about 50% of denture wearers. It is also associated with patients who wear orthodontic appliances or an obturator for cleft palate. It is sometimes called 'denture sore mouth', which is a misnomer as the patient is usually unaware of the condition. The affected area presents as a red, swollen, inflamed mucosa, commonly involving the palatal mucosa beneath the fitting surface of both complete and partial upper dentures (Fig. 26.12). The lower ridge is seldom affected. The palatal lesions have been categorized into three types depending on severity:

- Type 1 as localized pinpoint hyperaemia;
- Type 2 as diffuse erythema and oedema of the denture-bearing area of palatal mucosa;
- Type 3 as inflamed hyperplastic epithelium.

The factors that predispose to denture-related candidosis are largely local, such as trauma, poor denture hygiene, and carbohydrate-rich diets. Occasionally other factors such as xerostomia, iron and folate deficiency, and diabetes mellitus may be involved.

The samples required for the laboratory diagnosis of erythematous candidosis are described in Fig. 26.9. The treatment of erythematous candidosis requires the prescription of antifungal agents and correction of the factors involved in its aetiology; for example consider amending current antibiotic or steroid drug treatment, correcting any haematological deficiencies, and introducing denture hygiene regimens. However, the correction of factors may not always be possible and a prolonged use of antifungal drugs may be required. In denture-related candidosis the fitting surface of the denture is the main reservoir for *Candida* spp. and patients should be encouraged to clean the fitting surface thoroughly with a toothbrush each night and soak the denture overnight in an antiseptic solution such as dilute hypochlorite for acrylic dentures or 2% chlorhexidine for metal dentures. Patients should also be discouraged from wearing dentures during sleep. In addition, antifungal therapy (see Fig. 26.7) should be instituted and topical therapy prolonged for at least 3–4 weeks.

Angular cheilitis

This disease can be associated with any type of oral candidosis but is most frequently seen as a complication of denture-related candidosis in edentulous patients. However, dentate young adults can also present with this condition. As with all forms of oral candidosis, angular cheilitis has a multifactorial aetiology (Fig. 26.13), though the relative importance of the different factors remains uncertain. Maceration of the epithelium at the angles of the mouth by saliva trapped in mucosal folds appears to be an important factor, especially in denture-related forms of the disease.

The clinical signs vary from areas of inflammation at the angles of the mouth to ulcerated and crusted fissures (Fig. 26.14). The presence of distinctive yellow crusts, not unlike the typical lesions of impetigo, may suggest involvement of *Staphylococcus aureus*. Since the lesions are usually only mildly irritating, most patients do not seek medical or dental treatment. The importance of *Candida* spp., *S. aureus*, and β-haemolytic streptococci (*Streptococcus agalactiae*) in the aetiology of the lesions is not clear but in many cases the use of specific antimicrobial agents leads to considerable

THE PATHOGENESIS OF ANGULAR CHEILITIS

Inadequate dentures with reduced vertical dimension

⇩

Skin creasing with saliva leakage and maceration at the angles of the mouth

Iron or Vitamin B12 deficiency → **Host defences compromised** ← Trauma

Candida spp. (mouth) → → ← *S. aureus* (nose/mouth)

⇩

Angular cheilitis

Fig. 26.13 Factors involved in the pathogenesis of angular cheilitis.

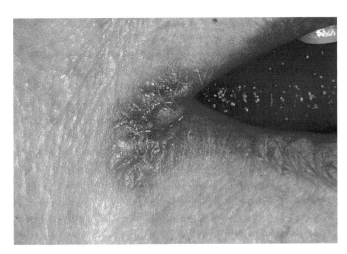

Fig. 26.14 Angular cheilitis. This may be candidal, staphylococcal, or a mixed fungal and bacterial infection.

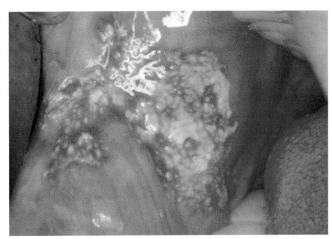

Fig. 26.15 Chronic hyperplastic candidosis. The commissure is a common site.

improvement in the condition. The source of these micro-organisms is mainly from the mouth, or also the nose in the case of *S. aureus*.

Details of the laboratory diagnosis of angular cheilitis are illustrated in Fig. 26.9.

Elimination of the reservoirs of infection and the factors that predispose to the disease is necessary for successful management. If intraoral candidosis is present, the appropriate topical antifungal therapy should be employed together with antifungal ointment applied to the affected angles of the mouth (Fig. 26.7). If *S. aureus* is isolated then an antistaphylococcal preparation, e.g. neomycin/chlorhexidine should be prescribed. If *S. aureus* is present in the anterior nares, mupirocin should be applied to that site to help eliminate nasal strains of staphylococci. Alternatively, miconazole gel, which has both antifungal and antistaphylococcal activity, can be used in mixed infections or when the infecting micro-organisms are unknown.

If the disease does not resolve with normal treatment then both patient compliance and the possible presence of underlying systemic disease should be taken into account. In addition, the possibility of chronic nose–mouth transfer of staphylococci should be considered. Patients with angular cheilitis attend work normally, but the presence of toxigenic strains of *S. aureus* in such lesions could result in outbreaks of staphylococcal infections linked to the patient's occupation. Examples would include wound infections due to defects in cross-infection control measures by nurses and other health-care personnel, or staphylococcal enteritis linked to food handlers.

Chronic hyperplastic candidosis (candidal leukoplakia)

This form of candidosis usually presents as individual lesions on the oral mucosa of the cheek near the commissure, at the angles of the mouth, or on the surface of the tongue. The white patches cannot be rubbed off, in contrast to the lesions of pseudomembranous candidosis, and are indistinguishable from leukoplakias due to other causes (Fig. 26.15). The presence of speckled, red-white areas in the lesion has clinical importance, since areas with this appearance have a higher chance of malignant transformation. Histologically, the surface epithelium is parakeratinized and markedly hyperplastic, with candidal hyphae invading the parakeratinized layer at right angles to the surface but remaining relatively superficial (Fig. 26.16). The role of *C. albicans* in the aetiology of these epithelial changes remains unresolved. *Candida* spp. may be a co-factor in epithelial hyperplasia, play a part in the malignant transformation of cells, or simply superinfect an already thickened area of abnormal epithelium. The fact that prolonged antifungal therapy leads to resolution of some of these lesions suggests that candida may play a causative role in at least some cases of this clinical entity. An accurate diagnosis of candidal

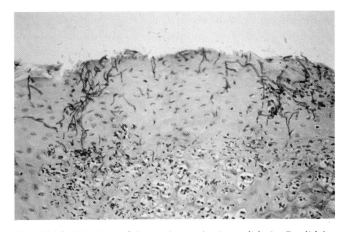

Fig. 26.16 Histology of chronic hyperplastic candidosis. Candidal hyphae can be seen superficially, together with microabscesses in the depth of the epithelium.

leukoplakia is important, since 5–11% of the lesions can become malignant.

After the laboratory diagnosis is made (see Fig. 26.9), general measures to reduce predisposing factors, for example tobacco smoking, folic acid or iron deficiency, should be instituted. Long-term antifungal therapy should be prescribed (see Fig. 26.7) until the lesions are removed by surgery, cryotherapy, or laser, depending on which procedure is most appropriate. Long-term review of patients is essential due to the risk of malignant change.

Miscellaneous oral candidoses

There are a number of oral and perioral lesions in which *Candida* spp. seem to play a major role, mainly on the basis that clinically they respond well to antifungal therapy. These include cheilocandidosis, juvenile juxtavermillion candidosis, chronic oral multifocal candidosis, and median rhomboid glossitis.

Chronic mucocutaneous candidosis (CMC)

This is a rare group of disorders characterized by persistent superficial candidal infection of the mouth, other mucosal surfaces, the skin, and nails. The oral lesions resemble those of chronic hyperplastic candidosis and can involve any part of the mucosa. The clinical patterns of presentation can be classified in a number of ways but four main subgroups are identified, based on clinical features and age of onset (Fig. 26.17). Chronic mucocutaneous candidosis must be confirmed by taking swabs and smears from the lesions and by histological examination of biopsies. In addition, appropriate clinical and laboratory investigations should be performed to define the extent of immunological or endocrine dysfunction.

Chronic mucocutaneous candidosis is probably the most difficult candidal infection to eradicate. Due to the complex aetiology of these conditions, the management is a combination of different approaches designed to remove predisposing factors and reduce the numbers of, if not eradicate, *Candida* spp. While attempts have been made to correct immune defects, for example with *Candida*-specific transfer factor, few appear to have long-term benefit, although the endocrinopathies associated with the disease do respond to conventional endocrine therapies. Essentially all systemic antifungal drugs are effective in chronic mucocutaneous candidosis.

Oral manifestations of systemic mycoses

Oral manifestations have been described for a wide range of systemic fungal infections (Fig. 26.18). Many are caused by dimorphic fungi and are extremely rare in Europe but are endemic in different parts of the Americas. In most instances the oral lesions are secondary to the primary infections, typically granulomatous lesions found in the lungs and on the skin. The oral lesions may, however, be the initial presenting sign of the disease, as is the case for histoplasmosis. In general, the main habitat for these organisms is the soil and infection is usually acquired by inhalation, with the primary lesions occurring in the lungs. In the majority of cases these heal without causing illness, but in progressive disease, sometimes related to lung cavitation, infection disseminates to the skin, mucous membranes, and internal organs. The lesions tend to be chronic granulomas, and diagnosis is by direct demonstration of the yeast-like form of the fungus in smears of sputum or in biopsy specimens. Culture and identification of pathogens from clinical samples is useful in diagnosis, as is serology in certain infections. An accurate diagnosis of this disease is important, since 5–11% of the lesions can become malignant (e.g. histoplasmosis and South American blastomycosis). Many of the dimorphic fungi are sensitive to amphotericin B but azole drugs, for example fluconazole, are replacing amphotericin for the treatment of some infections.

CHRONIC MUCOCUTANEOUS CANDIDOSIS (CMC) SYNDROMES	
Type	**Features**
Familial CMC	First decade — persistent candidosis: mouth, nails, skin. Iron deficiency
Diffuse CMC (Candida granuloma)	First 5 years — chronic candidosis: mouth, nails, skin, pharynx Susceptible to bacterial infections
Candidosis–endocrinopathy syndrome	Hypothyroidism, hypoadrenocorticism, and mild chronic hyperplastic candidosis involving the mouth
Candidosis–thymoma syndrome	Haematological disorders Pseudomembranous or hyperplastic candidosis: mouth, skin, nails

Fig. 26.17 Chronic mucocutaneous candidosis (CMC) syndromes.

ORAL MANIFESTATIONS OF SELECTED SYSTEMIC MUCOSES			
	Histoplasmosis	**Paracoccidiomycosis**	**Mucormycosis**
Organism	*Histoplasma capsulatum*	*Paracoccidioides brasiliensis*	*Mucor* spp.
Type of fungus	Dimorphic	Dimorphic	Filamentous
Main sites affected	Oral mucosa, tongue, palate, gingiva, periapical area	Hard and soft palate, gingiva, tongue	Extension from maxillary sinus through palate into the mouth
Major manifestations	Nodular, indurated or granular masses of tissue destruction with bone erosion	Papules or vesicles leading to ulcers. Extensive local destruction	Sloughing ulcers with grey eschar and exposed bone (especially maxilla). Unilateral facial pain
Frequency of oral infection	40% of cases	Common	Common

Fig. 26.18 Oral manifestations of selected systemic mycoses.

Key facts

- Fungi are eukaryotic and possess a defined nucleus and other cellular inclusions.

- Fungi grow either as ovoid cells or as thin filamentous hyphal elements.

- The most common oral fungal infection is candidosis, caused by *Candida* spp., particularly *C. albicans*.

- About 50% of the population are symptomless oral carriers of *Candida* spp., but only a small proportion of individuals have the signs and symptoms of infection.

- The pathogenesis of oral candidosis involves a complex interaction between host defence mechanisms and fungal virulence factors.

- The common forms of oral candidosis are pseudo-membranous, erythematous (including HIV-associated infection and denture-related candidosis), hyperplastic, and angular cheilitis.

- Laboratory investigations are often required for a definitive diagnosis of oral candidosis.

- Treatment consists of correcting predisposing factors and prescribing oral or systemic antifungal agents.

- The development of resistance in *Candida* spp. to azole drugs, such as fluconazole, may follow prolonged treatment and has been linked to treatment failure.

- Oral lesions caused by fungi other than *Candida* spp. are rare and are usually secondary to primary infections of the lungs.

Further reading

Bennett, JE, Hoy, RJ, and Peterson, PK (ed.). (1992). *New strategies in fungal disease.* Churchill Livingstone, Edinburgh.

Kibber, CC, MacKenzie, DWR, and Odds, FC (ed.). (1996). *Principles and practice of clinical mycology.* Wiley, Chichester.

Odds, FC (1988). *Candida and candidosis* (2nd edn). Baillière Tindall, London.

Richardson, MD and Warnock, DW (1997). *Fungal infection – diagnosis and management* (2nd edn). Blackwell, Oxford.

Samaranayake, LP and MacFarlane, TW (ed.). (1990). *Oral candidosis.* Wright, London.

Scully, C, El-Kabir, M, and Samaranayake, LP (1994). Candida and oral candidosis: a review. *Critical Reviews in Oral Biology and Medicine*, **5**, 125–57.

Wray, D and Bagg, J (1997). *Pocket reference to oral candidosis.* Science Press, London.

27

Bacterial and viral infections of the oral mucosa

- Bacterial infections of the oral mucosa
- Viral infections of the oral mucosa

Bacterial and viral infections of the oral mucosa

The important fungal infections of the oral mucosa are described in Chapter 26. This chapter will describe the bacterial and viral infections of the oral mucosa important to dentists.

Bacterial infections of the oral mucosa

Specific bacterial infections of the oral mucosa are uncommon in the USA and Europe and are often manifestations of systemic diseases, for example syphilis, gonorrhoea, or tuberculosis. Such infections are seen more frequently in many developing countries.

Gonorrhoea

The microbiology of this sexually transmitted disease, caused by *Neisseria gonorrhoeae* (*N. gonorrhoeae*), has been discussed in Chapter 14. When lesions are present in the oral cavity (Fig. 27.1) they are found most frequently in the pharynx, though any part of the oral mucosa may be affected. The main risk factor for gonococcal pharyngitis is orogenital sexual contact. Thus, the oral lesions are more commonly associated with a primary infection of the mouth than with the spread of *N. gonorrhoeae* from a distant site.

ORAL GONORRHOEA	
Primary infection	Orogenital contact
Commonest site	Pharynx
Clinical features	Oral lesions variable — inflammation, oedema, vesiculation, ulceration, pseudomembranes
	Submandibular lymphadenopathy
	Pain
Diagnosis	Culture
Treatment	Penicillin or tetracycline

Fig. 27.1 The features of oral infection with *Neisseria gonorrhoeae*.

Clinical features

Patients complain of an initial burning sensation in the mouth. Within 1–2 days the mouth becomes acutely painful and the submandibular lymph nodes enlarge. The intraoral lesions have a variable appearance, showing signs of inflammation, oedema, vesiculation, ulceration, and pseudomembranes. Oral functions such as speech and swallowing become very painful.

Diagnosis

In view of the variable clinical appearances of the oral lesions of gonorrhoea, laboratory tests are essential. Direct examination of a Gram-stained smear from oral lesions may show the presence of Gram-negative intracellular diplococci, though the large numbers of commensal *Neisseria* spp. in the mouth are a complicating factor. Swabs taken from the lesions should be placed in bacteriological transport medium and sent rapidly to the laboratory for culture on an appropriate semi-selective medium such as Thayer–Martin agar. Isolates can be identified on the basis of a positive oxidase test followed by carbohydrate utilization or fluorescent antibody tests. Evidence of urogenital infection should be sought.

Treatment

Oropharyngeal gonorrhoea should be treated with intramuscular procaine penicillin or with oral tetracycline.

Syphilis

Clinical features

Syphilis may have a variety of oral manifestations (Fig. 27.2).

As described in Chapter 14, the clinical course of syphilis can be divided into three main stages, all of which may have oral features:

1. The characteristic lesion of primary syphilis is the chancre (Fig. 27.3). Extragenital chancres occur most commonly on the lip, though intraoral chancres may also be seen. They are usually a result of transmission of *Treponema pallidum* by orogenital sexual practices. These lesions are highly infectious, contain many motile spirochaetes, and heal 1–5 weeks after appearing. There is enlargement of the regional lymph nodes.

SYPHILIS	
Oral manifestations	
Primary syphilis	Chancre — typically on lip
Secondary syphilis	Mucous patches on mucosa
	'Snail track' ulcers
	Rubbery, enlarged cervical lymph nodes
Tertiary syphilis	Gumma — often of palate
	Glossitis
	Syphilitic leukoplakia
Diagnosis	Serological
Treatment	Penicillin or tetracycline

Fig. 27.2 The oral manifestations at each stage of syphilis.

2. About 6 weeks later the secondary stage of syphilis begins. The oral lesions are glistening, greyish-white patches on the oral mucosa, some of which may combine to produce so-called 'snail track ulcers'. The cervical lymph nodes are enlarged and rubbery. Secondary syphilitic lesions are infectious and heal within 6 weeks.

3. Tertiary syphilis appears 3–10 years after initial infection and, as a result of modern treatment, is now seen very rarely. The gumma is the characteristic lesion, in which ulceration of an initial raised lesion is followed by necrosis. In the mouth the most common site is the hard palate and from this site there may be perforation into the nasal cavity. Atrophic glossitis and syphilitic leukoplakia on the dorsum of the tongue are other late stage features, rarely seen today.

Diagnosis

Laboratory tests are essential to the diagnosis of syphilis (Chapter 14). Due to the presence of endogenous spirochaetes, dark-ground microscopy is of limited value for diagnosing syphilitic oral lesions. The diagnosis is usually based on serological investigations.

Treatment

Penicillin is the treatment of choice for all stages of syphilis, but tetracycline can be used for penicillin-allergic patients.

Tuberculosis

World-wide, 1.7 billion people are infected with *Mycobacterium tuberculosis*. There are 10 million new cases annually and the disease causes 3 million deaths per year. Whilst 95% of cases occur in developing countries, there has been a recent resurgence of tuberculosis in Europe and North America, particularly among the homeless and those who are HIV-infected. This elevated prevalence includes an increase in extrapulmonary tuberculosis.

Figure 27.4 summarizes the key features of oral tuberculosis. Primary infections of the oral mucosa are rare in humans and oral lesions are usually secondary to a primary lung infection (Chapter 16).

Clinical features

The clinical presentation of tuberculous lesions of the oral mucosa is varied, but ulceration and pain are common. The tongue is affected most commonly, but lesions have been reported at all intraoral sites. Lesions are found more commonly in the posterior part of the mouth, possibly related to the distribution of lymphoid tissue.

Tuberculous lymphadenitis commonly affects the cervical lymph nodes. The swelling, which may be up to several centimetres in diameter, is initially firm but mobile. Later it becomes fixed, with abscess and sinus formation. The atypical mycobacteria, for example *Mycobacterium avium-intracellulare*, are frequently involved in cervical lymphadenitis among children (see Fig. 25.6), while *M. tuberculosis* is more common in adults.

Diagnosis

Tuberculous lesions of the oral mucosa are difficult to diagnose, and a biopsy is usually undertaken. If tuberculosis is suspected at the time of biopsy, half of the specimen should be placed in

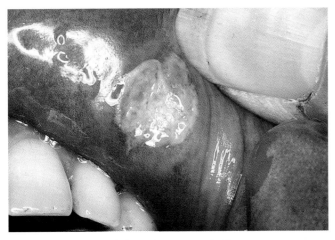

Fig. 27.3 Primary syphilis (a chancre) on the lip.

ORAL TUBERCULOSIS	
Clinical features	Primary infection usually in lungs
	Oral lesions variable — ulceration and pain are common
	Tongue is most common site
	Cervical lymphadenopathy
Diagnosis	Biopsy, culture, and skin testing
Treatment	Combination chemotherapy with antituberculous drugs

Fig. 27.4 Features of the oral lesions of tuberculosis.

normal saline for culture, and the remainder placed in formol saline for histological examination. Mycobacteria are cultured on Lowenstein–Jensen medium. Extended incubation for up to 3 months is necessary before colonies appear.

Histological examination of the formalin-fixed tissue will reveal caseating granulomata and Ziehl–Neelsen stained sections may show the presence of acid- and alcohol-fast bacilli.

The Mantoux test is sometimes helpful in diagnosing the oral lesions of tuberculosis, and differential testing may be of value for diagnosing cervical lymphadenitis in children. Appropriate radiographic examination, including a chest radiograph, is obligatory in all patients with oral tuberculosis.

Treatment

All patients with tuberculosis must be referred to an experienced physician for evaluation and treatment. Combinations of antituberculous drugs, for example rifampicin, isoniazid, ethambutol, and pyrazinamide are used. In the case of multidrug-resistant strains of *M. tuberculosis*, drug treatment should be guided by local knowledge of the sensitivity patterns until formal sensitivity testing has been completed. The atypical mycobacteria are frequently resistant to standard antituberculous drug regimens and in children with cervical lymphadenitis caused by these organisms, surgical excision of the node is usually a more appropriate treatment.

Viral infections of the oral mucosa

Viral infections of the oral mucosa are common. The viruses most frequently involved are listed in Fig. 27.5 and will be dealt with in turn.

Herpes group viruses

Figure 27.6 lists the currently recognized members of the human herpesvirus family. All are enveloped, icosahedral viral particles with a double-stranded DNA genome. They are renowned for establishing latent infections (Chapter 5), with the result that clinical presentations may vary depending on whether the infection is primary or a reactivation (secondary). Long-term intermittent shedding of herpesviruses into saliva is also important in relation to the spread of infection in the community and to cross-infection in the clinical setting.

Herpes simplex virus infections

PRIMARY HERPETIC GINGIVOSTOMATITIS

Primary herpetic gingivostomatitis is the most common viral infection of the mouth. It is usually caused by herpes simplex virus (HSV) type I, though a small number of cases are caused by HSV type II which is the usual isolate from genital herpes. The virus is spread by direct contact with infected saliva or reactivation lesions (see below). The incubation period is about 5 days. Infection in early childhood often results in a subclinical infection, but in older children and adults the symptoms are more severe. Initially there is a fever, together with enlarged cervical lymph nodes and intraoral pain. Vesicles then develop on the oral mucosa, particularly the gingiva, tongue, and buccal mucosa. These vesicles are intraepithelial and rupture quickly to form superficial ulcers with erythematous margins on greyish-yellow bases (Fig. 27.7). The mouth is painful, making eating and

---

VIRAL INFECTIONS OF ORAL MUCOSA

- Herpes simplex virus
- Varicella zoster virus
- Epstein–Barr virus
- Group A coxsackieviruses
- Measles virus
- Papillomaviruses

Fig. 27.5 Major viruses which infect the oral mucosa.

HUMAN HERPESVIRUSES

Virus	Examples of disease associations
Herpes simplex virus type I	Gingivostomatitis; herpes labialis
Herpes simplex virus type II	Genital herpes
Varicella zoster virus	Chickenpox; shingles
Epstein–Barr virus	Infectious mononucleosis
Cytomegalovirus	Severe infections in the immunocompromised
Human herpesvirus 6	Exanthem subitum
Human herpesvirus 7	Not known
Human herpesvirus 8	Kaposi's sarcoma

Fig. 27.6 The currently recognized human herpesviruses.

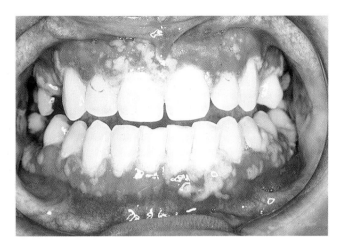

Fig. 27.7 Clinical photograph of primary herpetic gingivostomatitis. Lesions are evident on the gingivae but other sites are also commonly involved.

swallowing difficult. The lips may also be swollen and covered in a blood-stained crust.

Bed rest, maintenance of fluid intake, and provision of antipyretics are important elements of treatment. In the immunocompetent, the lesions are self-limiting and heal within 10 days without scarring. The prescribing of aciclovir at an early stage in the infection may shorten its course and reduce the severity of symptoms.

SECONDARY (REACTIVATION) HERPES SIMPLEX INFECTION

About one-third of patients who have been infected with HSV develop secondary infections later in life, due to reactivation of the virus lying latent in the trigeminal ganglion. A number of factors have been associated with reactivation of HSV, including sun exposure and menstruation. The most common lesion is herpes labialis, also known as a 'cold sore' (Fig. 27.8). These lesions appear on the mucocutaneous junction of the lip or on the skin adjacent to the nostril. There is a premonitory burning sensation for 24 hours before the vesicles develop, rupture, crust over, and heal within 10–14 days. Treatment with the topical application of 5% aciclovir cream, starting during the premonitory burning sensation, may reduce the severity of the lesions.

Intraoral reactivation lesions have been described, but are rare. They present as small clusters of lesions, typically involving the palatal mucosa.

DIAGNOSIS OF HSV INFECTIONS IN THE MOUTH

HSV can be grown readily in a wide range of tissue-culture systems and viral culture is a very sensitive diagnostic tool. However, it takes at least 24 hours to produce a result. Smears prepared from lesional tissue can be stained with fluorescent monoclonal antibodies to HSV types I and II, to allow a rapid diagnosis and provide a useful additional test. Serology can be used in the diagnosis of primary HSV infections, by detecting either a fourfold rise in IgG antibody titre between the acute and convalescent specimens, or by demonstrating specific IgM antibodies. However, serological methods do not permit rapid diagnosis and their value is therefore limited in the clinical situation.

HSV IN THE IMMUNOSUPPRESSED

Like many of the herpesviruses, HSV is an important pathogen in the immunosuppressed patient. The oral lesions in this group usually represent reactivation of latent virus as a consequence of the altered host–parasite relationship. The clinical presentation is often atypical (Fig. 27.9) and a high index of suspicion is required for a diagnosis to be made. Treatment should be commenced urgently with systemic aciclovir, and laboratory tests employed to confirm the clinical diagnosis.

Varicella zoster virus infections

Primary infection with varicella zoster virus (VZV) causes chickenpox and the reactivation disease is shingles.

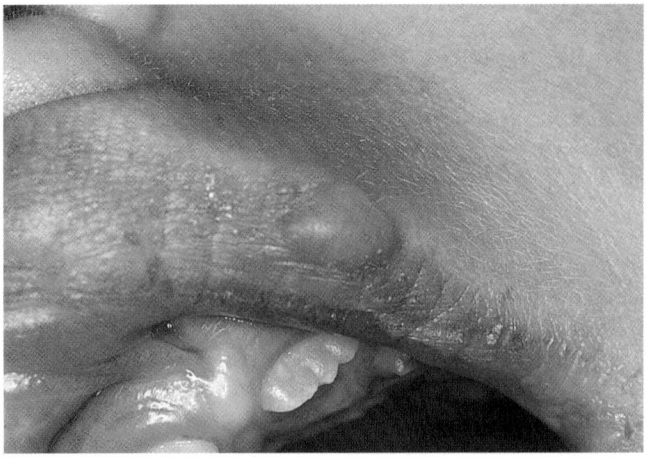

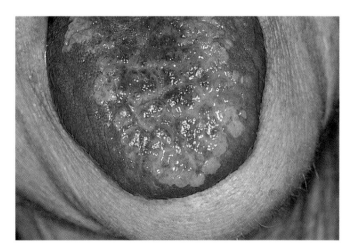

Fig. 27.8 Herpes labialis, a reactivation of herpes simplex virus. The lesions are initially vesicular, as illustrated, but rapidly burst and crust over, before healing without scarring.

Fig. 27.9 Reactivation of herpes simplex virus in a patient with terminal cancer.

CHICKENPOX

This is one of the common infectious diseases of childhood. The virus is spread by direct contact or droplet spread. Infection is established initially in the upper respiratory tract from where haematogenous spread occurs to other parts of the body. The characteristic skin rash begins as pink maculopapules which become vesicular and itchy. They appear first on the back, then on the chest, abdomen, face, and scalp. The diagnosis of chickenpox is usually made clinically.

Before development of the skin rash, oral lesions may be detectable, especially on the hard palate, pillars of the fauces, and uvula. The oral lesions are small ulcers, 2–4 mm in diameter, surrounded by an erythematous halo.

SHINGLES

Shingles results from the reactivation of VZV lying latent in sensory ganglia. It is more common in older individuals and recurrent shingles may be a marker of underlying immune suppression, for example in patients with lymphoma. Local severe pain and paraesthesia commonly precede the appearance of the skin eruption by several days, and the diagnosis is extremely difficult to make at this early stage. The lesions present as a localized eruption involving an area of skin supplied by one or more sensory ganglia, known as a dermatome. Groups of vesicles are present on an erythematous base, and the distribution is strictly unilateral (see Fig. 13.17). The vesicles dry within a few days to form scabs which separate and heal without scarring. Subsequently a proportion of patients, particularly the elderly, may suffer from an intractable form of facial pain known as postherpetic neuralgia.

The trigeminal nerve is involved in about 15% of cases. If the maxillary or mandibular divisions are affected, then the lesions of shingles may affect both skin and oral mucosa (Figs 27.10 (a), (b)). The severe prodromal pain may be misdiagnosed as toothache, until the vesicular eruption appears.

A diagnosis of shingles is usually made clinically. However, if necessary the diagnosis can be confirmed by submitting vesicle fluid for electron microscopy and virus isolation, smears for immunofluorescence, and serum for the detection of specific IgM antibodies.

High-dose aciclovir (800 mg, five times daily) should be prescribed as soon as possible. Ideally, this treatment should commence before the skin eruption appears, though this is often precluded by the difficulties of diagnosis in the early stages.

Epstein–Barr virus infection

Epstein–Barr virus (EBV) is associated with a range of pathologies in the oral cavity (Fig. 27.11). Most importantly it is responsible for infectious mononucleosis (glandular fever). EBV establishes a latent infection in oropharyngeal epithelial cells and is intermittently shed into the saliva of healthy carriers as well as those suffering or convalescing from infectious mononucleosis. Saliva is, therefore, the main route of transmission of this virus.

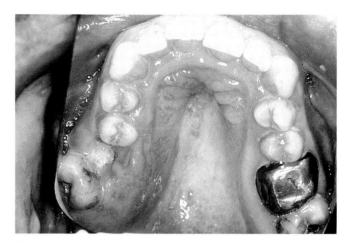

(a)

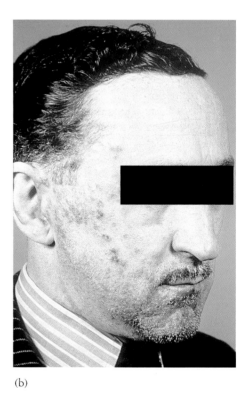

(b)

Fig. 27.10 Shingles (reactivation of varicella zoster virus) involving (a) oral mucosa and (b) skin of the face. The strictly unilateral distribution of the lesions is clearly evident.

INFECTIOUS MONONUCLEOSIS

The infection is commonest in children and young adults. In many cases, particularly among children, the disease is subclinical.

In those with clinical disease, the classic features are lymph node enlargement, fever, and pharyngeal inflammation. Intraorally, the throat may be painful and congested in the early stages. Clusters of fine petechial haemorrhages may be seen at the

---

EBV AND ORAL DISEASE

Infectious mononucleosis
  Cervical lymphadenopathy
  Pharyngeal inflammation
  Tonsillar pseudomembrane
  Palatal petechiae

Burkitt's lymphoma

Nasopharyngeal carcinoma

Oral hairy leukoplakia

Fig. 27.11 The various forms of oral disease associated with Epstein–Barr virus.

junction of the hard and soft palate. Later, a white pseudomembrane may develop on the tonsil.

The diagnosis of infectious mononucleosis is made by laboratory tests. A blood film and differential white cell count will demonstrate the lymphocytosis and 'atypical' mononuclear cells (Downey cells) characteristic of infectious mononucleosis. Final confirmation is made on the basis of serological demonstration of antibodies to EBV-related antigens. The Paul–Bunnel test has been used for many years to detect the presence of the heterophile antibody, produced in most patients with infectious mononucleosis, which causes the agglutination of red cells from species other than humans. The original test has been replaced in many laboratories by a more convenient slide agglutination test called the 'monospot' test, which is based on the same principle. In specialized laboratories, tests for specific EBV antibodies are undertaken, particularly to early antigen (EA) and viral capsid antigen (VCA).

EBV AND OTHER ORAL MUCOSAL DISORDERS

EBV is an oncogenic virus and plays a role in the pathogenesis of Burkitt's lymphoma, an aggressive tumour of the jaws seen in certain parts of the world where malaria is endemic. It is also linked to nasopharyngeal carcinoma, particularly in Southern China.

Finally, EBV is of interest to dentists because of its association with oral hairy leukoplakia in patients with HIV infection (Chapter 19) and other forms of immunosuppression.

Other herpesvirus infections

Cytomegalovirus (CMV) infection is widespread and usually asymptomatic in the immunocompetent host, though it may cause CMV mononucleosis, a disease similar to that caused by EBV. However, it is an important cause of serious disease in the newborn and in the immunosuppressed, for example those with HIV infection. Like all herpesviruses it is able to remain latent and may become reactivated when patients become immunosuppressed. CMV is the commonest infectious cause of congenital abnormalities. It causes a potentially fatal congenital infection called cytomegalic inclusion disease, with widely disseminated organ involvement including salivary gland enlargement. It is also a major pathogen in transplant patients, particularly following bone marrow transplantation, in which interstitial pneumonitis, a lung infection, is a serious complication. There have been several reports of CMV-related oral ulcerative lesions in those with AIDS and in transplant patients.

Human herpesvirus 6 (HHV-6) infects most infants between the ages of 6 and 11 months. It is usually asymptomatic, though a small proportion develop a mild febrile disease called exanthem subitum. The virus is commonly shed in the saliva of both

---

COXSACKIEVIRUS INFECTIONS

Hand, foot, and mouth disease

Cause	Coxsackie A (usually type A16)
Clinical features	Localized epidemics
	Mainly children
	Intraoral vesicles and ulcers (any site)
	Skin lesions: palmar surfaces of hands
	plantar surfaces of feet
	Mild illness, lasting 5—8 days
Treatment	Supportive

Herpangina

Cause	Coxsackie A (types A2, A4, A5, A6, A8)
Clinical features	Fever and sore throat
	Pharyngeal hyperaemia
	Vesicles and ulcers in pharynx and back of mouth
	Mild illness, lasting 3—4 days
Treatment	Supportive

Fig. 27.12 Clinical features of hand, foot, and mouth disease and herpangina.

children and adults and saliva is the main route of transmission. There are no clear associations between HHV-6 infection and disease in adults.

Human herpesvirus 8 has been described very recently and is believed to play a role in the aetiology of Kaposi's sarcoma. This tumour is an important oral manifestation of HIV infection (Chapter 19).

Coxsackievirus infections

Members of the group A coxsackieviruses are responsible for hand, foot, and mouth disease and for herpangina, both of which have oral manifestations (Fig. 27.12).

Hand, foot, and mouth disease

This infection occurs in small localized epidemics, particularly among children. The disease is usually very mild. An early symptom is facial pain, together with tenderness along the path of the parotid duct and small vesicles around the duct opening. There is a variable degree of systemic upset. The oral lesions appear as bright-red macules which become vesicular and burst, resulting in small shallow ulcers with an erythematous margin. Any intraoral site may be affected.

The palmar surfaces of the hands and plantar surfaces of the feet are also involved. The diagnosis is usually clinical, but the virus can be isolated from saliva, vesicle fluid, or faeces if laboratory confirmation is required. A significant rise in neutralizing antibody titre is also evident during the course of the illness.

Herpangina

This systemic viral infection, which lasts for 3–4 days, is most common in children. Clinically, there is a sudden onset of fever and sore throat followed by the appearance of oral and pharyngeal lesions. Other symptoms may include anorexia, vomiting, and abdominal pains.

Intraorally, small papulovesicular lesions develop on the mucosa of the anterior pillars of the fauces, hard and soft palate, tongue, uvula, pharyngeal wall, and tonsils (Fig. 27.13).

This typical distribution at the back of the mouth is useful diagnostically.

As described for hand, foot, and mouth disease, laboratory confirmation of the diagnosis may be made by viral culture or serology.

Morbillivirus infection

Measles virus

Measles is one of the common childhood infections. The virus is spread by droplet infection.

The disease begins with a catarrhal stage. The buccal mucosa during this stage is erythematous and after about 2 days tiny, bluish-white spots surrounded by red margins appear on the buccal mucosa opposite the molar teeth. These are called Koplik's spots and last for only 1–2 days. As the red, maculopapular skin rash appears, 3–4 days after the catarrhal stage, the Koplik's spots disappear. The skin rash lasts for 2–3 days and then fades, after which recovery is rapid.

Papillomavirus infections of the oral mucosa

More than 70 types of the human papillomavirus (HPV) have been identified. They give rise to warty lesions of skin and mucous membranes. Most of these lesions are benign, but some malignant lesions, for example carcinoma of the cervix, have been associated with certain types of HPV (Chapter 14).

The common wart (verruca vulgaris) frequently affects skin and may be seen on the lips or intraorally (Fig. 27.14), particularly in children when they may be associated with autoinoculation from the fingers. The lesions are typically white, because of the surface keratinization. Common warts are usually associated with HPV types 2 or 4.

Venereal warts (condyloma acuminatum) may also be seen intraorally and form soft, pink papillary lesions. These are usually associated with HPV types 6, 11, and 16.

Fig. 27.13 Oral lesions in herpangina.

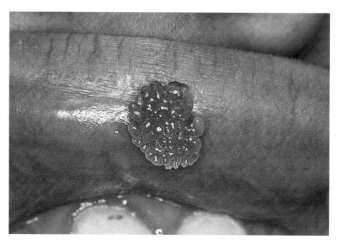

Fig. 27.14 A common wart, verruca vulgaris, on the upper labial mucosa.

Key facts

- Most bacterial infections of the oral mucosa are manifestations of systemic diseases.

- Oral infection with *Neisseria gonorrhoea* may occur following orogenital contact, resulting in gonococcal stomatitis.

- Oral manifestations may be a feature of primary syphilis (chancre), secondary syphilis (snail track ulcers), and tertiary syphilis (gumma, atrophic glossitis, syphilitic leukoplakia).

- Oral lesions of tuberculosis are usually secondary to primary infection in the lungs. A chest radiograph is obligatory.

- Ulceration, pain, and lymphadenitis are common features of oral tuberculosis.

- Eight human herpesviruses are currently recognized.

- Human herpesviruses can cause serious disease in the immunosuppressed patient.

- Herpes simplex virus type I causes herpetic gingivostomatitis (primary infection) and herpes labialis (reactivation infection).

- Primary infection with varicella zoster virus causes chickenpox.

- Reactivation of latent varicella zoster virus causes shingles, a unilateral eruption involving well-defined dermatomes.

- Epstein–Barr virus may cause infectious mononucleosis, in which there is lymph node enlargement, fever, and pharyngeal inflammation.

- Epstein–Barr virus is also associated with Burkitt's lymphoma, nasopharyngeal carcinoma, and oral hairy leukoplakia.

- Coxsackie A viruses cause hand, foot, and mouth disease and herpangina.

- Papillomaviruses cause common and venereal warts, which may affect the oral cavity.

Further reading

Bagg, J (1994). Virology and the mouth. *Reviews in Medical Microbiology*, 5, 209–16.

Bagg, J, Sweeney, MP, Harvey-Wood, K, and Wiggins, A (1995). Possible role of *Staphylococcus aureus* in severe oral mucositis among elderly dehydrated patients. *Microbial Ecology in Health and Disease*, 8, 51–6.

Cleator, GM and Klapper, PE (1994). The Herpesviridae. In *Principles and practice of clinical virology* (3rd edn) (ed. AJ Zuckerman, JE Banatvala, and JR Pattison), Chapter 1. Wiley, Chichester.

Greenberg, MS (1996). Herpesvirus infections. *Dental Clinics of North America*, 40, 359–68.

MacFarlane, TW and Helnarska, S (1976). The microbiology of angular cheilitis. *British Dental Journal*, 140, 403–6.

Scully, C and Samaranayake, LP (1992). *Clinical virology in oral medicine and dentistry*. Cambridge University Press, Cambridge.

28

Cross-infection control in dentistry

- Introduction
- Universal infection control
- Occupationally acquired infections
- Health-care workers infected with blood-borne viruses

Cross-infection control in dentistry

Introduction

In recent years there has been heightened professional and public awareness of the potential for cross-infection in the dental surgery. To a large extent this has followed the discovery of human immunodeficiency virus (HIV) as the cause of AIDS. However, many other micro-organisms pose a potential threat and in many cases they are more infectious than HIV.

The possible routes of cross-infection in the dental surgery are summarized in Fig. 28.1. It has been recognized for many years that dentists may acquire occupational infections, for example hepatitis B, from patients they are treating. Transmission of these infections may occur by direct contact with the patient or indirectly through contact with contaminated instruments or surfaces. More recently, there has been considerable interest in the possible risk of patients becoming infected from health-care workers who are themselves carriers of blood-borne viruses (see below).

Many items of modern dental equipment, particularly high-speed handpieces and ultrasonic scalers, produce massive aerosols during use. As some micro-organisms – including many respiratory tract pathogens – are transmitted by droplet spread, aerosols are, therefore, an important potential mode of spread of infection in dentistry.

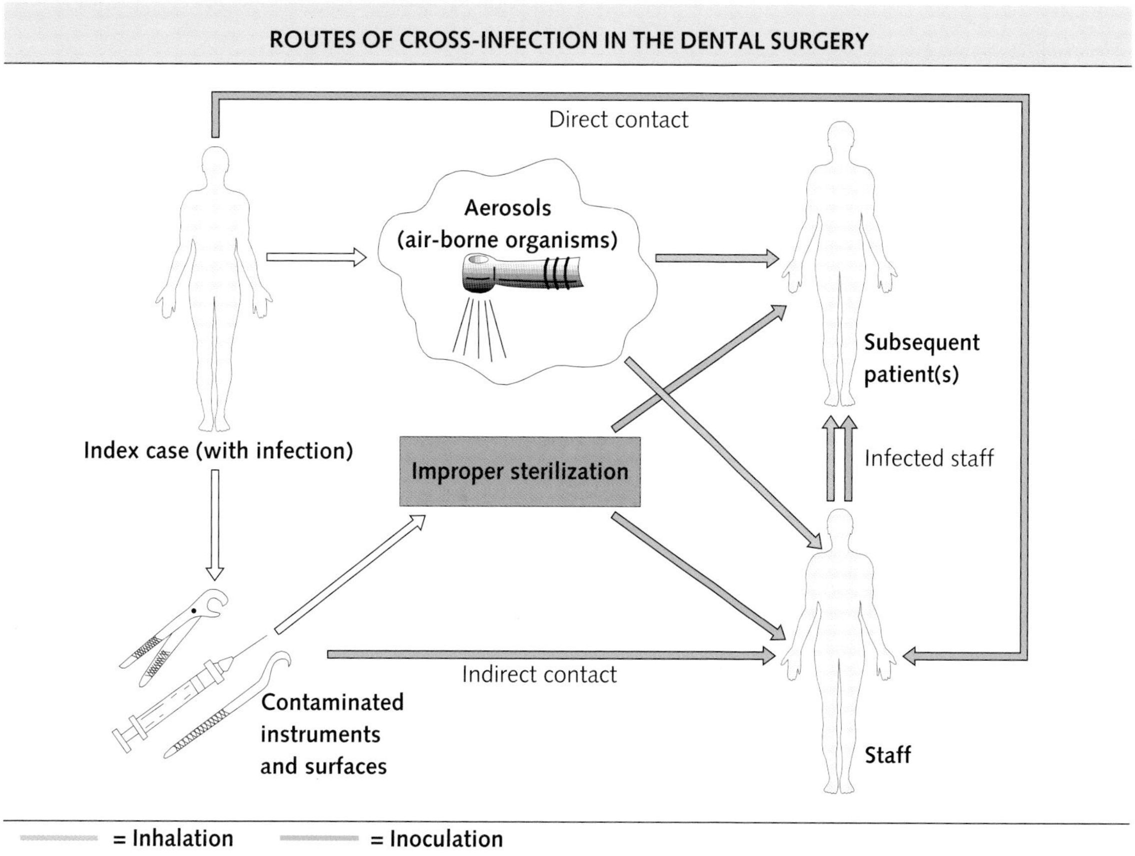

ROUTES OF CROSS-INFECTION IN THE DENTAL SURGERY

Direct contact

Aerosols (air-borne organisms)

Subsequent patient(s)

Index case (with infection)

Improper sterilization

Infected staff

Indirect contact

Contaminated instruments and surfaces

Staff

======== = Inhalation   ======== = Inoculation

Fig. 28.1 The potential routes of transmission of micro-organisms in the dental surgery. (Redrawn from Samaranayake 1989; with permission from George Warman Publications (UK).)

Finally, there is a risk that patients may become infected from instruments or other items contaminated during treatment of a previous patient. Effective sterilization of instruments, which is central to all infection control policies, will prevent this route of transmission.

Universal infection control

In the light of the multiple routes of transmission noted above, there are some key principles which underpin modern infection control procedures in dentistry (Fig. 28.2). First, whilst there is widespread concern about blood-borne viruses such as HIV, dentists regularly encounter a wide range of pathogenic micro-organisms in the clinical setting, such as common respiratory tract viruses. Thus attention must also be given to preventing the spread of both rare and common infections.

Second, there are many potential sources of infection (Fig. 28.3), most of them unrecognized. Carriers of hepatitis B virus, who frequently appear clinically well and are unaware of their carrier status, are a good example. Thus, any patient, regardless of background or medical history, must be considered a potential carrier.

The response to these concepts is the adoption of universal infection control, whereby every patient is treated as a potential carrier. The infection control protocol adopted must be sufficiently stringent to reduce the risk of contamination of patients or staff to a level which is highly unlikely to cause infection. It also follows that known carriers of HIV or other blood-borne viruses will pose no additional risk, and can be treated safely under the same operating conditions.

Key elements of universal infection control

The important elements of modern, universal infection control protocols are summarized in Fig. 28.4. These will now be dealt with individually.

Medical history

The collection of an accurate medical history is part of good clinical practice and is helpful in the identification of immuno-compromised patients. However, whilst a medical history may provide useful information in respect of previous infectious

---

UNIVERSAL INFECTION CONTROL

- Many different pathogens pose a problem
- There are many, usually unknown, sources of infection
- Any patient may be a carrier
- Routine procedures must be effective
- All blood is potentially infectious

THE SAME CROSS-INFECTION CONTROL PROCEDURES MUST BE USED FOR ALL PATIENTS (UNIVERSAL INFECTION CONTROL)

Fig. 28.2 The principles of universal infection control.

INFECTION CONTROL PROCEDURES

- Medical history
- Cleaning of instruments
- Sterilization of instruments
- Use of disposables
- Decontamination of surgery surfaces
- Protective workwear
- Avoidance of needlestick and other sharps injuries
- Immunization of staff
- Effective aspiration and ventilation
- Safe waste disposal
- Disinfection of laboratory items
- Effective training for staff

Fig. 28.4 The key elements of modern, universal infection control policies.

SOURCES OF INFECTION	
Patients in the acute phase of an infection	EASILY RECOGNIZED Examples: influenza and common cold
Patients in the prodromal phase of an infection	NOT EASILY RECOGNIZED Examples: measles, mumps and chickenpox
Healthy carriers of pathogenic organisms	NOT EASILY RECOGNIZED Includes convalescent carriers and asymptomatic carriers Examples: HIV, hepatitis B and C, herpes viruses

Fig. 28.3 Potential sources of infection from patients and staff.

diseases, the clinician must be aware that it does not allow one to categorize patients into 'high risk' and 'low risk' from the viewpoint of infectivity to staff and other patients.

Cleaning instruments

Cleaning used dental instruments to remove visible deposits is an essential step prior to their sterilization (Chapter 10). This cleaning may be achieved by hand scrubbing in soap or detergent, but ultrasonic baths are very useful for many items, particularly endodontic instruments. Heavy duty protective gloves should be worn during instrument cleaning, and care taken to avoid sharps injuries.

Sterilizing instruments

Sterilization measures are considered in detail in Chapter 10. After clinical use all dental instruments, including dental handpieces, must be sterilized before they are used to treat a subsequent patient. Most dental instruments are heat-stable and the sterilization method of choice is the autoclave. The two common cycles are 121°C for 15 minutes or 134°C for 3 minutes, with the latter favoured in the United Kingdom. The bench-top autoclaves used by dentists are usually of the downward displacement type, with reliance placed on the incoming steam to remove air from the chamber. It is critical that the steam makes physical contact with the surfaces of all the instruments to be sterilized, and care must be taken not to overload the autoclave and impede steam penetration. In the United Kingdom at present, it is recommended that instruments should not be wrapped before sterilization in a downward displacement autoclave because of the risk of air pockets inhibiting steam penetration. A chemical indicator strip (Fig. 28.5) should be placed in the centre of the load as a check on the effectiveness of each autoclave cycle.

Hot air ovens are microbiologically acceptable for sterilization purposes, but not recommended. The higher temperature and longer cycle (160°C for 60 minutes) make them more damaging to instruments and logistically less attractive.

Chemical agents such as aldehydes are inappropriate for the routine sterilization of dental items and equipment. They are unreliable and some are toxic or corrosive (Chapter 10).

Using disposables

Disposable items, such as plastic mouth-rinse beakers, saliva ejectors, and impression trays, are generally recommended. However, there is a cost implication, and some practitioners have found it more economical in the long term to purchase multiple-sterilizable items, for example stainless-steel beakers. Disposable items should always be used once only and then discarded.

Needles cannot be reliably cleaned and sterilized and must always be discarded into a sharps bin after use on a single patient. Similarly, a local anaesthetic cartridge must never be used for the treatment of more than one patient.

Decontaminating surgery surfaces

The surfaces around a dental chair frequently become contaminated with saliva and blood during patient treatment sessions (Fig. 28.6). This contamination can be reduced by good operating technique but cannot be prevented entirely.

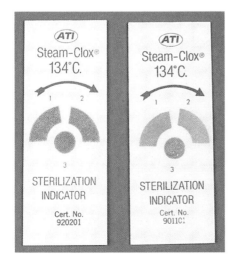

Fig. 28.5 Chemical indicator strips (unused on the left and used on the right) for monitoring the effectiveness of sterilization. The colour change to the two top panels on the used strip indicates a satisfactory autoclave run. A strip should routinely be placed in the centre of each autoclave load.

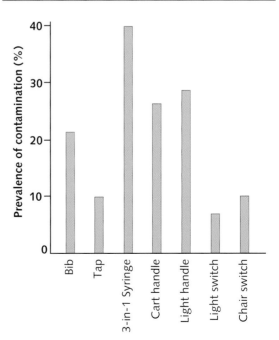

Fig. 28.6 Graph illustrating the prevalence of blood contamination on dental surgery surfaces following periodontal treatment. Blood was detected by the Kastle–Meyer technique, a sensitive forensic test for haemoglobin. (Adapted from McColl *et al.* 1994; with permission from the *British Dental Journal*.)

There are two main approaches to the problem. One is the use of disposable, impervious surface barriers. Sites likely to become contaminated, such as light switches, are covered with a plastic film, or equivalent, which is removed and replaced between each patient.

The second approach is to clean the exposed surfaces with a disinfectant between each patient. At present it is difficult to recommend an appropriate disinfectant for this purpose, though many are available commercially.

Whichever method is adopted, cross-infection control is enhanced by a process called zoning, in which particular areas of the working surfaces are identified as 'clean' or 'dirty' zones. The use of sterilizable tray systems is also recommended.

Between clinical sessions, all work surfaces, even those that appear uncontaminated, should be cleaned with an appropriate detergent.

In the event of an overt spillage of blood or other body fluid, it should be soaked into an absorbent cloth and a disinfectant such as hypochlorite (10 000 p.p.m. available chlorine) applied. Alternatively, commercially available spillage granules may be employed.

Protective workwear

All dental staff should wear long-sleeved clinical jackets to protect outdoor clothes from contamination. Operating gloves must be worn routinely by all dental personnel with direct patient contact and those handling body fluids, tissues, or objects contaminated with them. A new pair of gloves should be worn for each patient. Eye protection should be worn by dentists and close support staff, together with a well-fitting surgical face mask which should be changed at least hourly.

Avoiding needlestick injuries

Occupationally acquired infections with hepatitis B and C viruses and with HIV have been recorded following needlestick injuries and related sharps accidents (see below). Figure 28.7 shows the prevalence of needlestick injuries among 100 dental surgeons. Whilst some of these injuries are unavoidable, most are essentially preventable and great care must be taken when handling and disposing of all sharps.

Needles should never be resheathed after use, unless a safe resheathing device is used. Care must also be taken not to injure other staff, for example when sharp instruments are being passed between dentist and dental nurse. Unsheathed needles must never be left exposed where others may injure themselves. All contaminated sharp items must be discarded into a sharps box (see below) and staff must never put their hands into the opening of the box.

Immunizing staff

Vaccination against hepatitis B virus (Chapter 18) is now a requirement in the United Kingdom for all clinical dental per-

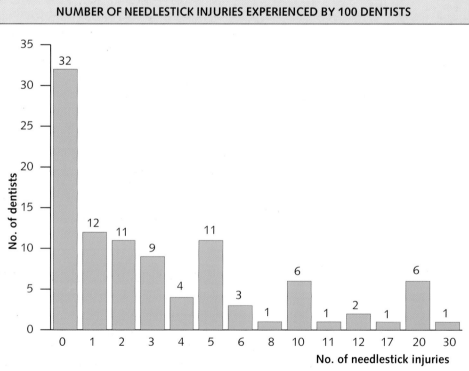

Fig. 28.7 Graph illustrating the numbers of needlestick injuries experienced in their careers by 100 general dental practitioners working in Wales, UK. Avoiding such injuries is an essential element of occupational hygiene for dentists.

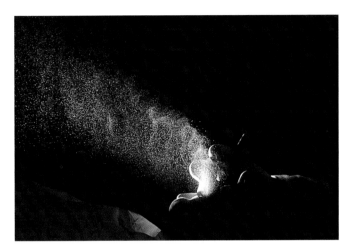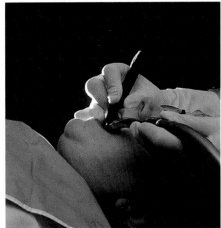

Fig. 28.8 The massive aerosols produced by modern dental equipment (left) can be largely controlled by the use of high-volume aspiration (right).

sonnel. Although not required in the USA, it is certainly recommended for all dental workers. Dentists' employers are required to offer (and pay for) the vaccine series to dental office personnel. In addition, the vaccine is recommended for all newborns and unvaccinated 12-year-olds in the USA. This vaccine provides protection from one of the most important and serious occupational infections of health-care workers.

Immunization against other infectious diseases such as tuberculosis (in the UK), tetanus, and poliomyelitis is also recommended and non-pregnant female dental personnel of childbearing age should be protected against rubella (Chapter 8).

Effective aspiration and ventilation

Some micro-organisms, for example respiratory tract viruses such as influenza virus and the bacterium *Mycobacterium tuberculosis*, are spread by the respiratory route. The copious aerosols produced by modern dental treatment (Fig. 28.8) therefore pose a threat.

Aerosols can be well controlled by the use of high-volume aspiration (Fig. 28.8). Aspiration equipment must be properly cleaned, maintained, and serviced and should be externally vented. Attention to good, general surgery ventilation is also important if acceptable air quality is to be maintained. In addition, performing dental treatment under rubber dam reduces the number of organisms liberated into the atmosphere.

Safe waste disposal

The dentist has a responsibility to ensure the safe disposal of all contaminated waste generated in the surgery. It must never be discarded through the domestic waste system and arrangements must be made with a local authority or private contractor for final collection and disposal. In the USA, regulated waste includes contaminated sharps, liquid blood and other body fluids, tissues (e.g. extracted teeth), non-sharp solid waste that is saturated or caked with body fluid (e.g. a dripping wet cotton roll), and microbiological materials contaminated with body fluid.

All sharp items must be consigned to a rigid, puncture-resistant container (sharps box), which should never be filled to more than two-thirds of its capacity. It should be securely closed and fastened before uplift for incineration.

Soft waste contaminated with blood or saliva should be placed into sturdy, impervious, sealed bags and clearly labelled as infective waste.

Disinfecting laboratory items

Items such as dental impressions and denture 'try-ins' are contaminated with saliva and, on occasions, visible blood. This contamination poses a potential threat to dental technicians, who should wear gloves when handling work received directly from a clinic. After removal from the mouth, all impressions and other items of laboratory work should be rinsed under running water and treated with an appropriate disinfecting agent, such as hypochlorite, before submission to the laboratory.

Effective training for staff

Good training of all dental staff engaged in patient care is an important element of infection control. In practice, it is the dental nurse who undertakes many of the necessary day-to-day duties, and a thorough understanding of the issues by this individual is essential. A written infection control policy should be available and procedures reviewed from time to time.

Occupationally acquired infections

The main concern of health-care workers relates to the risk of infection with blood-borne viruses, notably HIV. Hepatitis B remains the major infectious occupational hazard for dentists and other health-care workers, who are up to ten times more likely to become infected than members of the general population. Figure 28.9 summarizes the relative risks of infection with HIV and hepatitis B virus. Hepatitis B virus is far more infectious

OCCUPATIONAL INFECTION WITH HIV AND HBV		
	HIV	HBV
Minimum volume of blood to transmit infection	0.1 ml	0.00004 ml
Risk of infection following needlestick injury from a seropositive patient	0.3%	7 – 30%

Fig. 28.9 The relative risks of infection with HIV and hepatitis B virus following needlestick injuries from patients infected with the respective viruses. The risk of infection with hepatitis B virus depends on whether the source patient is a high-risk carrier (HBeAg-positive).

than HIV, and it is fortunate that most health-care workers respond to the hepatitis B vaccine, thereby gaining protection. Up to September 1993 there had only been 64 documented cases world-wide of occupationally acquired HIV infection in health-care workers, most of which followed sharps accidents with large-bore needles.

The occupational risk of infection with hepatitis C virus is not yet clear, but several recent studies suggest that the overall risk is low. However, well-documented seroconversions following needlestick accidents have been reported and emphasize the importance of avoiding such injuries.

Other infections may be occupationally acquired by dentists. Figure 13.16 shows an herpetic whitlow contracted by a dentist from a patient with an oral herpes simplex virus infection. There is also a documented occupational risk of infection with respiratory tract viruses and, among many groups of health-care workers, with *Mycobacterium tuberculosis*.

Management of sharps injuries

This is an important issue in the prevention of occupationally acquired infections with blood-borne viruses. The principles of management are summarized in Fig. 28.10. All such events should be officially recorded in an accident book. Immediate first aid involves cleaning the wound and allowing it to bleed under running water, without scrubbing or manipulation, and the application of a waterproof dressing. After arranging completion of the patient's treatment, medical advice should be sought.

Ideally, blood should be taken from the health-care worker at the time of the accident and the anti-HBs antibody titre measured. Residual serum is stored so that it is available in the future for HIV and hepatitis C virus antibody testing if necessary.

Although the concept of approaching the source patient is controversial (but required in the USA), ideally blood should also be collected from this individual. Appropriate discussion and counselling are obviously essential, but if consent is given the blood can be screened for hepatitis markers and HIV antibody. Such information can be very reassuring to a health-care worker who

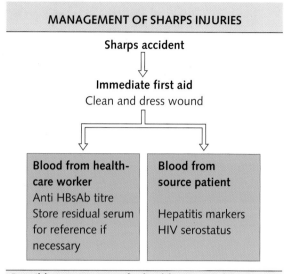

Fig. 28.10 Flow chart summarizing the management of needlestick and related sharps accidents.

has sustained an injury, but no pressure should be exerted on the patient to donate the appropriate sample.

Immediate treatment for the health-care worker may include passive immunization for a hepatitis B vaccine non-responder, or a vaccine booster for those whose anti-HBs antibody titre has waned. The administration of prophylactic AZT for those who have sustained an injury from a known HIV-positive patient has been controversial, but recent evidence suggests that, in combination with other antiretroviral drugs, it may significantly reduce the risk of infection.

Health-care workers infected with blood-borne viruses

There is strong epidemiological evidence that health-care workers who are high-risk carriers of hepatitis B virus (HBe-antigen positive) may transmit hepatitis B to patients if they undertake exposure-prone procedures. Exposure-prone procedures are those in which there is a risk that injury to the worker may result in the exposure of the patient's open tissues to the worker's blood. The majority of dental treatment procedures fall into this category, and dentists or dental hygienists who are HBeAg-positive are not permitted to continue clinical practice in the UK. In the USA these persons are asked to seek the advice of an expert review panel which will recommend the conditions under which the person may continue to practise. Those who are HBsAg-positive but not HBeAg-positive are permitted to continue with exposure-prone procedures, providing they have not been associated with spread of infection to patients.

Apart from the case in which a Florida dentist with AIDS apparently transmitted HIV to several patients, there is only one other report of an HIV-infected health-care worker transmitting the virus to a patient. This involved an HIV-seropositive orthopaedic surgeon in France who apparently transmitted HIV to a patient during hip surgery in 1992. At the time, the surgeon was asymptomatic and unaware of his infection. Thus, currently available data suggest that the risk of transmission of HIV to patients from HIV-infected health-care workers is extremely low. Nevertheless, in the United Kingdom, health-care workers who are known to be HIV seropositive are not permitted to undertake exposure-prone procedures.

There are only two known cases worldwide in which hepatitis C virus has been transmitted from seropositive health-care workers (both cardiothoracic surgeons) to patients. There is no current restriction on clinical activities of HCV-infected health-care workers unless they have been associated with transmission to a patient.

References and further reading

ADA Council on Scientific Affairs and ADA Council on Dental Practice. (1996). Infection control recommendations for the dental office and the dental laboratory. *Journal of the American Dental Association*, 127, 672–80.

British Dental Association Advisory Service. (1996). *The control of cross-infection in dentistry*. Advice Sheet A12.

Chenoweth, CE and Gobetti, JP (1997). Postexposure chemoprophylaxis for occupational exposure to HIV in the dental office. *Journal of the American Dental Association*, 128, 1135–9.

Garfunkel, AA and Galili, D (1996). Dental health care workers at risk. *Dental Clinics of North America*, 40, 277–91.

McColl, E, Bagg, J, Winning, S (1994). The detection of blood on dental surgery surfaces and equipment following dental hygiene treatment. *British Dental Journal*, 176, 65–7.

Miller, CH (1996). Infection control. *Dental Clinics of North America*, 40, 437–56.

Samaranayake, LP (1989). Cross infection control in dentistry: 1 General concepts and surgery attire. *Dental Update*, 16, 58–63.

UK Health Departments. (1997). Guidelines on post-exposure prophylaxis for health care workers occupationally exposed to HIV. Department of Health, London.

Key facts

- A wide range of micro-organisms pose a potential cross-infection hazard in the dental surgery.

- There are many unrecognized carriers of pathogens in the community.

- Modern clinical procedures are based on universal infection control, in which all patients are treated as potential carriers.

- Cleaning is an essential prerequisite to effective sterilization of instruments.

- The autoclave is the most appropriate method for sterilizing heat-stable dental instruments.

- Disposable items are generally recommended, and needles and local anaesthetic cartridges must always be discarded between patients.

- Contamination of surgery surfaces should be controlled by the use of surface barriers, cleaning and disinfecting agents, and a consideration of zoning techniques.

- Protective workwear (gloves, eye protection, and face mask) should be worn routinely by dental personnel.

- Avoid needlestick and related sharps injuries.

- Treat all sharps injuries promptly according to the local protocol.

- Maintain staff vaccination schedules, especially against hepatitis B.

- Use effective high-volume aspiration to control aerosols.

- Dispose of clinical waste safely.

- Disinfect contaminated laboratory items before they leave clinical areas.

- Ensure staff are well trained in cross-infection control measures.

- Hepatitis B is the most significant infectious occupational hazard for dentists.

- The risk of infection with HIV following a needlestick injury from a known HIV-seropositive patient is between 0.2% and 0.3%.

Index